Evaluation and Testing in Nursing Education

FOURTH EDITION

MARILYN H. OERMANN, PhD, RN, ANEF, FAAN

KATHLEEN B. GABERSON, PhD, RN, CNOR, CNE, ANEF

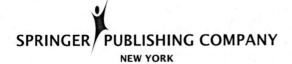

SPRINGER PUBLISHING COMPANY

NEW YORK

Springer Publishing Company, LLC
11 West 42nd Street
New York, NY 10036
www.springerpub.com

Acquisitions Editor: Margaret Zuccarini
Composition: diacriTech

ISBN: 978-0-8261-9555-5
e-book ISBN: 978-0-8261-9556-2
Instructor's Materials: 978-0-8261-7494-9

Instructor's Materials: Instructors may request supplements by emailing textbook@springerpub.com

12 13 14 15 / 5 4 3 2 1

The author and the publisher of this Work have made every effort to use sources believed to be reliable to provide information that is accurate and compatible with the standards generally accepted at the time of publication. Because medical science is continually advancing, our knowledge base continues to expand. Therefore, as new information becomes available, changes in procedures become necessary. We recommend that the reader always consult current research and specific institutional policies before performing any clinical procedure. The author and publisher shall not be liable for any special, consequential, or exemplary damages resulting, in whole or in part, from the readers' use of, or reliance on, the information contained in this book. The publisher has no responsibility for the persistence or accuracy of URLs for external or third-party Internet websites referred to in this publication and does not guarantee that any content on such websites is, or will remain, accurate or appropriate.

Library of Congress Cataloging-in-Publication Data

Oermann, Marilyn H.
  Evaluation and testing in nursing education / Marilyn H. Oermann, PhD, RN, ANEF, FAAN, Kathleen B. Gaberson, PhD, RN, CNOR, CNE, ANEF —Fourth edition.
       pages cm
  Includes bibliographical references and index.
  ISBN 978-0-8261-9555-5—ISBN 978-0-8261-9556-2 (e-book)
  1. Nursing—Examinations. 2. Nursing—Ability testing. 3. Nursing—Study and teaching—Evaluation.
  I. Gaberson, Kathleen B. II. Title.
  RT73.7.O47 2013
  610.73—dc23

                                                 2012040041

Special discounts on bulk quantities of our books are available to corporations, professional associations, pharmaceutical companies, health care organizations, and other qualifying groups. If you are interested in a custom book, including chapters from more than one of our titles, we can provide that service as well.
For details, please contact:
Special Sales Department, Springer Publishing Company, LLC
11 West 42nd Street, 15th Floor, New York, NY 10036-8002
Phone: 877-687-7476 or 212-431-4370; Fax: 212-941-7842
E-mail: sales@springerpub.com

Printed in the United States of America by Bang Printing.

To nurse educators and students preparing for a future role as a teacher in nursing

Contents

Preface

All teachers at some time or another need to assess learning. The teacher may write test items; prepare tests and analyze their results; develop rating scales and clinical evaluation methods; and plan other strategies for assessing learning in the classroom, clinical practice, online courses, simulation, and other settings. Often teachers are not prepared to carry out these tasks as part of their instructional role. This fourth edition of *Evaluation and Testing in Nursing Education* is a resource for teachers in nursing education programs and health care agencies, a textbook for graduate students preparing for their roles as nurse educators, a guide for nurses in clinical practice who teach others and are responsible for evaluating their learning and performance, and a resource for other health professionals involved in assessment, measurement, testing, and evaluation. Although the examples of test items and other types of assessment methods provided in this book are nursing-oriented, they are easily adapted to assessment in other health fields.

The purposes of this book are to describe concepts of assessment, testing, and evaluation in nursing education and prepare teachers for carrying these out as part of their roles. The book presents qualities of effective assessment procedures; how to plan for testing, assemble and administer tests, and analyze test results; how to write all types of test items and develop assessment methods; and how to assess higher level cognitive skills and learning. There is a new chapter in this edition on online testing and assessment of learning. The book describes the evaluation of written assignments in nursing; the processes to follow for clinical evaluation and how to evaluate clinical performance; the social, ethical, and legal issues associated with assessment and testing; the fundamentals of grading; and program assessment. The content is useful for teachers in any setting who are involved in evaluating others, whether they are students, nurses, or other types of health care personnel.

Chapter 1 addresses the purposes of assessment, testing, measurement, and evaluation in nursing education. Differences between formative and summative evaluation and between norm-referenced and criterion-referenced measurements are explored. Because effective assessment requires a clear description of *what* and *how* to assess, the chapter describes the use of objectives for developing test items, provides examples of objectives at different taxonomic levels, and describes how test items would be developed at each of these levels. Some teachers, however, do not use objectives as the basis for testing but instead develop test items and other assessment methods from the content of the course. For this reason Chapter 1 also includes an explanation of how to plan assessment using that process.

In Chapter 2, qualities of effective assessment procedures are discussed. The concept of assessment validity, the role of reliability, and their effects on the interpretive quality of assessment results are described. Teachers must gather evidence to support their inferences about scores obtained on a measure. Although this evidence traditionally has been classified as content, criterion-related, and construct validity, validity now is considered a unitary concept. Current ways of thinking about reliability and its relationship to validity are explained. Also discussed in Chapter 2 are important practical considerations that might affect the choice or development of tests and other instruments.

Chapter 3 describes the steps involved in planning for test construction, enabling the teacher to make good decisions about what and when to test, test length, difficulty of test items, item formats, and scoring procedures. An important focus of the chapter is how to develop a test blueprint and then use it for writing test items; examples are provided to clarify this process for the reader. Broad principles important in developing test items regardless of the specific type are described in the chapter.

There are different ways of classifying test items. One way is to group them according to how they are scored—objectively or subjectively. Another way is to group them by the type of response required of the test-taker—selected- or constructed-response—which is how we organized the chapters. Selected-response items require the test-taker to select the correct or best answer from options provided by the teacher. These items include true–false, matching exercises, multiple-choice, and multiple-response. Constructed-response items ask the test-taker to supply an answer rather than choose from options already provided. These items include short answer (fill-in-the-blank) and essay (short and extended). Chapters 4 through 6 discuss these test items.

A true–false item consists of a statement that the student judges as true or false. In some forms, students also correct the response or supply a rationale as to why the statement is true or false. True–false items are most effective for recall of facts and specific information but may also be used to test the student's comprehension of the content. Chapter 4 describes how to construct true–false items and different variations, for example, correcting false statements or providing a rationale for the response, which allows the teacher to assess if the learner understands the content. Chapter 4 also explains how to develop matching exercises. These consist of two parallel columns in which students match terms, phrases, sentences, or numbers from one column to the other. Principles for writing each type of item are presented, accompanied by sample items.

In Chapter 5 the focus is on writing multiple-choice and multiple-response items. Multiple-choice items, with one correct answer, are used widely in nursing and other fields. This format of test item includes an incomplete statement or question, followed by a list of options that complete the statement or answer the question. Multiple-response items are designed similarly, although more than one answer may be correct. Both of these formats of test items may be used for assessing learning at the recall, comprehension, application, and analysis levels, making them adaptable for a wide range of content and learning outcomes. There are three parts in a multiple-choice item, each with its own set of principles for development: (a) stem, (b) answer, and (c) distractors. In Chapter 5 we discuss how to write each of these parts and provide many examples. We also describe principles for writing multiple-response items, including the format used on the NCLEX®.

With true–false, matching, multiple-choice, and multiple-response items, the test-taker chooses the correct or best answer from the options provided by the teacher. In contrast, with constructed-response items, the test-taker supplies an answer rather than selecting from the options already provided. These items include short answer and essay questions. Short-answer items can be answered by a word, phrase, or number. One format presents a question that students answer in a few words or phrases. With the other format, completion or fill-in-the-blank, students are given an incomplete sentence that they complete by inserting a word or words in the blank space. On the NCLEX, candidates may be asked to perform a calculation and type in the number or to put a list of responses in proper order. In this chapter we describe how to write different formats of short-answer items. We also explain how to develop and score essay items. With essay items, students construct responses based on their understanding of the content. Essay items provide an opportunity for students to select content to discuss, present ideas in their own words, and develop an original and creative response to a question. We provide an extensive discussion on scoring essay responses.

There is much debate in nursing education about students developing higher level thinking skills and clinical judgment. With higher level thinking, students apply concepts, theories, and other forms of knowledge to new situations; use that knowledge to solve patient and other types of problems; and arrive at rational and well thought-out decisions about actions to take. The main principle in assessing higher level learning is to develop test items and other assessment methods that require students to apply knowledge and skills in a *new* situation; the teacher can then assess whether the students are able to use what they have learned in a different context. Chapter 7 presents strategies for assessing higher levels of learning in nursing. Context-dependent item sets or interpretive exercises are discussed as one format of testing appropriate for assessing higher level cognitive skills. Suggestions for developing these are presented in the chapter, including examples of different items. Other methods for assessing cognitive skills in nursing also are presented in this chapter: case method and study, unfolding cases, discussions using higher level questioning, debate, media clips, and short written assignments.

Chapter 8 focuses on developing test items that prepare students for licensure and certification examinations. The chapter begins with an explanation of the NCLEX test plans and their implications for nurse educators. Examples are provided of items written at different cognitive levels, thereby avoiding tests that focus only on recall and memorization of facts. The chapter also describes how to write questions about clinical practice or the nursing process and provides sample stems for use with those items. The types of items presented in the chapter are similar to those found on the NCLEX and many certification tests. When teachers incorporate these items on tests in nursing courses, students acquire experience with this type of testing as they progress through the program, preparing them for taking licensure and certification examinations as graduates.

Through papers and other written assignments, students develop an understanding of the content they are writing about. Written assignments with feedback from the teacher also help students improve their writing ability, an important outcome in any nursing program from the beginning level through graduate study. Chapter 9 provides guidelines for assessing formal papers and other written assignments in nursing courses. The chapter includes criteria for assessing the quality of papers, an example of a scoring rubric, and suggestions for assessing and grading written assignments.

Chapter 10 explains how to assemble and administer a test. In addition to preparing a test blueprint and skillful construction of test items, the final appearance of the test and the way in which it is administered can affect the validity of its results. In Chapter 10, test design rules are described; suggestions for reproducing the test, maintaining test security, administering it, and preventing cheating are presented in this chapter as well. As more courses and programs are offered through distance education, teachers are faced with how to prevent cheating on an assessment when they cannot directly observe their students; we discuss different approaches that can be used for this purpose.

Online education in nursing has developed rapidly and will likely continue to expand in the future. Chapter 11, a new chapter in this edition, discusses assessment of learning in online courses, including testing and appraising course assignments to determine if course outcomes have been met. The chapter begins with a discussion of online testing. To deter cheating and promote academic integrity, faculty members can use a variety of both low- and high-technology solutions. Multiple solutions are presented with guidelines for implementing them in a course. Course assignments may require adjustment for online learning to suit the electronic medium, and this is discussed in the chapter. We have included a sample rubric for an online discussion board assignment and evaluation criteria.

After administering the test, the teacher needs to score it, interpret the results, and then use the results to make varied decisions. Chapter 12 discusses the processes of obtaining scores and performing test and item analysis. It also suggests ways in which teachers can use posttest discussions to contribute to student learning and seek student feedback that can lead to test item improvement. The chapter begins with a discussion of scoring tests, including weighting items and correcting for guessing, then proceeds to item analysis. How to calculate the difficulty index and discrimination index and analyze each distractor are described; performing an item analysis by hand is explained with an illustration for teachers who do not have computer software for this purpose. Teachers often debate the merits of adjusting test scores by eliminating items or adding points to compensate for real or perceived deficiencies in test construction or performance. We discuss this in the chapter and provide guidelines for faculty in making these decisions. A section of the chapter also presents suggestions and examples of developing a test-item bank. Many publishers also offer test-item banks that relate to the content contained in their textbooks; we discuss why faculty members need to be cautious about using these items for their own examinations.

Chapter 13 describes the process of clinical evaluation in nursing. It begins with a discussion of the outcomes of clinical practice in nursing programs and then presents essential concepts underlying clinical evaluation. In this chapter we discuss fairness in evaluation, how to build feedback into the evaluation process, and how to determine *what* to evaluate in clinical courses.

Chapter 14 builds on concepts of clinical evaluation examined in the preceding chapter. Many evaluation methods are available for assessing competencies in clinical practice. We discuss observation and recording observations in notes about performance, checklists, and rating scales; simulations, standardized patients, and Objective Structured Clinical Examinations; written assignments useful for clinical evaluation such as journals, concept maps, case analyses, and short papers; portfolio assessment and how to set up a portfolio system for clinical evaluation, including an electronic portfolio; and other methods such as conference, group projects, and self-evaluation. The chapter includes a sample form for evaluating student participation in clinical conferences and a rubric for peer evaluation of participation in group projects. Because most nursing education programs use rating scales for clinical evaluation, we have included a few examples for readers to review. We also include an example of an instrument for evaluating student performance in simulation.

Chapter 15 explores social, ethical, and legal issues associated with testing and evaluation. Social issues such as test bias, grade inflation, effects of testing on self-esteem, and test anxiety are discussed. Ethical issues include privacy and access to test results. By understanding and applying codes for the responsible and ethical use of tests, teachers can assure the proper use of assessment procedures and the valid interpretation of test results. We include several of these codes in the Appendices. We also discuss selected legal issues associated with testing.

In Chapter 16, the discussion focuses on how to interpret the meaning of test scores. Basic statistical concepts are presented and used for criterion- and norm-referenced interpretations of teacher-made and standardized test results.

Grading is the use of symbols, such as the letters A through F or pass–fail, to report student achievement. Grading is for summative purposes, indicating how well the student met the outcomes of the course and clinical practicum. To represent valid judgments about student achievement, grades should be based on sound evaluation practices, reliable test results, and multiple assessment methods. Chapter 17 examines the uses of grades in nursing programs, criticisms of grades, types of grading systems, assigning letter grades, selecting a grading framework, and calculating grades with each of these frameworks. We also discuss grading clinical practice, using pass–fail and other systems for grading, and provide guidelines for the teacher to follow when students are on the verge of failing a clinical practicum.

Program assessment is the process of judging the worth or value of an educational program. With the demand for high-quality programs, the development of newer models for the delivery of higher education, such as distance education, and public calls for accountability, there has been a greater emphasis on systematic and ongoing program evaluation. Thus, Chapter 18 presents an overview of program assessment models and discusses evaluation of selected program components, including curriculum, outcomes, and teaching. Assessment of online programs, courses, and teaching also is included in the chapter.

In addition to this text, we have provided an *Instructor's Manual* that includes a sample course syllabus, chapter summaries and student learning activities, and chapter-based PowerPoint presentations. To obtain your electronic copy of these materials, faculty should contact Springer Publishing Company at textbook@springerpub.com.

The authors thank Anna N. Vioral, MSN, MEd, RN, OCN, for writing Chapter 11 on online testing and assessment of learning, in collaboration with Kathy Gaberson. Anna also prepared the new content on assessment of online courses, programs, and teaching in Chapter 18. Anna is an Oncology Quality and Education specialist at West Penn Allegheny Health System and Adjunct Faculty at Duquesne University School of Nursing, Pittsburgh, Pennsylvania. She also is a doctoral student in the PhD Nursing Program at Indiana University of Pennsylvania.

We wish to acknowledge Margaret Zuccarini, our editor at Springer, for her enthusiasm and patience. We also thank Springer Publishing Company for its continued support of nursing education.

Marilyn H. Oermann
Kathleen B. Gaberson

PART I

Basic Concepts of

Assessment

ONE

Assessment and the Educational Process

In all areas of nursing education and practice, the process of assessment is important to obtain information about student learning, judge performance and determine competence to practice, and arrive at other decisions about students and nurses. Assessment is integral to monitoring the quality of educational and health care programs. By evaluating outcomes achieved by students, graduates, and patients, the effectiveness of programs can be measured and decisions can be made about needed improvements.

Assessment provides a means of ensuring accountability for the quality of education and services provided. Nurses, like other health professionals, are accountable to their patients and society in general for meeting patients' health needs. Along the same lines, nurse educators are accountable for the quality of teaching provided to learners, outcomes achieved, and overall effectiveness of programs that prepare graduates to meet the health needs of society. Educational institutions also are accountable to their governing bodies and society in terms of educating graduates for present and future roles. Through assessment, nursing faculty members and other health professionals can collect information for evaluating the quality of their teaching and programs as well as documenting outcomes for others to review. All educators, regardless of the setting, need to be knowledgeable about assessment, testing, measurement, and evaluation.

ASSESSMENT

Educational assessment involves collecting information to make decisions about learners, programs, and educational policies. Are students learning the important concepts in the course and developing the clinical competencies? With information collected through assessment, the teacher can determine relevant instructional strategies to meet students' learning needs and help them improve performance. Assessment that provides information about learning needs is diagnostic; teachers use that information to decide on the appropriate content, learning activities, and clinical practice for students to meet the desired learning outcomes.

Assessment also generates feedback for students, which is particularly important in clinical practice as students develop their performance skills and learn to think through complex clinical situations. Feedback from assessment similarly informs the teacher and provides data for deciding how best to teach certain content and skills; in this way assessment enables teachers to improve their educational practices and how they teach students.

Another important purpose of assessment is to provide valid and reliable data for determining students' grades. Although nurse educators continually assess students' progress in meeting the outcomes of learning and developing the clinical competencies, they also need to measure students' achievement in the course. Grades serve that purpose. Assessment strategies provide the data for faculty to determine if students achieved the outcomes and developed the essential clinical competencies. Grades are symbols, for instance, the letters A through F, for reporting student achievement.

Assessment also generates information for decisions about courses, the curriculum, and the nursing program, and for developing educational policies in the nursing education program. Other uses of assessment information are to select students for admission to an educational institution and a nursing program and place students in appropriate courses.

There are many assessment strategies that teachers can use to obtain information about students' learning and performance. These methods include tests that can be developed with different types of items, papers, other written assignments, projects, small-group activities, oral presentations, portfolios, observations of performance, and conferences. Each of those assessment strategies as well as others will be presented in this book.

Nitko and Brookhart (2011) identified five principles for effective assessment. These principles should be considered when deciding on the assessment strategy and its implementation in the classroom, online course, laboratory, or clinical setting.

1. *Identify the learning targets (outcomes, objectives, or competencies) to be assessed.* These provide the basis for the assessment: the teacher determines if students are meeting or have met the outcomes, objectives, and clinical competencies. The clearer the teacher is about *what* to assess, the more effective will be the assessment.

2. *Match the assessment technique to the learning target.* The assessment strategy needs to provide information about the particular outcome, objective, or competency being assessed. If the objective relates to analyzing issues in the care of patients with chronic pain, a true–false item about a pain medication would not be appropriate. An essay item, however, in which students analyze a scenario about an adult with chronic pain and propose multiple approaches for pain management would provide relevant information for deciding whether students achieved that outcome.

3. *Meet the students' needs.* Students should be clear about what is expected of them. The assessment strategies, in turn, should provide feedback to students about their progress and achievement in demonstrating those expectations, and should guide the teacher in determining the instruction needed to improve performance.

4. *Use multiple assessment techniques.* It is unlikely that one assessment strategy will provide sufficient information about achievement of the objectives. A test that contains mainly recall items will not provide information on students' ability to apply concepts to practice or analyze clinical situations. In most courses multiple assessment strategies are needed to determine if the outcomes were met.

5. *Keep in mind the limitations of assessment when interpreting the results.* One test, one paper, or one observation in clinical practice may not be a true measure of the student's learning and performance. Many factors can influence the assessment, particularly in the clinical setting, and the information collected in the assessment is only a sample of the student's overall achievement and performance.

TESTS

A test is a set of items to which students respond in written or oral form, typically during a fixed period of time. Nitko and Brookhart (2011) defined a test as an instrument or a systematic procedure for describing characteristics of a student. Tests are typically scored based on the number or percentage of answers that are correct and are administered similarly to all students. Although students often dread tests, information from tests enables faculty to make important decisions about students.

Tests are used frequently as an assessment strategy. They can be used to assess students' knowledge and skills prior to instruction, which enables the teacher to gear instruction to the learners' needs. Test results indicate gaps in learning and performance that should be addressed first as well as knowledge and skills already acquired. With this information teachers can better plan their instruction. When teachers are working with large groups of students, it is difficult to gear the instruction to meet each student's needs. However, the teacher can use diagnostic quizzes and tests to reveal content areas in which individual learners may lack knowledge and then suggest remedial learning activities. Not only do the test results guide the teacher, but they also serve as feedback to students about their learning needs. In some nursing programs students take commercially available tests as they progress through the curriculum to identify gaps in their learning and prepare them for taking the National Council Licensure Examination for Registered Nurses (NCLEX-RN®) or National Council Licensure Examination for Practical Nurses (NCLEX-PN®).

Tests are commonly used to determine students' grades in a course, but in most nursing courses they are not the only assessment strategy. Faculty members ($N = 1573$) in prelicensure nursing programs reported that papers, collaborative group projects, and case study analyses were used more frequently for assessment in their courses than were tests. However, tests were weighted most heavily in determining the students' course grades (Oermann, Saewert, Charasika, & Yarbrough, 2009).

Tests are used for selecting students for admission to nursing programs. Admission tests provide norms that allow comparison of the applicant's performance with that of other applicants. Tests also may be used to place students into appropriate courses. Placement tests, taken after students have been admitted, provide data for determining which courses they should complete in their programs of study. For example, a diagnostic test of statistics may determine whether a nursing student is required to take a statistics course prior to beginning graduate study.

By reviewing test results teachers can identify content areas that students learned and did not learn in a course. With this information, faculty can modify the instruction to better meet student learning needs in future courses. Last, testing may be an integral part of the curriculum and program evaluation in a nursing education program. Students may complete tests to measure program outcomes rather than to document what was learned in a course. Test results for this purpose often suggest areas of the curriculum for revision and may be used for accreditation reports.

MEASUREMENT

Measurement is the process of assigning numbers to represent student achievement or performance according to certain rules, for instance, answering 85 out of 100 items correctly on a test. The numbers or scores indicate the degree to which a learner possesses a certain characteristic or trait (Nitko & Brookhart, 2011). Measurement is important for reporting the achievement of learners on nursing and other tests, but not all outcomes important in nursing practice can be measured by testing. Many outcomes are evaluated qualitatively through other means, such as observations of performance.

Although measurement involves assigning numbers to reflect learning, these numbers in and of themselves have no meaning. Scoring 15 on a test means nothing unless it is referenced or compared with other students' scores or to a predetermined standard. Perhaps 15 was the highest or lowest score on the test, compared with other students. Or the student might have set a personal goal of achieving 15 on the test; thus meeting this goal is more important than how others scored on the test. Another interpretation is that a score of 15 might be the standard expected of this particular group of learners. To interpret the score and give it meaning, having a reference point with which to compare a particular test score is essential.

In clinical practice, how does a learner's performance compare with that of others in the group? Did the learner meet the outcomes of the clinical course and develop the essential competencies regardless of how other students in the group performed in clinical practice? Answers to these questions depend on the basis used for interpreting clinical performance, similar to interpreting test scores.

Norm-Referenced Interpretation

There are two main ways of interpreting test scores and other types of assessment results: norm-referencing and criterion-referencing. In norm-referenced interpretation, test scores and other assessment data are compared to those of a norm group. Norm-referenced interpretation compares a student's test scores with those of others in the class or with some other relevant group. The student's score may be described as below or above average or at a certain rank in the class. Problems with norm-referenced interpretations, for example, "grading on a curve," are that they do not indicate what the student can and cannot do, and the interpretation of a student's performance can vary widely depending on the particular comparison group selected.

In clinical settings, norm-referenced interpretations compare the student's clinical performance with those of a group of learners, indicating that the student has more or less clinical competence than others in the group. A clinical evaluation instrument in which student performance is rated on a scale of below to above average reflects a norm-referenced system. Again, norm-referenced clinical performance does not indicate whether a student has developed desired competencies, only whether a student performed better or worse than other students.

Criterion-Referenced Interpretation

Criterion-referenced interpretation, on the other hand, involves interpreting scores based on preset criteria, not in relation to the group of learners. With this type of measurement, an individual score is compared to a preset standard or criterion. The concern is how well the student performed and what the student can do regardless of the performance of other learners. Criterion-referenced interpretations may (a) describe the specific learning tasks a student can perform, for example, define medical terms; (b) indicate the percentage of tasks performed or items answered correctly, for example, define correctly 80% of the terms; and (c) compare performance against a set standard and decide whether the student met that standard, for example, met the medical terminology competency (Miller, Linn, & Gronlund, 2009). Criterion-referenced interpretation determines how well the student performed at the end of the instruction in comparison with the outcomes and competencies to be achieved.

With criterion-referenced clinical evaluation, student performance is compared against preset criteria. In some nursing courses these criteria are the outcomes of the course to be met by students. In other courses they are the competencies to be demonstrated in clinical practice, which are then used as the standards for evaluation. Rather than comparing the performance of the student to others in the group, and indicating that the student was above or below the average of the group, in criterion-referenced clinical evaluation, performance is measured against the objectives or competencies to be demonstrated. The concern with criterion-referenced clinical evaluation is whether students achieved the outcomes of the course or demonstrated the essential competencies, not how well they performed in comparison to the other students.

EVALUATION

Evaluation is the process of making judgments about student learning and achievement, clinical performance, employee competence, and educational programs, based on assessment data. In nursing education, evaluation typically takes the form of judging student attainment of the educational outcomes of the course and knowledge gained in the course, and the quality of student performance in the clinical setting. With this evaluation, learning needs are identified, and additional instruction can be provided to assist students in their learning and in developing competencies for practice. Similarly, evaluation of employees provides information on their performance at varied points in time as a basis for judging their competence.

Evaluation extends beyond a test score or clinical rating. In evaluating learners, teachers judge the merits of the learning and performance based on data. Evaluation involves making value judgments about learners; in fact, *value* is part of the word "evaluation." Questions such as "How *well* did the student perform?" and "Is the student *competent* in clinical practice?" are answered by the evaluation process. The teacher collects and analyzes data about the student's performance, then makes a value judgment about the quality of that performance.

In terms of educational programs, evaluation includes collecting information *prior* to developing the program, *during* the process of program development to provide a basis for ongoing revision, and *after* implementing the program to determine its effectiveness. With program evaluation, faculty members collect data about their students, alumni, curriculum, and other dimensions of the program for the purposes of documenting the program outcomes, judging the quality of the program, and making sound decisions about curriculum revision. As educators measure outcomes for accreditation and evaluate their courses and curricula, they are engaging in program evaluation. Although many of the concepts described in this book are applicable to program evaluation, the focus instead is on evaluating learners, including students in all types and levels of nursing programs and nurses in health care settings. The term *students* is used broadly to reflect both of these groups of learners.

Formative Evaluation

Evaluation fulfills two major roles: it is both formative and summative. Formative evaluation judges students' progress in meeting the desired outcomes and developing clinical competencies. With formative evaluation the teacher judges the quality of the achievement while students are still in the process of learning (Nitko & Brookhart, 2011). Formative evaluation occurs throughout the instructional process and provides feedback for determining where further learning is needed.

With formative evaluation the teacher assesses student learning and performance, gives them prompt and specific feedback about the knowledge and skills that still need to be acquired, and plans further instruction to enable students to fill their gaps in learning. Considering that formative evaluation is diagnostic, it typically is not graded. Teachers should remember that the purpose of formative evaluation is to determine where further learning is needed. In the classroom, formative information may be collected by teacher observation and questioning of students, diagnostic quizzes, small-group activities, written assignments, and other activities that students complete in and out of class. These same types of strategies can be used to assess student learning in online and other courses offered for distance education.

In clinical practice, formative evaluation is an integral part of the instructional process. The teacher continually makes observations of students as they learn to provide patient care, questions them about their understanding and clinical decisions, discusses these observations and judgments with them, and guides them in how to improve performance. With formative evaluation the teacher gives feedback to learners about their progress in achieving the goals of clinical practice and how they can further develop their knowledge and competencies.

Summative Evaluation

Summative evaluation, on the other hand, is end-of-instruction evaluation designed to determine what the student has learned. With summative evaluation the teacher judges the quality of the student's achievement in the course, not the progress of the learner in meeting the outcomes. As such, summative evaluation occurs at the end of the learning process, for instance, the end of a course, to determine the student's grade and competencies. Although formative evaluation occurs on a continual basis throughout the learning experience, summative evaluation is conducted on a periodic basis, for instance, every few weeks or at the midterm and final evaluation periods. This type of evaluation is "final" in nature and serves as a basis for grading and other high-stakes decisions.

Summative evaluation typically judges broader content areas than formative evaluation, which tends to be more specific in terms of the content evaluated. Strategies used commonly for summative evaluation in the classroom and online courses are tests, papers, and other projects. In clinical practice, rating scales, written assignments, portfolios, projects completed about clinical experiences, and other performance measures may be used.

Both formative and summative evaluation are essential components of most nursing courses. However, because formative evaluation represents feedback to learners with the goal of improving learning, it should be the major part of any nursing course. By providing feedback on a continual basis and linking that feedback with further instruction, the teacher can assist students in developing the knowledge and skills they lack.

Evaluation and Instruction

Figure 1.1 demonstrates the relationship between evaluation and instruction. The intended learning outcomes are the knowledge, skills, and competencies students are to achieve. Following assessment to determine gaps

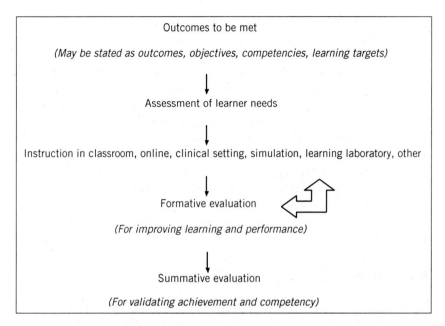

Figure 1.1   Relationship of evaluation and instruction.

in learning and performance, the teacher selects teaching strategies and plans clinical activities to meet those needs. This phase of the instructional process includes developing a plan for learning, selecting learning activities, and teaching learners in varied settings.

The remaining components of the instructional process relate to evaluation. Because formative evaluation focuses on judging student *progress* toward achieving the outcomes and demonstrating competency in clinical practice, this type of evaluation is displayed with a feedback loop to instruction. Formative evaluation provides information about further learning needs of students and where additional instruction is needed. Summative evaluation, at the end of the instruction, determines whether the outcomes have been achieved and competencies developed.

OBJECTIVES FOR ASSESSMENT AND TESTING

The desired learning outcomes or objectives play an important role in teaching students in varied settings in nursing. They provide guidelines for student learning and instruction and a basis for evaluating learning. This does not mean that the teacher is unconcerned about learning that occurs but is not expressed as outcomes. Many students will acquire knowledge, values, and skills beyond those expressed in the objectives, but the assessment strategies planned by the teacher and the evaluation that is done in a course should focus on the outcomes to be met by students.

The learning targets, the knowledge, skills, and performances students are to learn, may be stated as *outcomes*, *objectives*, or *competencies* to be met by students. They can include the acquisition of knowledge and higher-level cognitive skills, development of values, and performance of psychomotor and technological skills. Regardless of the terms used in a particular nursing program, the outcomes, objectives, and competencies provide the basis for assessing learning in the classroom, online environment, practice laboratories, and clinical setting. The next section of the chapter explains how to write objectives as a framework for assessment, but this same process can be used in determining outcomes or clinical competencies to be met by students.

Writing Objectives

In earlier years teachers developed highly specific objectives that included a description of the learner, behaviors the learner would exhibit at the end of the instruction, conditions under which the behavior would be demonstrated, and the standard of performance. An example of this format for an objective is: Given assessment data, the student identifies in writing two patient problems with supporting rationale. It is clear from this example that highly specific instructional objectives are too prescriptive for use in nursing. The complexity of learning expected in a nursing program makes it difficult to use such a system for specifying the objectives. Nursing students need to gain complex knowledge and skills and learn to problem solve and think critically; those outcomes cannot be specified as detailed and prescriptive objectives. In addition, specific objectives limit flexibility in planning teaching methods and in developing assessment strategies. For these reasons, a general format for writing objectives is sufficient to express the learning outcomes and to provide a basis for assessing learning in nursing courses.

A general objective similar to the earlier outcome is: The student identifies patient problems based on the assessment. This general objective, which is open-ended, provides flexibility for the teacher in developing instruction to meet the objective and for assessing student learning. The outcome could be met and evaluated through varied activities in which students analyze assessment data, presented in a lecture, written scenario, videoclip, or simulation, and then identify the patient's problems. Students might work in groups, reviewing various assessments and discussing possible problems, or they might analyze scenarios presented online. In the clinical setting, patient assignments, conferences, discussions with students, and reviews of cases provide other strategies for learners to identify patient problems from assessment data and for evaluating student competency. Generally stated objectives, therefore, provide sufficient guidelines for instruction and evaluation of student learning.

The objectives are important in developing assessment strategies that collect data on the knowledge and competencies to be acquired by learners. In evaluating the sample objective cited earlier, the method selected— for instance, a test—needs to examine student ability to identify patient problems from assessment data. The objective does not specify the number of problems, type of problem, complexity of the assessment data, or other variables associated with the clinical situation; there is opportunity for the teacher to develop various types of test questions and assessment methods as long as they require the learner to identify patient-related problems based on the given data.

Clearly written objectives guide the teacher in selecting assessment methods such as tests, observations in the clinical setting, written assignments, and others. When the chosen method is testing, the objective in turn suggests the type of test item, for instance, true–false, multiple choice, or essay. In addition to guiding decisions about assessment methods, the objective gives clues to faculty about teaching methods and learning activities to assist students in meeting the objective. For the sample objective, teaching methods might include: readings, lecture, discussion, case analysis, simulation, role play, videoclip, clinical practice, postclinical conference, and other approaches that present assessment data and ask students to identify patient problems.

Objectives that are useful for test construction and for designing other assessment methods meet four general principles. First, the objective should represent the outcome expected of the learner at the end of the instruction. Second, it should be measurable. Terms such as *identify*, *describe*, and *analyze* are specific and may be measured; words such as *understand* and *know*, in contrast, represent a wide variety of behaviors, some simple and others complex, making these terms difficult to assess. The student's knowledge might range from identifying and naming through synthesizing and evaluating. Sample behaviors useful for writing objectives are presented in Table 1.1.

Third, the objectives should be as general as possible to allow for their achievement with varied course content. For instance, instead of stating that the student will identify physiological problems from the assessment of acutely ill patients, indicating that the learner will identify patient problems from assessment data provides more flexibility for the teacher in designing assessment methods that reflect different types of problems a patient might experience based on varied data sets presented in the course. Fourth, the teaching method should be omitted from the objective to provide greater

☐Table 1.1

SAMPLE VERBS FOR TAXONOMIC LEVELS

Cognitive Domain	Affective Domain	Psychomotor Domain
Knowledge	Receiving	Imitation
Define	Acknowledge	Follow example of
Identify	Ask	Imitate
Label	Reply	
List	Show awareness of	Manipulation
Name		Assemble
Recall	Responding	Carry out
State	Act willingly	Follow procedure
	Assist	
Comprehension	Is willing to	Precision
Defend	Support	Demonstrate skill
Describe	Respond	Is accurate in
Differentiate	Seek	
Draw conclusions	opportunities	Articulation
Explain		Carry out (accurately
Give examples	Valuing	and in reasonable
Interpret	Accept	time frame)
Select	Assume	Is skillful
Summarize	responsibility	
	Participate in	Naturalization
Application	Respect	Is competent
Apply	Support	Carry out
Demonstrate use of	Value	competently
Modify		Integrate skill within
Operate	Organization of Values	care
Predict	Argue	
Produce	Debate	
Relate	Declare	
Solve	Defend	
Use	Take a stand	
Analysis	Characterization by	
Analyze	Value	
Compare	Act consistently	
Contrast	Stand for	
Detect		
Differentiate		
Identify		
Relate		
Select		

Table 1.1 *(continued)*

Cognitive Domain	Affective Domain	Psychomotor Domain
Synthesis		
Compile		
Construct		
Design		
Develop		
Devise		
Generate		
Plan		
Produce		
Revise		
Synthesize		
Write		
Evaluation		
Appraise		
Assess		
Critique		
Discriminate		
Evaluate		
Judge		
Justify		
Support		

flexibility in how the instruction is planned. For example, in the objective "Uses effective communication techniques in a simulated patient–nurse interaction," the teacher is limited to evaluating communication techniques through simulations rather than through interactions the student might have in the clinical setting. The objective would be better if stated as "Uses effective communication techniques with patients."

TAXONOMIES OF OBJECTIVES

The need for clearly stated objectives or learning targets, *what* the student should achieve at the end of the instruction, becomes evident when the teacher translates them into test items and other methods of assessment. Test items need to adequately assess the objective, for instance, to identify, describe, apply, and analyze, as it relates to the content area. Objectives may be written to reflect three domains of learning, cognitive, affective, and psychomotor, each with its own taxonomy, although in nursing education typically only the cognitive taxonomy is used for this purpose. The taxonomies classify the objectives into various levels of complexity (Nitko & Brookhart, 2011).

Cognitive Domain

The cognitive domain deals with knowledge and intellectual skills. Learning within this domain includes the acquisition of facts and specific information, use of knowledge in practice, and higher level cognitive skills. The most widely used cognitive taxonomy was developed in 1956 by Bloom, Englehart, Furst, Hill, and Krathwohl. It includes six levels of cognitive learning, increasing in complexity: knowledge, comprehension, application, analysis, synthesis, and evaluation. This taxonomy suggests that knowledge, such as recall of specific facts, is less complex and demanding intellectually than the higher levels of learning. Evaluation, the most complex level, requires judgments based on varied criteria.

In an update of the taxonomy by Anderson and Krathwohl (2001), the names for the levels of learning were reworded as verbs, for example, the "knowledge" level was renamed "remember," and synthesis and evaluation were reordered. In the adapted taxonomy, the highest level of learning is "create," which is the process of synthesizing elements to form a new product.

One advantage in considering this taxonomy when writing objectives and test items is that it encourages the teacher to think about higher levels of learning expected as a result of the instruction. If the course goals reflect application of knowledge in clinical practice and complex thinking, these higher levels of learning should be reflected in the objectives and assessment rather than focusing only on the recall of facts and other information.

In using the taxonomy, the teacher decides first on the level of cognitive learning intended and then develops objectives and assessment methods for that particular level. Decisions about the taxonomic level at which to gear instruction and assessment depend on the teacher's judgment in considering the background of the learner; placement of the course and learning activities within the curriculum to provide for the progressive development of knowledge and competencies; and complexity of the content in relation to the time allowed for teaching. If the time for teaching and evaluation is limited, the objectives may need to be written at a lower level. The taxonomy provides a continuum for educators to use in planning instruction and evaluating learning outcomes, beginning with recall of facts and information and progressing toward understanding, using concepts and theories in practice, analyzing situations, synthesizing from different sources to develop new products, and evaluating materials and situations based on internal and external criteria.

A description and sample objective for each of the six levels of learning in Bloom's cognitive taxonomy follow.

1. *Knowledge*: Recall of facts and specific information: Memorization of specifics

   Defines the term *systole*.

2. *Comprehension*: Understanding: Ability to describe and explain the material

   Describes the blood flow through the heart.

3. *Application*: Use of information in a new situation: Ability to use knowledge in a new situation

   Applies evidence on family-based interventions when caring for acutely ill children.

4. *Analysis*: Ability to break down material into component parts and identify the relationships among them

   Analyzes the organizational structure of the community health agency and its impact on client services.

5. *Synthesis*: Ability to develop and combine elements to form a new product

   Develops nursing guidelines for assessment, education, and referral of patients with postpartum depression.

6. *Evaluation*: Ability to make value judgments based on internal and external criteria and determine the extent to which materials and objects meet criteria

   The learner evaluates the quality of nursing research studies and their applicability to practice.

This taxonomy is useful in developing test items because it helps the teacher gear the item to a particular cognitive level. For example, if the objective focuses on application, the test question should measure whether the student can use the concept in a new situation, which is the intent of learning at that level. However, the taxonomy alone does not always determine the level of complexity of the item because one other consideration is how the information was presented in the instruction. For example, a test item at the application level requires use of previously learned concepts and theories in a new situation. Whether or not the situation is new for each student, however, is not known. Some students may have had clinical experience with that situation or been exposed to it through another learning activity. As another example, a question written at the comprehension level may actually be at the knowledge level if the teacher used that specific explanation in class and students only need to recall the explanation to answer the item.

Marzano and Kendall (2007, 2008) developed a taxonomy for writing objectives and designing assessment. Their taxonomy addresses three domains of knowledge—information, mental procedures, and psycho-motor procedures—and six levels of processing. The levels of processing begin with retrieval, the lowest cognitive level, which is recalling information without understanding it and performing procedures accurately but without understanding their rationale. At the second level, comprehension, the learner understands information and its critical elements. The third level is analysis, which involves identifying consequences of information, deriving generalizations, analyzing errors, classifying, and identifying similarities and differences. The next level—knowledge utilization—is the ability to use information to conduct investigations, generate and test hypotheses, solve problems, and make decisions. Level 5 is metacognition, during which the learner explores the accuracy of information and her or his own clarity of understanding, develops goals, and monitors progress in meeting these goals. The highest level, self-system thinking, occurs when students identify their own motivations to learn, emotional responses to learning, and beliefs about the ability to improve competence, and then examine the importance of the information, mental procedure, or psycho-motor procedure to them.

Affective Domain

The affective domain relates to the development of values, attitudes, and beliefs consistent with standards of professional nursing practice. Although affective learning outcomes are important in preparing students for professional practice, there is limited literature on this domain and its assessment in nursing students (Miller, 2010). Developed by Krathwohl, Bloom, and Masia (1964), the taxonomy of the affective domain includes five levels organized around the principle of increasing involvement of the learner and internalization of a value. The principle on which the affective taxonomy is based relates to the movement of learners from mere awareness of a value, for instance, confidentiality, to internalization of that value as a basis for their own behavior.

There are two important dimensions in evaluating affective outcomes. The first relates to the student's knowledge of the values, attitudes, and beliefs that are important in guiding decisions in nursing. Prior to internalizing a value and using it as a basis for decision making and behavior, the student needs to know what are important values in nursing. There is a cognitive base, therefore, to the development of a value system. Evaluation of this dimension focuses on acquisition of knowledge about the values, attitudes, and beliefs consistent with professional nursing practice. A variety of test items and assessment methods are appropriate to evaluate this knowledge base.

The second dimension of affective evaluation focuses on whether or not students have accepted these values, attitudes, and beliefs and are internalizing them for their own decision making and behavior. Assessment at these higher levels of the affective domain is more difficult because it requires observation of student behavior over time to determine whether there is commitment to act according to professional values. Test items are not appropriate for these levels as the teacher is concerned with the use of values in practice and the motivation to carry them out consistently in patient care.

A description and sample objective for each of the five levels of learning in the affective taxonomy follow:

1. *Receiving*: Awareness of values, attitudes, and beliefs important in nursing practice. Sensitivity to a patient, clinical situation, and problem.

   Expresses an awareness of the need for maintaining confidentiality of patient information.

2. *Responding*: Learner's reaction to a situation. Responding voluntarily to a given phenomenon reflecting a choice made by the learner.

   Shares willingly feelings about caring for a dying patient.

3. *Valuing*: Internalization of a value. Acceptance of a value and the commitment to using that value as a basis for behavior.

   Supports the rights of patients to make their own decisions about care.

4. *Organization*: Development of a complex system of values. Creation of a value system.

   Forms a position about issues relating to the cost effectiveness of interventions.

5. *Characterization by a value*: Internalization of a value system providing a philosophy for practice.

   Acts consistently to involve patients and families in decision making about care.

Psychomotor Domain

Psychomotor learning involves the development of motor skills and competency in the use of technology. This domain includes activities that are movement oriented, requiring some degree of physical coordination. Motor skills have a cognitive base, which involves the principles underlying the skill. They also have an affective component reflecting the values of the nurse while carrying out the skill, for example, respecting the patient while performing the procedure.

In developing psychomotor skills, learners progress through three phases of learning: cognitive (understanding what needs to be done), associative (gradually improving performance until movements are consistent), and autonomous (performing the skill automatically) (Schmidt & Lee, 2005). To progress through these levels, students need to practice the skill repetitively and receive specific, informative feedback on their performance: this is called deliberate practice (Ericsson, 2004; Issenberg, McGaghie, Petrusa, Gordon, & Scalese, 2005; McGaghie, Issenberg, Petrusa, & Scalese, 2006, 2010). An understanding of motor skill development guides teachers in planning the instruction of skills in nursing, building in sufficient practice to gain expertise (Oermann, 2011; Oermann, Kardong-Edgren, & Odom-Maryon, 2011).

Different taxonomies have been developed for the evaluation of psychomotor skills. One taxonomy useful in nursing education specifies five levels in the development of psychomotor skills. The lowest level is imitation learning; here the learner observes a demonstration of the skill and imitates that performance. In the second level, the learner performs the skill following written guidelines. By practicing skills the learner refines the ability to perform them without errors (precision) and in a reasonable time frame (articulation) until they become a natural part of care (naturalization) (Dave, 1970; Gaberson & Oermann, 2010). A description of each of these levels and sample objectives follows:

1. *Imitation*: Performance of a skill following demonstration by teacher or through multimedia; imitative learning

   Follows the example for changing a dressing.

2. *Manipulation*: Ability to follow instructions rather than needing to observe the procedure or skill

   Suctions a patient according to the accepted procedure.

3. *Precision*: Ability to perform a skill accurately, independently, and without using a model or set of directions

Takes vital signs accurately.

4. *Articulation*: Coordinated performance of a skill within a reasonable time frame

   Demonstrates skill in suctioning patients with varying health problems.

5. *Naturalization*: High degree of proficiency; integration of skill within care

   Competently carries out skills needed for care of technology-dependent children in their homes.

In another taxonomy, psychomotor skills levels begin with "never performed the skill" and progress through "minimal," "able to perform with support," "able to perform independently," and "experienced" levels, ending with "mastered," meaning that the learner performs the skill automatically (Ferris, 2010; Ferris & Aziz, 2005). This taxonomy has been used in engineering education but also could be adapted for the instruction and assessment of psychomotor skills in nursing.

Assessment methods for psychomotor skills provide data on knowledge of the principles underlying the skill and ability to carry out the procedure in simulations and with patients. Most of the evaluation of performance is done in the clinical setting and in learning and simulation laboratories; however, test items may be used for assessing principles associated with performing the skill.

Integrated Framework

One other framework that could be used to classify objectives was developed by Miller et al. (2009, pp. 54–55). This framework integrates the cognitive, affective, and psychomotor domains into one list and can be easily adapted for nursing education:

1. *Knowledge* (knowledge of terms, facts, concepts, and methods)
2. *Understanding* (understanding concepts, methods, written materials, and problem situations)
3. *Application* (of factual information, concepts, methods, and problem-solving skills)
4. *Thinking skills* (critical and scientific thinking)
5. *General skills* (laboratory, performance, communication, and other skills)

6. *Attitudes* (and values, for example, reflecting standards of nursing practice)
7. *Interests* (personal, educational, and occupational)
8. *Appreciations* (literature, art, and music; scientific and social achievements)
9. *Adjustments* (social and emotional)

USE OF OBJECTIVES FOR ASSESSMENT AND TESTING

As described earlier, the taxonomies provide a framework for the teacher to plan instruction and design assessment strategies at different levels of learning, from simple to complex in the cognitive domain, from awareness of a value to developing a philosophy of practice based on a value system in the affective domain, and increasing psychomotor competency, from imitation of the skill to performance as a natural part of care. These taxonomies are of value in assessing learning and performance to gear tests and other strategies to the level of learning anticipated from the instruction. If the outcome of learning is application, then test items also need to be at the application level. If the outcome of learning is valuing, then the assessment methods need to examine students' behaviors over time to determine if they are committed to practice reflecting these values. If the outcome of skill learning is precision, then the assessment needs to focus on accuracy in performance, not the speed with which the skill is performed. The taxonomies, therefore, provide a useful framework to assure that test items and assessment methods are at the appropriate level for the intended learning outcomes.

In developing test items and other types of assessment methods, the teacher first identifies the outcome, objective, or competency to be evaluated, then designs test items or other methods to collect information to determine if the student has achieved it. For the objective "Identifies characteristics of premature ventricular contractions" the test item would examine student ability to recall those characteristics. The expected performance is at the knowledge level: recalling facts about premature ventricular contractions, not understanding them nor using that knowledge in clinical situations.

Some teachers choose not to use objectives as the basis for testing and evaluation and instead develop test items and other assessment methods from the content of the course. With this process the teacher identifies explicit content areas to be evaluated; test items then sample knowledge of this content. If using this method, the teacher should refer to the course outcomes and placement of the course in the curriculum for decisions about the level of complexity of the test items and other assessment methods.

Throughout this book, multiple types of test items and other assessment methods are presented. It is assumed that these items were developed from specific outcomes, objectives, or competencies, depending on the format used in the nursing program, or from explicit content areas. Regardless of whether the teacher uses objectives or content domains as the framework for assessment, test items and other strategies should evaluate the learning outcome intended from the instruction. The key is linking the objectives to the teaching strategies in the course and the evaluation of students (Cannon & Boswell, 2012).

SUMMARY

Assessment is the collection of information for making decisions about learners, programs, and educational policies. With information collected through assessment, the teacher can determine the progress of students in a course, provide feedback to them about continued learning needs, and plan relevant instructional strategies to meet those needs and help students improve performance. Assessment provides data for making judgments about learning and performance, which is the process of evaluation, and for arriving at grades of students in courses.

A test is a set of items each with a correct answer. Tests are a commonly used assessment strategy in nursing programs. Measurement is the process of assigning numbers to represent student achievement or performance according to certain rules, for instance, answering 20 out of 25 items correctly on a quiz. There are two main ways of interpreting assessment results: norm-referencing and criterion-referencing. In norm-referenced interpretation, test scores and other assessment data are interpreted by comparing them to those of other individuals. Norm-referenced clinical evaluation compares students' clinical performance with those of a group of learners, indicating that the learner has more or less clinical competence than other students. Criterion-referenced interpretation, on the other hand, involves interpreting scores based on preset criteria, not in relation to a group of learners. With criterion-referenced clinical evaluation, student performance is compared with a set of criteria to be met.

Evaluation is an integral part of the instructional process in nursing. Through evaluation, the teacher makes important judgments and decisions about the extent and quality of learning. Evaluation fulfills two major roles: formative and summative. Formative evaluation judges students' progress in meeting the outcomes of learning and developing competencies for practice. It occurs throughout the instructional process and provides feedback for determining where further learning is needed. Summative evaluation, on the other hand, is end-of-instruction evaluation designed to determine what the student has learned in the classroom, an online course, or clinical practice. Summative evaluation judges the quality of the student's achievement in the course, not the progress of the learner in meeting the outcomes.

The learning outcomes or objectives play a role in teaching students in varied settings in nursing. They provide guidelines for student learning and instruction and a basis for assessing learning and performance. These learning targets may be stated as the outcomes, objectives, or competencies to be met by students. Evaluation serves to determine the extent and quality of the student's learning and performance in relation to these outcomes. Some teachers choose not to use objectives or learning outcomes as the basis for testing and evaluation and instead develop their assessment strategies from the content of the course. With this process the teacher identifies explicit content areas to be evaluated; test items and other strategies determine how well students have learned that content. The important principle is that the assessment relates to the expected learning outcomes of the course.

REFERENCES

Anderson, L. W., & Krathwohl, D. R. (Eds.). (2001). *A taxonomy for learning, teaching, and assessing: A revision of Boom's taxonomy of educational objectives.* New York, NY: Longman.

Bloom, B. S., Englehart, M. D., Furst, E. J., Hill, W. H., & Krathwohl, D. R. (1956). *Taxonomy of educational objectives: The classification of educational goals. Handbook I: Cognitive domain.* White Plains, NY: Longman.

Cannon, S., & Boswell, C. (2012). *Evidence-based teaching in nursing: A foundation for educators.* Sudbury, MA: Jones & Bartlett Learning.

Dave, R. H. (1970). Psychomotor levels. In R. J. Armstrong (Ed.), *Developing and writing behavioral objectives.* Tucson, AZ: Educational Innovators.

Ericsson, K. A. (2004). Deliberate practice and the acquisition and maintenance of expert performance in medicine and related domains. *Academic Medicine, 79*(10), S70–S81.

Ferris, T. L. J. (2010). Bloom's taxonomy of educational objectives: A psychomotor skills extension for engineering education. *International Journal of Engineering Education, 26,* 699–707.

Ferris T. L. J., & Aziz, S. M. (2005). A psychomotor skills extension to Bloom's taxonomy of education objectives for engineering education. Paper presented at Exploring Innovation in Education and Research Conference, Tainan, Taiwan.

Gaberson, K. B., & Oermann, M. H. (2010). *Clinical teaching strategies in nursing* (3rd ed.). New York, NY: Springer Publishing.

Issenberg, S. B., McGaghie, W. C., Petrusa, E. R., Gordon, D. L., & Scalese, R. J. (2005). Features and uses of high-fidelity medical simulations that lead to effective learning: A BEME systematic review. *Medical Teacher, 27*(1), 10–28.

Krathwohl, D., Bloom, B., & Masia, B. (1964). *Taxonomy of educational objectives. Handbook II: Affective domain.* New York, NY: Longman.

Marzano, R. J., & Kendall, J. S. (2007). *The new taxonomy of educational objectives* (2nd ed.). Thousand Oaks, CA: Corwin Press.

Marzano, R. J., & Kendall, J. S. (2008). *Designing and assessing educational objectives: Applying the new taxonomy*. Thousand Oaks, CA: Corwin Press.

McGaghie, W. C., Issenberg, S. B., Petrusa, E. R., & Scalese, R. J. (2006). Effect of practice on standardised learning outcomes in simulation-based medical education. *Medical Education, 40*, 792–797.

McGaghie, W. C., Issenberg, S. B., Petrusa, E. R., & Scalese, R. J. (2010). A critical review of simulation-based medical education research: 2003–2009. *Medical Education, 44*, 50–63.

Miller, C. (2010). Improving and enhancing performance in the affective domain of nursing students: Insights from the literature for clinical educators. *Contemporary Nurse, 35*(1), 2–17.

Miller, M. D., Linn, R. L., & Gronlund, N. E. (2009). *Measurement and assessment in teaching* (10th ed.). Upper Saddle River, NJ: Prentice Hall.

Nitko, A. J., & Brookhart, S. M. (2011). *Educational assessment of students* (6th ed.). Upper Saddle River, NJ: Pearson Education.

Oermann, M. H. (2011). Toward evidence-based nursing education: Deliberate practice and motor skill learning. *Journal of Nursing Education, 50*(2), 63–64.

Oermann, M. H., Kardong-Edgren, S., & Odom-Maryon, T. (2011). Effects of monthly practice on nursing students' CPR psychomotor skill performance. *Resuscitation, 82*, 447–453.

Oermann, M. H., Saewert, K. J., Charasika, M., & Yarbrough, S. S. (2009). Assessment and grading practices in schools of nursing: Findings of the Evaluation of Learning Advisory Council Survey. *Nursing Education Perspectives, 30*(4), 274–278.

Schmidt, R. A., & Lee, T. D. (2005). *Motor control and learning: A behavioral emphasis* (4th ed.). Champaign, IL: Human Kinetics.

TWO

Qualities of Effective

Assessment Procedures

How does a teacher know if a test or another assessment instrument is good? If assessment results will be used to make important educational decisions, teachers must have confidence in their interpretations of test scores. Good assessments produce results that can be used to make appropriate inferences about learners' knowledge and abilities. In addition, assessment tools should be practical and easy to use.

Two important questions have been posed to guide the process of constructing or proposing tests and other assessments:

1. To what extent will the interpretation of the scores be appropriate, meaningful, and useful for the intended application of the results?
2. What are the consequences of the particular uses and interpretations that are made of the results? (Miller, Linn, & Gronlund, 2009)

This chapter will explain the concept of assessment validity, the role of reliability, and their effects on the interpretive quality of assessment results. It will also discuss important practical considerations that might affect the choice or development of tests and other instruments.

ASSESSMENT VALIDITY

Definitions of validity have changed over time. Early definitions, formed in the 1940s and early 1950s, emphasized the validity of an assessment tool itself. Tests were characterized as valid or not, apart from consideration of how they were used. It was common in that era to support a claim of validity with evidence that a test correlated well with another "true" criterion. The concept of validity changed, however, in the 1950s through the 1970s to focus on evidence that an assessment tool is valid for a specific purpose. Most measurement textbooks of that era classified validity by three types—content, criterion-related, and construct—and suggested that validation of a test should include more than one approach. In the 1980s, the understanding of validity shifted again, to an emphasis on providing evidence to support the particular inferences that teachers make from assessment results. Validity was defined in terms of the appropriateness and usefulness of the inferences made from assessments, and assessment validation was seen as a process of collecting evidence to support those inferences. The usefulness of the validity "triad" also was questioned; increasingly, measurement experts recognized that construct validity was the key element and unifying concept of validity (Goodwin, 1997; Goodwin & Goodwin, 1999).

The current philosophy of validity continues to focus not on assessment tools themselves or on the appropriateness of using a test for a specific purpose, but on the meaningfulness of the interpretations that teachers make of assessment results. Tests and other assessment instruments yield scores that teachers use to make inferences about how much learners know or what they can do. Validity refers to the adequacy and appropriateness of those interpretations and inferences and how the assessment results are used (Miller et al., 2009). The emphasis is on the consequences of measurement: Does the teacher make accurate interpretations about learners' knowledge or ability based on their test scores? Assessment experts increasingly suggest that in addition to collecting evidence to support the accuracy of inferences made, evidence also should be collected about the intended and unintended consequences of the use of a test (Goodwin, 1997; Goodwin & Goodwin, 1999; Nitko & Brookhart, 2011).

Validity does not exist on an all-or-none basis (Miller et al., 2009); there are degrees of validity depending on the purpose of the assessment and how the results are to be used. A given assessment may be used for many different purposes, and inferences about the results may have greater validity for one purpose than for another. For example, a test designed to measure knowledge of perioperative nursing standards may produce results that have high validity for the purpose of determining certification for perioperative staff nurses, but the results may have low validity for assigning grades to students in a perioperative nursing elective course. Additionally, validity evidence may change over time, so that validation of inferences must not be considered a onetime event.

Validity now is considered a unitary concept (Miller et al., 2009; Nitko & Brookhart, 2011). The concept of validity in testing is described in the *Standards for Educational and Psychological Testing* prepared by a joint committee of the American Educational Research Association (AERA), American Psychological Association (APA), and National Council on Measurement in Education (NCME). The most recent *Standards* (1999) no longer includes the view that there are different types of validity—for example, construct, criterion-related, and content.

Instead, there are a variety of sources of evidence to support the validity of the interpretation and use of assessment results. The strongest case for validity can be made when evidence is collected regarding four major considerations for validation:

1. content
2. construct
3. assessment-criterion relationships
4. consequences (Miller et al., 2009, p. 74)

Each of these considerations will be discussed as they can be used in nursing education settings.

Content Considerations

The goal of content validation is to determine the degree to which a sample of assessment tasks accurately represents the domain of content or abilities about which the teacher wants to interpret assessment results. Tests and other assessment measures usually contain only a sample of all possible items or tasks that could be used to assess the domain of interest. However, interpretations of assessment results are based on what the teacher believes to be the universe of items that could have been generated. In other words, when a student correctly answers 83% of the items on a women's health nursing final examination, the teacher usually infers that the student probably would answer correctly 83% of all items in the universe of women's health nursing content. The test score thus serves as an indicator of the student's true standing in the larger domain. Although this type of generalization is commonly made, it should be noted that the domains of achievement in nursing education involve complex understandings and integrated performances, about which it is difficult to judge the representativeness of a sample of assessment tasks (Miller et al., 2009).

A superficial conclusion could be made about the match between a test's appearance and its intended use by asking a panel of experts to judge whether the test appears to be based on appropriate content. This type of judgment, sometimes referred to as face validity, is not sufficient evidence of content representativeness and should not be used as a substitute for rigorous appraisal of sampling adequacy (Miller et al., 2009).

Efforts to include suitable content on an assessment can and should be made during its development. This process begins with defining the universe of content. The content definition should be related to the purpose for which the test will be used. For example, if a test is supposed to measure a new staff nurse's understanding of hospital safety policies and procedures presented during orientation, the teacher first defines the universe of content by outlining the knowledge about policies that the staff nurse needs to function satisfactorily. The teacher then uses professional judgment to write or select test items that satisfactorily represent this desired content domain. A system for documenting this process, the construction of a test blueprint or table of specifications, will be described in Chapter 3.

If the teacher needs to select an appropriate assessment for a particular use, for example, choosing a standardized achievement test, content validation is also of concern. A published test may or may not be suitable for the intended use in a particular nursing education program or with a specific group of learners. The ultimate responsibility for appropriate use of an assessment and interpretation of results lies with the teacher (Miller et al., 2009; AERA, APA, & NCME, 1999; see APA Table 6.1). To determine the extent to which an existing test is suitable, experts in the domain review the assessment, item by item, to determine if the items or tasks are relevant and satisfactorily represent the defined domain, represented by the table of specifications, and the desired learning outcomes. Because these judgments admittedly are subjective, the trustworthiness of this evidence depends on clear instructions to the experts and estimation of rater reliability.

Construct Considerations

Construct validity has been proposed as the "umbrella" under which all types of assessment validation belong (Goodwin, 1997; Goodwin & Goodwin, 1999). Content validation determines how well test scores represent a given domain and is important in evaluating assessments of achievement. When teachers need to make inferences from assessment results to more general abilities and characteristics, however, such as critical thinking or communication ability, a critical consideration is the construct that the assessment is intended to measure (Miller et al., 2009).

A construct is an individual characteristic that is assumed to exist because it explains some observed behavior. As a theoretical construction, it cannot be observed directly, but it can be inferred from performance on an assessment. Construct validation is the process of determining the extent to which assessment results can be interpreted in terms of a given construct or set of constructs. Two questions, applicable to both teacher-constructed and published assessments, are central to the process of construct validation:

1. How adequately does the assessment represent the construct of interest (construct representation)?
2. Is the observed performance influenced by any irrelevant or ancillary factors (construct relevance)? (Miller et al., 2009)

Assessment validity is reduced to the extent that important elements of the construct are underrepresented in the assessment. For example, if the construct of interest is clinical problem-solving ability, the validity of a clinical performance assessment would be weakened if it focused entirely on problems defined by the teacher, because the learner's ability to recognize and define clinical problems is an important aspect of clinical problem solving (Gaberson & Oermann, 2010).

The influence of factors that are unrelated or irrelevant to the construct of interest also reduces assessment validity. For example, students for whom English is a second language may perform poorly on an assessment of clinical problem solving, not because of limited ability to recognize, identify, and solve problems, but because of unfamiliarity with language or cultural colloquialisms used by patients or teachers (Bosher & Bowles, 2008; Bosher, 2009). Another potential construct-irrelevant factor is writing skill. For example, the ability to communicate clearly and accurately in writing may be an important outcome of a nursing education program, but the construct of interest for a course writing assignment is clinical problem solving. To the extent that student scores on that assignment are affected by spelling or grammatical errors, the construct-relevant validity of the assessment is reduced. Testwiseness, performance anxiety, and learner motivation are additional examples of possible construct-irrelevant factors that may undermine assessment validity (Miller et al., 2009).

Construct validation for a teacher-made assessment occurs primarily during its development by collecting evidence of construct representation and construct relevance from a variety of sources. Test manuals for published tests should include evidence that these methods were used to generate evidence of construct validity. Methods used in construct validation include:

1. *Defining the domain to be measured.* The assessment specifications should clearly define the meaning of the construct so that it is possible to judge whether the assessment includes relevant and representative tasks.

2. *Analyzing the process of responding to tasks required by the assessment.* The teacher can administer an assessment task to the learners (for example, a multiple-choice item that purportedly assesses critical thinking) and ask them to think aloud while they perform the test (for example, explain how they arrived at the answer they chose). This method may reveal that students were able to identify the correct answer because the same example was used in class or in an assigned reading, not because they were able to analyze the situation critically.

3. *Comparing assessment results of known groups.* Sometimes it is reasonable to expect that scores on a particular measure will differ from one group to another because members of those groups are known to possess different

levels of the ability being measured. For example, if the purpose of a test is to measure students' ability to think critically about pediatric clinical problems, students who achieve high scores on this test would be assumed to be better critical thinkers than students who achieve low scores. To collect evidence in support of this assumption, the teacher might design a study to determine if student scores on the test are correlated with their scores on a standardized test of critical thinking in nursing. The teacher could divide the sample of students into two groups based on their standardized test scores: those who scored high on the standardized test in one group and those whose standardized test scores were low in the other group. Then the teacher would compare the teacher-made test scores of the students in both groups. If the teacher's hypothesis is confirmed (that is, if the students with high standardized test scores obtained high scores on the teacher-made test), this evidence could be used as partial support for construct validation (Miller et al., 2009).

Group-comparison techniques also have been used in studies of test bias or test fairness. Approaches to detection of test bias have looked for differential item functioning (DIF) related to test-takers' race, gender, or culture. If test items function differently for members of groups with characteristics that do not directly relate to the variable of interest, differential validity of inferences from the test scores may result. Issues related to test bias will be discussed more fully in Chapter 15.

4. *Comparing assessment results before and after a learning activity.* It is reasonable to expect that assessments of student performance would improve during instruction, whether in the classroom or in the clinical area, but assessment results should not be affected by other variables such as anxiety or memory of the preinstruction assessment content. For example, evidence that assessment scores improve following instruction but are unaffected by an intervention designed to reduce students' test anxiety would support the assessment's construct validity (Miller et al., 2009).

5. *Correlating assessment results with other measures.* Scores produced by a particular assessment should correlate well with scores of other measures of the same construct but show poor correlation with measures of a different construct. For example, teachers' ratings of students' performance in pediatric clinical settings should correlate highly with scores on a final exam testing knowledge of nursing care of children, but may not correlate satisfactorily with their classroom or clinical performance in a women's health course. These correlations may be used to support the claim that a test measures the construct of interest (Miller et al., 2009).

Assessment-Criterion Relationship Considerations

This approach to obtaining validity evidence focuses on predicting future performance (the criterion) based on current assessment results. For example, nursing faculties often use scores from a standardized comprehensive exam given in the final academic semester or quarter to predict whether prelicensure students are likely to be successful on the NCLEX® (the criterion measure). Obtaining this type of evidence involves a predictive validation study (Miller et al., 2009).

If teachers want to use assessment results to estimate students' performance on another assessment (the criterion measure) at the same time, the validity evidence is concurrent, and obtaining this type of evidence requires a concurrent validation study. This type of evidence may be desirable for making a decision about whether one test or measurement instrument may be substituted for another, more resource-intensive one. For example, a staff development educator may want to collect concurrent validity evidence to determine if a checklist with a rating scale can be substituted for a less efficient narrative appraisal of a staff nurse's competence.

Teachers rarely conduct formal studies of the extent to which the scores on assessments that they have constructed are correlated with criterion measures. In some cases, adequate criterion measures are not available; the test in use is considered to be the best instrument that has been devised to measure the ability in question. If better measures were available, they might be used instead of the test being validated. However, for tests with high-stakes outcomes, such as licensure and certification, this type of validity evidence is crucial. Multiple criterion measures often are used so that the strengths of one measure may offset the weaknesses of others (Miller et al., 2009).

The relationship between assessment scores and those obtained on the criterion measure usually is expressed as a correlation coefficient. A desired level of correlation between the two measures cannot be recommended because the correlation may be influenced by a number of factors, including test length, variability of scores in the distribution, and the amount of time between measures. The teacher who uses the test must use good professional judgment to determine what magnitude of correlation is considered adequate for the intended use of the assessment for which criterion-related evidence is desired.

Consideration of Consequences

Incorporating concern about the social consequences of assessment into the concept of validity is a relatively recent trend. Assessment has both intended and unintended consequences. For example, the faculties of many undergraduate nursing programs have adopted programs of achievement testing that are designed to assess student performance throughout the nursing curriculum. The intended positive consequence of such testing is to identify students at risk of failure on the NCLEX, and to use this information to design remediation programs to increase student learning. Unintended negative consequences, however, may include increased student anxiety, decreased time for instruction relative to increased time allotted for testing, and tailoring instruction to more closely match the content of the tests while focusing less intently on other important aspects of the curriculum that will not be tested on the NCLEX. The intended consequence of using standardized comprehensive exam scores to predict success on the NCLEX may be to motivate students whose assessment results predict failure to remediate and prepare more thoroughly for the licensure exam. But an unintended consequence might be that students whose comprehensive exam scores predict NCLEX success may decide not to prepare further for that important exam, risking a negative outcome.

Ultimately, assessment validity requires an evaluation of interpretations and use of assessment results. The concept of validity thus has expanded to include consideration of the consequences of assessment use and how results are interpreted to students, teachers, and other stakeholders. An adequate consideration of consequences must include both intended and unintended effects of assessment, particularly when assessment results are used to make high-stakes decisions (Miller et al., 2009).

Influences on Validity

A number of factors affect the validity of assessment results, including characteristics of the assessment itself, the administration and scoring procedures, and the test-takers. Teachers should be alert to these factors when constructing assessments or choosing published ones (Miller et al., 2009).

Characteristics of the Assessment

Many factors can prevent the assessment items or tasks from functioning as intended, thereby decreasing the validity of the interpretations from the assessment results. Such factors include unclear directions, ambiguous statements, inadequate time limits, oversampling of easy-to-assess aspects, too few assessment items, poor arrangement of assessment items, an obvious pattern of correct answers, and clerical errors in test construction (Miller et al., 2009). Ways to prevent test construction errors such as these will be addressed in the following chapters.

Assessment Administration and Scoring Factors

On teacher-made assessments, factors such as insufficient time, inconsistency in giving aid to students who ask questions during the assessment, cheating, and scoring errors may lower validity. On published assessments, an additional factor may be failure to follow the standard directions, including time limits (Miller et al., 2009).

Student Characteristics

Some invalid interpretations of assessment results are the result of personal factors that influence a student's performance on the assessment. For example, a student may have had an emotionally upsetting event such as an auto accident or death in the family just prior to the assessment, test anxiety may prevent the student from performing according to true ability level, or the student may not be motivated to exert maximum effort on the assessment. These and similar factors may modify student responses on the assessment and distort the results, leading to lower validity (Miller et al., 2009).

RELIABILITY

Reliability refers to the consistency of scores. If an assessment produces reliable scores, the same group of students would achieve approximately the same scores if the same assessment were given on another occasion. Each assessment produces a limited measure of performance at a specific time. If this measurement is reasonably consistent over time, with different raters, or with different samples of the same domain, teachers can be more confident in the assessment results. However, assessment results cannot be perfectly consistent because many extraneous factors may influence the measurement of performance. Scores may be inconsistent because:

1. the behavior being measured is unstable over time because of fluctuations in memory, attention, and effort; intervening learning experiences; or varying emotional or health status;
2. the sample of tasks varies from one assessment to another, and some students find one assessment to be easier than another because it contains tasks related to topics they know well;
3. assessment conditions vary significantly between assessments; or
4. scoring procedures are inconsistent (the same rater may use different criteria on different assessments, or different raters may not reach perfect agreement on the same assessment).

These and other factors introduce a certain but unknown amount of error into every measurement. Methods of determining assessment reliability, therefore, are means of estimating how much measurement error is present under varying assessment conditions. When assessment results are reasonably consistent, there is less measurement error and greater reliability (Miller et al., 2009).

For purposes of understanding sources of inconsistency, it is helpful to view an assessment score as having two components, a true score and an error score, represented by the following equation:

$$X = T + E$$

A student's actual assessment score (X) is also known as the observed or obtained score. That student's hypothetical true score (T) cannot be measured directly because it is the average of all scores the student would obtain if tested on many occasions with the same test. The observed score contains a certain amount of measurement error (E), which may be a positive or a negative value. This error of measurement, representing the difference between the observed score and the true score, results in a student's obtained score being higher or lower than his or her true score (Nitko & Brookhart, 2011). If it were possible to measure directly the amount of measurement error that occurred on each testing occasion, two of the values in this equation would be known (X and E), and we would be able to calculate the true score (T). However, we can only estimate indirectly the amount of measurement error, leaving us with a hypothetical true score. Therefore, teachers need to recognize that the obtained score on any test is only an estimate of what the student really knows about the domain being tested.

For example, Matt may obtain a higher score than Kelly on a community health nursing unit test because Matt truly knows more about the content than Kelly does. Test scores should reflect this kind of difference, and if the difference in knowledge is the only explanation for the score difference, no error is involved. However, there may be other potential explanations for the difference between Kelly's and Matt's test scores. Matt may have behaved dishonestly to obtain a copy of the test in advance; knowing which items would be included, he had the opportunity to use unauthorized resources to determine the correct answers to those items. In his case, measurement error would have increased Matt's obtained score. Kelly may have worked overtime the night before the test and may not have gotten enough sleep to allow her to feel alert during the test. Thus, her performance may have been affected by her fatigue and her decreased ability to concentrate, resulting in an obtained score lower than her true score. One goal of assessment designers therefore is to maximize the amount of score variance that explains real differences in ability and to minimize the amount of random error variance of scores.

The following points further explain the concept of assessment reliability (Miller et al., 2009):

1. *Reliability pertains to assessment results, not to the assessment instrument itself.* The reliability of results produced by a given instrument will vary depending on the characteristics of the students being assessed and the circumstances under which it is used. Reliability should be estimated with each use of the assessment instrument.

2. *A reliability estimate always refers to a particular type of consistency.* Assessment results may be consistent over different periods of time, or different samples of the domain, or different raters or observers. It is possible for assessment results to be reliable in one or more of these respects but not in others. The desired type of reliability evidence depends on the intended use of the assessment results. For example, if the faculty wants to assess students' ability to make sound clinical decisions in a variety of settings, a measure of consistency over time would not be appropriate. Instead, an estimate of consistency of performance across different tasks would be more useful.

3. *A reliability estimate always is calculated with statistical indices.* Consistency of assessment scores over time, among raters, or across different assessment measures involves determining the relationship between two or more sets of scores. The extent of consistency is expressed in terms of a reliability coefficient (a form of correlation coefficient) or a standard error of measurement. A reliability coefficient differs from a validity coefficient (described earlier) in that it is based on agreement between two sets of assessment results from the same procedure instead of agreement with an external criterion.

4. *Reliability is an essential but insufficient condition for validity.* Teachers cannot make valid inferences from inconsistent assessment results. Conversely, highly consistent results may indicate only that the assessment measured the wrong construct (although doing it very reliably). Thus, low reliability always produces a low degree of validity, but a high reliability estimate does not guarantee a high degree of validity. "In short, reliability merely provides the consistency that makes validity possible" (Miller et al., 2009, p. 108).

An example may help to illustrate the relationship between validity and reliability. Suppose that the author of this chapter was given a test of her knowledge of assessment principles. The author of a textbook on assessment in nursing education might be expected to achieve a high score on such a test. However, if the test were written in Mandarin Chinese, the author's score might be very low, even if she were a remarkably good guesser, because she cannot read Mandarin Chinese. If the same test were administered the following week, and every week for a month, her scores would likely be consistently low. Therefore, these test scores would be considered reliable because there would be a high correlation among scores

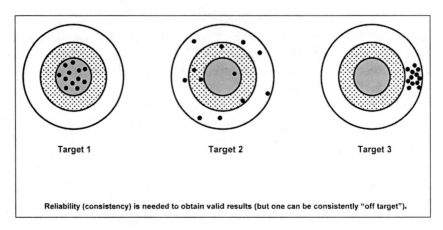

Reliability (consistency) is needed to obtain valid results (but one can be consistently "off target").

Figure 2.1   The relationship between reliability and validity.
Source: From M. D. Miller, R. L. Linn, & N. E. Gronlund (2009). *Measurement and assessment in teaching* (10th ed.). Boston, MA: Allyn and Bacon/Merrill Education. Copyright © 2009 by Pearson Education. Reprinted by permission of the publisher.

obtained on the same test over a period of several administrations. But a valid score-based interpretation of the author's knowledge of assessment principles could not be drawn because the test was not appropriate for its intended use.

Figure 2.1 uses a target-shooting analogy to further illustrate these relationships. When they design and administer assessments, teachers attempt to consistently (reliably) measure the true value of what students know and can do (hit the bull's eye); if they succeed, they can make valid inferences from assessment results. Target 1 illustrates the reliability of scores that are closely grouped on the bull's eye, the true score, allowing the teacher to make valid inferences about them. Target 2 displays assessment scores that are widely scattered at a distance from the true score; these scores are not reliable, contributing to a lack of validity evidence. Target 3 shows assessment scores that are reliable because they are closely grouped together, but they are still distant from the true score. The teacher would not be able to make valid interpretations of such scores (Miller et al., 2009).

Methods of Estimating Reliability

Because reliability is viewed in terms of different types of consistency, these types are determined by different methods: over time (stability), among different forms of the assessment (equivalence), within the assessment itself (internal consistency), and among different raters (consistency of ratings or interrater reliability). Each method of estimating reliability will be described in further detail.

Measure of Stability

Evidence of stability indicates whether students would achieve essentially the same scores if they took the same assessment at another time—a test–retest procedure. The correlation between the set of scores obtained on the first administration and the set obtained on the second yields a test–retest reliability coefficient. This type of reliability evidence is known as stability, and is appropriate for situations in which the trait being measured is expected to be stable over time. In general, the longer the period of time between administrations of the test, the lower the stability–reliability estimate (Nitko & Brookhart, 2011). In nursing education settings, the test–retest method of obtaining reliability information may have limited usefulness. If the same test items are used on both tests, the students' answers on the retest are not independent of their answers on the first test. That is, their responses to the second test may be influenced to some extent by recall of their previous responses or by discussion or individual review of content after taking the first test. In addition, if there is a long interval between testing occasions, other factors such as real changes in student ability as a result of learning may affect the retest scores. When selecting standardized tests, however, stability is an important consideration (Miller et al., 2009).

Measure of Equivalence

Equivalent-forms reliability, also known as alternate or parallel forms, involves the use of two or more forms of the same assessment, constructed independently but based on the same set of specifications. Both forms of the assessment are administered to the same group of students in close succession, and the resulting scores are correlated. A high reliability coefficient indicates that the two forms sample the domain of interest equally well, and that generalizations about student performance from one assessment to the other can be made with a high degree of validity. The equivalent-form estimates of reliability are widely used in standardized testing, primarily to assure test security, but the user cannot assume comparability of alternate forms unless the test manual provides information about equivalence (Miller et al., 2009). This method of reliability estimation is not practical for teacher-constructed assessments because most teachers do not find time to prepare two forms of the same test, let alone to assure that these forms indeed are equivalent (Nitko & Brookhart, 2011).

Measures of Internal Consistency

Internal consistency methods can be used with a set of scores from only one administration of a single assessment. Sometimes referred to as split-half or half-length methods, estimates of internal consistency reveal the extent to which consistent results are obtained from two halves of the same assessment.

The split-half technique consists of dividing the assessment into two equal subtests, usually by including odd-numbered items on one subtest and even-numbered items on the other. Then the subtests are scored separately, and the two subscores are correlated. The resulting correlation coefficient is an estimate of the extent to which the two halves consistently perform the same measurement. Longer assessments tend to produce more reliable results than shorter ones, in part because they tend to sample the content domain more fully. Therefore, a split-half reliability estimate tends to underestimate the true reliability of the scores produced by the whole assessment (because each subset includes only half of the total number of items). This underestimate can be corrected by using the Spearman-Brown prophecy formula, also called the Spearman-Brown double length formula, as represented by the following equation (Miller et al., 2009, p. 114):

Reliability of full assessment =

$$\frac{2 \times \text{correlation between half test scores}}{1 + \text{correlation between half test scores}}$$

Another method of estimating the internal consistency of a test is to use certain types of coefficient alpha. Coefficient alpha reliability estimates provide information about the extent to which the assessment tasks measure similar characteristics. When the assessment contains relatively homogenous material, the coefficient alpha reliability estimate is similar to that produced by the split-half method. In other words, coefficient alpha represents the average correlation obtained from all possible split-half reliability estimates. The Kuder-Richardson formulas are a specific type of coefficient alpha. Computation of Formula 20 (KR20) is based on the proportion of correct responses and the standard deviation of the total score distribution. If the assessment items are not expected to vary much in difficulty, the simpler Formula 21 (K-R21) can be used to approximate the value of K-R20, although in most cases it will produce a slightly lower estimate of reliability. To use either formula, the assessment items must be scored dichotomously, that is, right or wrong (Miller et al., 2009; Nitko & Brookhart, 2011). If the assessment items could receive a range of points, coefficient alpha should be used to provide a reliability estimate. The widespread availability of computer software for assessment scoring and test and item analysis makes these otherwise cumbersome calculations more feasible to obtain efficiently (Miller et al. 2009).

Measures of Consistency of Ratings

Depending on the type of assessment, error may arise from the procedures used to score a test. Teachers may need to collect evidence to answer the question, "Would this student have obtained the same score if a different person had scored the assessment or judged the performance?" The easiest method for collecting this evidence is to have two equally qualified persons score each student's paper or rate each student's performance. The two scores then are compared to produce a percentage of agreement or correlated to produce an index of scorer consistency, depending on whether agreement in an absolute sense or a relative sense is required. Achieving a high degree of interrater consistency depends on consensus of judgment among raters regarding the value of a given performance. Such consensus is facilitated by the use of scoring rubrics and training of raters to use those rubrics. Interrater consistency is important to ensure that differences in stringency or leniency of ratings between raters do not place some students at a disadvantage (Miller et al., 2009).

Factors That Influence the Reliability of Scores

From the previous discussion, it is obvious that various factors can influence the reliability of a set of test scores. These factors can be categorized into three main sources: the assessment instrument itself, the student, and the assessment administration conditions.

Assessment-related factors include the length of the test, the homogeneity of assessment tasks, and the difficulty and discrimination ability of the individual items. In general, the greater the number of assessment tasks (e.g., test items), the greater the score reliability. The Spearman-Brown reliability estimate formula can be used to estimate the effect on the reliability coefficient of adding assessment tasks. For example, if a 10-item test has a reliability coefficient of 0.40, adding 15 items (creating a test that is 2.5 times the length of the original test) would produce a reliability estimate of 0.625. Of course, adding assessment tasks to increase score reliability may be counterproductive after a certain point. After that point, adding tasks will increase the reliability only slightly, and student fatigue and boredom actually may introduce more measurement error. Score reliability also is enhanced by homogeneity of content covered by the assessment. Course content that is tightly organized and highly interrelated tends to make homogeneous assessment content easier to achieve. Finally, the technical quality of assessment items, their difficulty, and their ability to discriminate between students who know the content and students who don't also affects the reliability of scores. Moderately difficult items that discriminate well between high achievers and low achievers and that contain no technical errors contribute a great deal to score reliability. See Chapter 12 for a discussion of item difficulty and discrimination.

Student-related factors include the heterogeneity of the student group, test-taking ability, and motivation. In general, reliability tends to increase as the range of talent in the group of students increases. Therefore, in situations in which students are very similar to one another in ability, such as in graduate programs, assessments are likely to produce scores with somewhat lower reliability than desired. A student's test-taking skill and experience also may influence score reliability to the extent that the student is able to obtain a higher score than true ability would predict. The effect of motivation on reliability is proportional to the extent to which it influences individual students differently. If some students are not motivated to put forth their best efforts on an assessment, their actual achievement levels may not be accurately represented, and their relative achievement in comparison to other students will be difficult to judge.

Teachers need to control assessment administration conditions to enhance the reliability of scores. Inadequate time to complete the assessment can lower the reliability of scores because some students who know the content well will be unable to respond to all of the items. Cheating also contributes random errors to assessment scores when students are able to respond correctly to items to which they actually do not know the answer. Cheating, therefore, has the effect of raising the offenders' observed scores above their true scores, contributing to inaccurate and less meaningful interpretations of test scores.

Because a reliability coefficient is an indication of the amount of measurement error associated with a set of scores, it is useful information for evaluating the meaning and usefulness of those scores. Again, it is important to remember that the numerical value of a reliability coefficient is not a stable property of an assessment; it will fluctuate from one sample of students to another each time the assessment is administered. Teachers often wonder how high the reliability coefficient should be to ensure that an assessment will produce reliable results. The degree of reliability desired depends on a number of factors, including the importance of the educational decision being made, how far-reaching the consequences would be, and whether it is possible to confirm or reverse the judgment later. For irreversible decisions that would have serious consequences, like the results of the first attempt of the NCLEX, a high degree of reliability must be assured. For less important decisions, especially if later review can confirm or reverse them without serious harm to the student, less reliable methods may be acceptable. For teacher-made assessments, a reliability coefficient between 0.60 and 0.85 is desirable (Miller et al., 2009).

PRACTICALITY

Although reliability and validity are used to describe the ways in which scores are interpreted and used, practicality (also referred to as usability) is a quality of the assessment instrument itself and its administration procedures. Assessment procedures should be efficient and economical. An assessment is practical or usable to the extent that it is easy to administer and score, does not take too much time away from other instructional activities, and has reasonable resource requirements. Whether they develop their own tests and other measurement tools or use published instruments, teachers should focus on the following questions to help guide the selection of appropriate assessment procedures (Miller et al., 2009; Nitko & Brookhart, 2011):

1. *Is the assessment easy to construct and use?* Essay test items may be written more quickly and easily than multiple-choice items, but they will take more time to score. Multiple-choice items that assess a student's ability to think critically about clinical problems are time-consuming to construct, but they may be machine-scored quickly and accurately. The teacher must determine the best use of the time available for assessment construction, administration, and scoring. If a published test is selected for assessment of students' competencies just prior to graduation, is it practical to use? Does proper administration of the test require special training? Are the test administration directions easy to understand?

2. *Is the time needed to administer and score the assessment and interpret the results reasonable?* A teacher of a 15-week, 3-credit course wants to give a weekly 10-point quiz that would be reviewed immediately and self-scored by students; these procedures would take a total of 30 minutes of class time. Is this the best use of instructional time? The teacher may decide that there is enormous value in the immediate feedback provided to students during the test review, and that the opportunity to obtain weekly information about the effectiveness of instruction is also beneficial; to that teacher, 30 minutes weekly is time well spent on assessment. Another teacher, whose total instructional time is only 4 days, may find that administering more than one test consumes time that is needed for teaching. Evaluation is an important step in the instructional process, but it cannot replace teaching. Although students often learn from the process of preparing for and taking assessments, instruction is not the primary purpose of assessment, and assessment is not the most efficient or effective way to achieve instructional goals. On the other hand, reliability is related to the length of an assessment (i.e., the number of assessment tasks); it may be preferable to use fewer assessments of longer length rather than more frequent shorter assessments.

3. *Are the costs associated with assessment construction, administration, and scoring reasonable?* Although teacher-made assessments may seem to be less expensive than published instruments, the cost of the instructor's time spent in assessment development must be taken into consideration. Additional costs associated with the scoring of teacher-made assessments also must be calculated. What is the initial cost of purchasing test booklets for published instruments, and can test booklets be reused? What is the cost of answer sheets, and does that cost include scoring services? When considering the adoption of a computerized testing package, teachers and administrators must decide how the costs of the program will be paid and by whom (the educational program or the individual students).

4. *Can the assessment results be interpreted easily and accurately by those who will use them?* If teachers score their own assessments, will they obtain results that will help them to interpret the results accurately? For example, will they have test and item statistics that will help them make meaning out of the individual test scores? Scanners and software are available that will quickly score assessments that use certain types of answer sheets, but the scope of the information produced in the score report varies considerably. Purchased assessments that are scored by the publisher also yield reports of test results. Are these reports useful for their intended purpose? What information is needed or desired by the teachers who will make evaluation decisions, and is that information provided by the score-reporting service?

Examples of information on score reports include individual raw total scores, individual raw subtest scores, group mean and median scores, individual or group profiles, and individual standard scores. Will the teachers who receive the reports need special training to interpret this information accurately? Some assessment publishers restrict the purchase of instruments to users with certain educational and experience qualifications, in part so that the test results will be interpreted and used properly.

SUMMARY

Because assessment results often are used to make important educational decisions, teachers must have confidence in their interpretations of test scores. Assessment validity produces results that permit teachers to make accurate interpretations about a test-taker's knowledge or ability. Validity is not a static property of the assessment itself, but rather, it refers to the ways in which teachers interpret and use the assessment results. Validity is not an either/or judgment; there are degrees of validity depending on the purpose of the assessment and how the results are to be used. A single assessment may be used for many different purposes, and the results may have greater validity for one purpose than for another.

Teachers must gather a variety of sources of evidence to support the validity of their interpretation and use of assessment results. Four major considerations for validation are related to content, construct, assessment-criterion relationships, and the consequences of assessment. *Content considerations* focus on the extent to which the sample of assessment items or tasks represents the domain of content or abilities that the teacher wants to measure. Content validity evidence may be obtained during the assessment-development process as well as by appraising a completed assessment, as in the case of a purchased instrument. Currently, *construct considerations* are seen as the unifying concept of assessment validity, representing the extent to which score-based inferences about the construct of interest are accurate and meaningful. Two questions central to the process of construct validation concern how adequately the assessment represents the construct of interest (construct representation), and the extent to which irrelevant or ancillary factors influence the results (construct relevance). Methods used in construct validation include defining the domain to be measured, analyzing the task-response processes required by the assessment, comparing assessment results of known groups, comparing assessment results before and after a learning activity, and correlating assessment results with other measures. Procedures for collecting evidence using each of these methods were described.

Assessment-criterion relationship considerations for obtaining validity evidence focus on predicting future performance (the criterion) based on current assessment results. Obtaining this type of evidence involves a predictive validation study. If the assessment results are to be used to estimate students' performance on another assessment (the criterion measure) at the same time, the evidence is concurrent, and obtaining this type of evidence requires a concurrent validation study. Teachers rarely study the correlation of their own assessment results with criterion measures, but for tests with high-stakes outcomes, such as licensure and certification, this type of validity evidence is critical.

Ultimately, assessment validity requires an evaluation of interpretations and use of assessment results. The concept of validity thus has expanded to include *consideration of the consequences of assessment use* and how results are interpreted to students, teachers, and other stakeholders. Consideration of consequences must include both intended and unintended effects of assessment, particularly when assessment results are used to make high-stakes decisions.

A number of factors affect the validity of assessment results, including characteristics of the assessment itself, the administration and scoring procedures, and the test-takers. Each of these factors was discussed in some detail.

Reliability refers to the consistency of scores. Each assessment produces a limited measure of performance at a specific time. If this measurement is reasonably consistent over time, with different raters, or with different samples of the same domain, teachers can be more confident in the assessment results. Many extraneous factors may influence the measurement of performance, including instability of the behavior being measured, different samples of tasks in each assessment, varying assessment conditions between assessments, and inconsistent scoring procedures. These and other factors introduce error into every measurement. Methods of determining assessment reliability estimate how much measurement error is present under varying assessment conditions. When assessment results are reasonably consistent, there is less measurement error and greater reliability.

Several points are important to an understanding of the concept of assessment reliability. Reliability pertains to assessment results, not to the assessment instrument itself. A reliability estimate always refers to a particular type of consistency, and it is possible for assessment results to be reliable in one or more of these respects but not in others. A reliability estimate always is calculated with statistical indices that express the relationship between two or more sets of scores. Reliability is an essential but insufficient condition for validity; low reliability always produces a low degree of validity, but a high reliability estimate does not guarantee a high degree of validity. Each of these points was discussed in this chapter.

Because reliability is viewed in terms of different types of consistency, these types are determined by different methods: over time (stability), among different forms of the assessment (equivalence), within the assessment itself (internal consistency), and among different raters (consistency of ratings or interrater reliability). Measures of stability indicate whether students would achieve essentially the same scores if they took the same assessment at another time—a test–retest procedure. Measures of equivalence involve the use of two or more forms of the same assessment, based on the same set of specifications (equivalent or alternate forms). Both forms of the assessment are administered to the same group of students in close succession, and the resulting scores are correlated. A high reliability coefficient indicates that teachers can make valid generalizations about student performance from one assessment to the other. Equivalent-form estimates of reliability are widely used in standardized testing, but are not practical for teacher-constructed assessments. Measures of internal consistency (split-half or half-length methods) can be used with a set of scores from only one administration of a single assessment. Estimates of internal consistency reveal the extent to which consistent results are obtained from two halves of the same assessment, revealing the extent to which the test items are internally consistent or homogeneous. Measures of consistency of ratings determine the extent to which ratings from two or more equally qualified persons agree on the score or rating. Interrater consistency is important to ensure that differences in stringency or leniency of ratings between raters do not place some students at a disadvantage. Use of scoring rubrics and training of raters to use those rubrics facilitates consensus among raters.

Various factors can influence the reliability of a set of test scores. These factors can be categorized into three main sources: the assessment instrument itself, the student, and the assessment administration conditions. Assessment-related factors include the length of the assessment, the homogeneity of assessment content, and the difficulty and discrimination ability of the individual items. Student-related factors include the heterogeneity of the student group, test-taking ability, and motivation. Factors related to assessment administration include inadequate time to complete the test and cheating.

In addition, assessment tools should be practical and easy to use. Although reliability and validity are used to describe the ways in which scores are interpreted and used, practicality or usability is a quality of the instrument itself and its administration procedures. Assessment procedures should be efficient and economical. Teachers need to evaluate the following factors: ease of construction and use; time needed to administer and score the assessment and interpret the results; costs associated with assessment construction, administration, and scoring; and the ease with which assessment results can be interpreted simply and accurately by those who will use them.

REFERENCES

American Educational Research Association, American Psychological Association, & National Council on Measurement in Education. (1999). *Standards for educational and psychological testing*. Washington, DC: American Educational Research Association.
Bosher, S. D. (2009). Removing language as a barrier to success on multiple-choice exams. In S. D. Bosher & M. D. Pharris (Eds.), *Transforming nursing education: The culturally inclusive environment* (pp. 259–284). New York, NY: Springer Publishing.
Bosher, S., & Bowles, M. (2008). The effects of linguistic modification on ESL students' comprehension of nursing course test items. *Nursing Education Perspectives, 29*, 165–172.
Gaberson, K. B., & Oermann, M. H. (2010). *Clinical teaching strategies in nursing education* (3rd ed.). New York, NY: Springer Publishing.
Goodwin, L. D. (1997). Changing conceptions of measurement validity. *Journal of Nursing Education, 36*, 102–107.
Goodwin, L. D., & Goodwin, W. L. (1999). Measurement myths and misconceptions. *School Psychology Quarterly, 14*, 408–427.
Miller, M. D., Linn, R. L., & Gronlund, N. E. (2009). *Measurement and assessment in teaching* (10th ed.). Upper Saddle River, NJ: Prentice Hall.
Nitko, A. J., & Brookhart, S. M. (2011). *Educational assessment of students* (6th ed.). Upper Saddle River, NJ: Pearson Education.

PART II

Testing and Other

Assessment Methods

THREE ❑

Planning for Testing

It was Wednesday, and Paul Johnson was caught by surprise when he looked at his office calendar and realized that a test for the course he was teaching was only 1 week away, even though he was the person who had scheduled it! Thankful that he was not teaching this course for the first time, he searched his files for the test he had used last year. When he found it, his brief review showed that some of the content was outdated and that the test did not include items on the new content he had added this year. Because of a university policy that requires a minimum of 3 business days for the copy center to reproduce a test, Paul realized that he would have to finish the necessary revisions of the test and submit it for copying no later than Friday. He would be teaching in the clinical area on Thursday and teaching a class on Friday morning, and he was preparing to go out of town to attend a conference on Saturday.

He stayed up late on Wednesday night to revise the test, planning to proofread it on Thursday after he finished his clinical teaching responsibilities. But because of a family emergency, he was not able to proofread the test that night. Trusting that he had not made any serious clerical errors, he sent the test to the copy center before his class on Friday. When he returned to the office after his conference on Tuesday, he discovered that the photocopier in the copy center had been damaged by a lightening strike before his test had been copied, and had not been repaired or replaced. Paul picked up his test at the copy center that afternoon, but couldn't take it anywhere else to be copied that day because of a scheduled committee meeting. To complicate matters, the department secretary had called in sick that day, and Paul couldn't change his child-care arrangements to allow him to stay late at the office to finish copying the test. He came in very early on Wednesday morning to use the department photocopier, and finally finished the job just before the test was scheduled to begin.

51

With 5 minutes to spare, Paul rushed into the classroom and distributed the still-warm test booklets. As he was congratulating himself for meeting his deadline the first student raised a hand with a question: "On item three, is there a typo?" Then another student said, "I don't think that the correct answer for item six is there." A third student complained, "Item 9 is missing; the numbers jump from 8 to 10" and a fourth student stated, "There are 2 ds for item 10." Paul knew that it was going to be a long morning. But the worst was yet to come. As they were turning in their tests, students complained, "This test didn't cover the material that I thought it would cover," and "We spent a lot of class time analyzing case studies, but we were tested on memorization of facts." Needless to say, Paul did not look forward to the posttest discussion the following week.

Too often, teachers give little thought to the preparation of their tests until the last minute and then rush to get the job done. A test that is produced in this manner often contains items that are poorly chosen, ambiguous, and either too easy or too difficult, as well as grammatical, spelling, and other clerical errors. The solution lies in adequate planning for test construction before the item-writing phase begins, followed by careful critique of the completed test by other teachers. Exhibit 3.1 lists the steps of the test-construction process. This chapter describes the steps involved in planning for test construction; subsequent chapters will focus on the techniques of writing test items of various formats, assembling and administering the test, and analyzing the test results.

PURPOSE AND POPULATION

All decisions involved in planning a test are based on a teacher's knowledge of the purpose of the test and the relevant characteristics of the population of learners to be tested. The *purpose* for the test involves why it is to be given, what it is supposed to measure, and how the test scores will be used. For example, if a test is to be used to measure the extent to which students have met learning objectives to determine course grades, its primary purpose is summative. If the teacher expects the course grades to reflect real differences in the amount of knowledge among the students, the test must be sufficiently difficult to produce an acceptable range of scores. On the other hand, if a test is to be used primarily to provide feedback to staff nurses about their knowledge following a continuing education program, the purpose of the test is formative. If the results will not be used to make important personnel decisions, a large range of scores is not necessary, and the test items can be of moderate or low difficulty.

❏Exhibit 3.1

Checklist for Test Construction

- ❏ Define the purpose of the test.
- ❏ Describe the population to be tested.
- ❏ Determine the optimum length of the test.
- ❏ Specify the desired difficulty and discrimination levels of the test items.
- ❏ Determine the scoring procedure or procedures to be used.
- ❏ Select item formats to be used.
- ❏ Construct a test blueprint or table of specifications.
- ❏ Write the test items.
- ❏ Have the test items critiqued.
- ❏ Determine the arrangement of items on the test.
- ❏ Write specific directions for each item format.
- ❏ Write general directions for the test and prepare a cover sheet.
- ❏ Print or type the test.
- ❏ Proofread the test.
- ❏ Reproduce the test.
- ❏ Prepare a scoring key.
- ❏ Prepare students for taking the test.

A teacher's knowledge of the population that will be tested will be useful in selecting the item formats to be used, determining the length of the test and the testing time required, and selecting the appropriate scoring procedures. The term *population* is not used here in its research sense, but rather to indicate the general group of learners who will be tested. The students' reading levels, English-language literacy, visual acuity, health, and previous testing experience are examples of factors that might influence these decisions. For example, if the population to be tested is a group of five patients who have completed preoperative instruction for coronary bypass graft surgery, the teacher would probably not administer a test of 100 multiple-choice and matching items with a machine-scored answer sheet. However, this type of test might be most appropriate as a final course examination for a class of 75 senior nursing students.

TEST LENGTH

The length of the test is an important factor that is related to its purpose, the abilities of the students, the item formats to be used, the amount of testing time available, and the desired reliability of the test scores. As discussed in Chapter 2, the reliability of test scores generally improves as the length of the assessment increases, so the teacher should attempt to include as many items as possible to adequately sample the content. However, if the purpose of the test is to measure knowledge of a small content domain with a limited number of objectives, fewer items will be needed to achieve an adequate sampling of the content.

It should be noted that assessment length refers to the number of test items or tasks, not to the amount of time it would take the student to complete the test. Items that require the student to analyze a complex data set, draw conclusions, and supply or choose a response take more test administration time; therefore, fewer items of those types can be included on a test to be completed in a fixed time period. When the number of complex assessment tasks to be included on a test is limited by test administration time, it is better to test more frequently than to create longer tests that test less important learning goals (Miller, Linn, & Gronlund, 2009; Waltz, Strickland, & Lenz, 2005).

Because test length probably is limited by the scheduled length of a testing period, it is wise to construct the test so that the majority of the students working at their normal pace will be able to attempt to answer all items. This type of test is called a *power* test. A *speeded* test is one that does not provide sufficient time for all students to respond to all items. Although most standardized tests are speeded, this type of test generally is not appropriate for teacher-made tests in which accuracy rather than speed of response is important (Miller et al., 2009; Nitko & Brookhart, 2011).

DIFFICULTY AND DISCRIMINATION LEVEL

The desired difficulty of a test and its ability to differentiate among various levels of performance are related considerations. Both factors are affected by the purpose of the test and the way in which the scores will be interpreted and used. The difficulty of individual test items affects the average test score; the mean score of a group of students is equal to the sum of the difficulty levels of the test items. The difficulty level of each test item depends on the complexity of the task, the ability of the students who answer it, and the quality of the teaching. It also may be related to the perceived complexity of the item; if students perceive the task as too difficult, they may skip it, resulting in a lower percentage of students who answer the item correctly (Nitko & Brookhart, 2011). See Chapter 12 for a more detailed discussion of item difficulty and discrimination. In general, items on an assessment should have a fairly narrow range of difficulty around the average difficulty level (Waltz et al., 2005), but this rule has different applications depending on how the test results will be interpreted.

If test results are to be used to determine the relative achievement of students (i.e., norm-referenced interpretation), the majority of items on the test should be moderately difficult. The recommended difficulty level for selection-type test items depends on the number of choices allowed. The percentage of students who answer each item correctly should be about midway between 100% and the chance of guessing correctly (e.g., 50% for true–false items, 25% correct for four-alternative multiple-choice items). For example, a moderately difficult true–false item should be answered correctly by 75 to 85% of students (Nitko & Brookhart, 2011; Waltz et al., 2005). When the majority of items on a test are too easy or too difficult, they will not discriminate well between students with varying levels of knowledge or ability.

However, if the teacher wants to make criterion-referenced judgments, more commonly used in nursing education and practice settings, the overall concern is whether a student's performance meets a set standard rather than on the actual score itself. If the purpose of the assessment is to screen out the least capable students (e.g., those failing a course), it should be relatively easy for most test-takers. However, comparing performance to a set standard does not limit assessment to testing of lower level knowledge and ability; considerations of assessment validity should guide the teacher to construct tests that adequately sample the knowledge or performance domain.

When criterion-referenced test results are reported as percentage scores, their variability (range of scores) may be similar to norm-referenced test results, but the interpretation of the range of scores would be more narrow. For example, on a final exam in a nursing course the potential score range may be 0% to 100%, but the passing score is set at 80%. Even if there is wide variability of scores on the exam, the primary concern is whether the test correctly classifies each student as performing above or below the standard (e.g., 80%). In this case, the teacher should examine the difficulty level of test items and compare them between groups (students who met the standard and students who didn't). If item difficulty levels indicate a relatively easy or relatively difficult exam, criterion-referenced decisions will still be appropriate if the measure consistently classifies students according to the performance standard (Miller et al., 2009; Waltz et al., 2005).

It is important to keep in mind that the difficulty level of test items can only be estimated in advance, depending on the teacher's experience in testing this content and knowledge of the abilities of the students to be tested. When the test has been administered and scored, the actual difficulty index for each item can be compared with the expected difficulty, and items can be revised if the actual difficulty level is much lower or much higher than anticipated (Waltz et al., 2005). Procedures for determining how the test items actually perform are discussed in Chapter 12.

ITEM FORMATS

Some students may be particularly adept at answering essay items; others may prefer multiple-choice items. However, tests should be designed to provide information about students' knowledge or abilities, not about their skill in taking certain types of tests. A test with a variety of item formats provides students with multiple ways to demonstrate their competence (Nitko & Brookhart, 2011). All item formats have their advantages and limitations, which are discussed in later chapters.

Selection Criteria for Item Formats

Teachers should select item formats for their tests based on a variety of factors, such as the learning outcomes to be evaluated, the specific skill to be measured, and the ability level of the students. Some objectives are better measured with certain item formats. For example, if the instructional objective specifies that the student will be able to "discuss the comparative advantages and disadvantages of breast- and bottle-feeding," a multiple-choice item would be inappropriate because it would not allow the teacher to evaluate the student's ability to organize and express ideas on this topic. An essay item would be a better choice for this purpose. Essay items provide opportunities for students to formulate their own responses, drawing on prior learning, and to express their ideas in writing; these often are desired outcomes of nursing education programs.

The teacher's time constraints for constructing the test may affect the choice of item format. In general, essay items take less time to write than multiple-choice items, but they are more difficult and time-consuming to score. A teacher who has little time to prepare a test and therefore chooses an essay format, assuming that this choice is also appropriate for the objectives to be tested, must plan for considerable time after the test is given to score it.

In nursing programs, faculty members often develop multiple-choice items as the predominant, if not exclusive, item format because for a number of years, licensure and certification examinations contained only multiple-choice items. Although this type of test item provides essential practice for students in preparation for taking such high-stakes examinations, it negates the principle of selecting the most appropriate type of test item for the outcome and content to be evaluated. In addition, it limits variety in testing and creativity in evaluating student learning. Although practice with multiple-choice questions is critical, other types of test items and evaluation strategies also are appropriate for measuring student learning in nursing. In fact, although the majority of NCLEX® examination items currently are four-option multiple-choice, the item pools now contain other formats such as completion and multiple response (National Council of State Boards of Nursing, 2010). It is clear from this example that nurse educators should not limit their selection of item formats based on the myth that learners must be tested exclusively with the item format most frequently used on a licensure or certification test.

On the other hand, each change of item format on a test requires a change of task for students. Therefore, the number of different item formats to include on a test also depends on the length of the test and the level of the learner. It is generally recommended that teachers use no more than three item formats on a test. Shorter assessments, such as a 10-item quiz, may be limited to a single item format.

Objectively and Subjectively Scored Items

Another powerful and persistent myth is that some item formats evaluate students more objectively than do other formats. Although it is common to describe true–false, matching, and multiple-choice items as "objective," objectivity refers to the way items are scored, not to the type of item or their content (Miller et al., 2009). Objectivity means that once the scoring key is prepared, it is possible for multiple teachers on the same occasion or the same teacher on multiple occasions to arrive at the same score. Subjectively scored items, like essay items (and short-answer items, to a lesser extent), require the judgment of the scorer to determine the degree of correctness and therefore are subject to more variability in scoring.

Selected-Response and Constructed-Response Items

Another way of classifying test items is to identify them by the type of response required of the test-taker (Miller et al., 2009). *Selected-response* (or "choice") items require the test-taker to select the correct or best answer from among options provided by the teacher. In this category are item formats such as true–false, matching exercises, and multiple-choice. *Constructed-response* (or "supply") formats require the learner to supply an answer, and may be classified further as limited response (or short response) and extended response. These are the short answer and essay formats. Exhibit 3.2 depicts this schema for classifying test-item formats and the variations of each type.

☐Exhibit 3.2

Classification of Test Items by Type of Response

SELECTED-RESPONSE ITEM FORMATS ("CHOICE" ITEMS)	CONSTRUCTED-RESPONSE ITEM FORMATS ("SUPPLY" ITEMS)
True–false	Short-answer
Matching exercises	Completion or fill-in-the-blank
Multiple-choice	Restricted-response essay
Multiple-response	Extended-response essay

SCORING PROCEDURES

Decisions about what scoring procedure or procedures to use are somewhat dependent on the choice of item formats. Student responses to short-answer, numerical-calculation, and essay items, for instance, usually must be hand-scored, whether they are recorded directly on the test itself, on a separate answer sheet, or in a booklet. Answers to objective test items such as multiple-choice, true–false, and matching also may be recorded on the test itself or on a separate answer sheet. Scannable answer sheets greatly increase the speed of objective scoring procedures and have the additional advantage of allowing computer-generated item analysis reports to be produced. The teacher should decide if the time and resources available for scoring a test suggest that hand scoring or electronic scoring would be preferable. In any case, this decision alone should not influence the choice of test-item format.

TEST BLUEPRINT

Most people would not think of building a house without blueprints. In fact, the word "house" denotes diverse attributes to different individuals. For this reason, a potential homeowner would not purchase a lot, call a builder, and say only, "Build a house for me on my lot." The builder might think that a proper house consists of a two-story brick colonial with four bedrooms, three baths, and a formal dining room, whereas the homeowner had a three-bedroom ranch with two baths, an eat-in kitchen, and a great room with a fireplace in mind. Similarly, the word "test" might mean different things to different teachers; students and their teacher might have widely varied expectations about what the test will contain. The best way to avoid misunderstanding regarding the nature of a test and to ensure that the teacher will be able to make valid judgments about the test scores is to develop a test blueprint, also known as a test plan or a table of specifications, before "building" the test itself.

The elements of a test blueprint include (a) a list of the major topics or instructional objectives that the test will cover, (b) the level of complexity of the task to be assessed, and (c) the emphasis each topic will have, indicated by number or percentage of items or points. Exhibit 3.3 is an example of a test blueprint for a unit test on nursing care during normal pregnancy that illustrates each of these elements.

The row headings along the left margin of the example are the content areas that will be tested. In this case, the content is indicated by a general outline of topics. Teachers may find that a more detailed outline of content or a list of the relevant objectives is more useful for a given purpose and population. Some teachers combine a content outline and the related objectives; in this case, an additional column of objectives would be inserted before or after the content list.

The column headings across the top of the example are taken from the taxonomy of cognitive objectives (Bloom, Engelhart, Furst, Hill, & Krathwohl, 1956). Because the test blueprint is a tool to be used by the teacher, it can be modified in any way that makes sense to the user. Accordingly, the teacher who prepared this blueprint chose to use only selected levels of the taxonomy. Other teachers might include all levels or different levels of Bloom's taxonomy, or use a different taxonomy.

The body of the test blueprint is a grid formed by the intersections of content topics and cognitive levels. Each of the cells of the grid has the potential to represent one or more test items that might be developed. The numbers in the cells of the sample test blueprint represent the number of points on the test that will relate to it; some teachers prefer to indicate numbers of items or the percentage of points or items represented by each cell. The percentage is a better indicator of the amount of emphasis to be given to each content area (Miller et al., 2009), but the number of items or points may be more helpful to the teacher in writing actual test items. It is not necessary to write test items for each cell; the teacher's judgment concerning the appropriate emphasis and balance of content governs the decision about which cells should be filled and how many items should be written for each.

Rigorous classification of items into these cells also is unnecessary and, in fact, impossible; the way in which the content is actually taught may affect whether the related test items will be written at the application or comprehension level, for example. For this reason, the actual test may deviate slightly from the specifications for certain cells, but the overall balance of emphasis between the test and the actual instruction should be very similar (Miller et al., 2009; Nitko & Brookhart, 2011).

☐Exhibit 3.3

Example of a Test Blueprint for a Unit Test on Normal Pregnancy (75 Points)

CONTENT	K	C	Ap	An	Total #[b]
I. Conception and fetal development		2	3	3	8
II. Maternal physiological changes in pregnancy	2	3	1	2	8
III. Maternal psychological changes in pregnancy		2	2	3	7
IV. Social, cultural, and economic factors affecting pregnancy outcome		3	2	3	8
V. Signs and symptoms of pregnancy	2	2	2		6
VI. Antepartal nursing care		8	10	12	30
VII. Preparation for childbirth		4	1	3	8
TOTAL #[b]	4	24	21	26	75

The "LEVEL OF COGNITIVE SKILL[a]" header spans the K, C, Ap, An, and Total # columns.

[a]According to Bloom et al. (1956) taxonomy of cognitive objectives. Selected levels are included in this test blueprint and are represented by the following key:
K = Knowledge
C = Comprehension
Ap = Application
An = Analysis
[b]Number of points. Test blueprints also may include the number or the percentage of items.

Once developed, the test blueprint serves several important functions. First, it is a useful tool for guiding the work of the item writer so that sufficient items are developed at the appropriate level to test important content areas and objectives. Without a test blueprint, teachers often use ease of construction as a major consideration in writing test items, resulting in tests with a limited and biased sample of learning tasks that may omit outcomes of greater importance that are more difficult to measure (Miller et al., 2009). Using test blueprints also helps teachers to be accountable for the educational outcomes they produce. The test blueprint can be used as evidence for judging the validity of the resulting test scores. The completed test and blueprint may be reviewed by content experts who can judge whether the test items adequately represent the specified content domain, as described in the procedures for collecting content-related evidence in Chapter 2.

Another important use of the test blueprint is to inform students about the nature of the test and how they should prepare for it. Although the content covered in class and assigned readings should give students a general idea of the content areas to be tested, students often lack a clear sense of the cognitive levels at which they will be tested on this material. Although it might be argued that the instructional objectives might give students a clue as to the level at which they will be tested, teachers often forget that students are not as sophisticated in interpreting objectives as teachers are. Also, some teachers are good at writing objectives that specify a reasonable expectation of performance, but their test items may in fact test higher or lower performance levels. Students need to know the level at which they will be tested because that knowledge will affect how they prepare for the test, not necessarily how much they prepare. They should prepare differently for items that test their ability to apply information than for items that test their ability to synthesize information.

Some teachers worry that if the test blueprint is shared with students, they will not study the content areas that would contribute less to their overall test scores, preferring to concentrate their time and energy on the more important areas of emphasis. If this indeed is the outcome, is it necessarily harmful? Lacking any guidance from the teacher, students may unwisely spend equal amounts of time reviewing all content areas. In fact, professional experience reveals that some knowledge is more important for use in practice than other knowledge. Even if they are good critical thinkers, students may be unable to discriminate more important content from that which is less important because they lack the practice experience to make this distinction. Withholding information about the content emphasis of the test from students might be perceived as an attempt to threaten or punish them for perceived shortcomings such as failure to attend class, failure to read what was assigned, or failure to discern the teacher's priorities. Such a use of testing would be considered unethical.

The best time to share the test blueprint with students is at the beginning of the course or unit of study. If students are unfamiliar with the use of a test blueprint, the teacher may need to explain the concept as well as discuss how it might be useful to the students in planning their preparation for the test. Of course, if the teacher subsequently makes modifications in the blueprint after writing the test items, those changes also should be shared with the students (Nitko & Brookhart, 2011).

WRITING THE TEST ITEMS

After developing the test blueprint, the teacher should begin to write the test items that correspond to each cell. Regardless of the selected item formats, the teacher should consider some general factors that contribute to the quality of the test items.

General Rules for Writing Test Items

1. *Every item should measure something important.* If a test blueprint is designed and used as described in the previous section, each test item will measure an important objective or content area. Without using a blueprint, teachers often write test items that test trivial or obscure knowledge. Sometimes the teacher's intent is to determine whether the students have read assigned materials; however, if the content is not important information, it wastes the teacher's time to write the item and wastes the students' time to read it and respond to it. Similarly, it is not necessary to write "filler" items to meet a targeted number; a test with 98 well-written items that measure important objectives will work as well as or better than one with 98 good items and 2 meaningless ones. Although the reliability of test results is related to the length of the assessment, this rule presumes that items added to a test to increase the number of tasks would be of the same quality as those that are already a part of the test. Adding items that are so easy that every student will answer the questions correctly, or so difficult that every student will answer them incorrectly, will not improve the reliability estimate (Miller et al., 2009). In fact, students who know the content well might regard a test item that measures trivial knowledge with annoyance or even suspicion, believing that it is meant to trick them into answering incorrectly. There is no reason other than ease of mentally calculating a percentage score for setting an absolute target number of points on a test at 100.

2. *Every item should have a correct answer.* The correct answer should be one that would be agreed on by experts (Miller et al., 2009). This may seem obvious, but the rule is violated frequently because of the teacher's failure to make a distinction between fact and belief. In some cases, the correct or best answer to a test item might be a matter of opinion, and unless a particular authority is cited in the item, students might justifiably argue a different response than the one the teacher expected. For example, one answer to the question, "When does life begin?" might be "When the kids leave home and the dog dies." If the intent of the question was to measure understanding of when a fetus becomes viable, this is not the correct answer, although if the latter was the teacher's intent, the question was poorly worded. There are a variety of opinions and beliefs about the concept of viability; a better way to word this question is, "According to the standards of the American College of Obstetricians and Gynecologists, at what gestational age does a fetus become viable?" If a test item asks the student to state an opinion about an issue and to support that position with evidence, that is a different matter. That type of item should not be scored as correct or incorrect, but with variable credit based on the completeness of the response, rationale given for the position taken, or the soundness of the student's reasoning (Nitko & Brookhart, 2011).

3. *Use simple, clear, concise, precise, grammatically correct language.* Students who read the test item need to know exactly what task is required of them. Wording a test item clearly is often difficult because of the inherent abstractness and imprecision of language, and it is a challenge to use simple words and sentence structure when writing about highly technical and complex material. The teacher should include enough detail in the test item to communicate the intent of the item but without extraneous words or complex syntax that only serve to increase the reading time. Additionally, grammatical errors may provide unintentional clues to the correct response for the testwise but unprepared student and, at best, annoy the well-prepared student.

This rule is particularly important when testing students for whom English is a second language or non-native speakers (NNSs). Bosher and Bowles (2008) found that in a majority of cases, linguistic modification of test items improved NNSs' comprehension of nursing exam items. The process of linguistic modification or simplification maintains key content area vocabulary but reduces the semantic and syntactic complexity of written English. Linguistic structures such as passive voice constructions, long question phrases, conditional and subordinate clauses, negation, and grammatical errors are particularly difficult for NNSs to understand, and they require more time to read and process (Bosher & Bowles, 2008; Bosher, 2009). Although arguments might be made that no accommodation is made for NNSs on the NCLEX, consideration of measurement validity must take into account that any test that employs language is at least partially a measure of language skills (American Educational Research Association, American Psychological Association, & National Council on Measurement in Education, 1999; Miller et al., 2009).

The following item stem, adapted from an example given by Bosher and Bowles (2008), illustrates the effect of linguistic simplification:

Original stem: A patient with chronic pain treated over a period of months with an oral form of morphine tells you that she is concerned because she has had to gradually increase the amount of medication she takes to achieve pain control. Your response should include:

Linguistically simplified stem: A patient has chronic pain. She is treated over a period of months with an oral form of morphine. She tells the nurse that she is concerned because she has gradually needed more medication to achieve the same level of pain control. How should the nurse respond? (Bosher & Bowles, 2008, p. 168).

Note that the same content is emphasized, but that the revised example contains four short simple sentences and ends with a question to be answered rather than a completion format. Given growing concerns that even native English speakers are entering postsecondary programs with poorer reading skills, such linguistic modification should benefit all students.

4. *Avoid using jargon, slang, or unnecessary abbreviations.* Health care professionals frequently use jargon, abbreviations, and acronyms in their practice environment; in some ways, it allows them to communicate more quickly, if not more effectively, with others who understand the same language. Informal language in a test item, however, may fail to communicate the intent of the item accurately. Because most students are somewhat anxious when taking tests, they may fail to interpret an abbreviation correctly for the context in which it is used. For example, does MI mean myocardial infarction, mitral insufficiency, or Michigan? Of course, if the intent of the test item is to measure students' ability to define commonly used abbreviations, it would be appropriate to use the abbreviation in the item and ask for the definition, or give the definition and ask the student to supply the abbreviation. Slang almost always conveys the impression that the item-writer does not take the job seriously. As noted previously, slang, jargon, abbreviations, and acronyms contribute to linguistic complexity especially for NNSs. Additionally, growing alarm about health care errors attributed to poor communication, including the overuse of abbreviations, suggests that nurse educators should set positive examples for their students by using only abbreviations generally approved for use in clinical settings.

5. *Try to use positive wording.* It is difficult to explain this rule without using negative wording, but in general, avoid including words like *no*, *not*, and *except* in the test item. As noted previously, negation contributes to linguistic complexity that interferes with the test performance of NNSs. The use of negative wording is especially confusing in true–false items. If using a negative form is unavoidable, underline the negative word or phrase, or use bold text and all uppercase letters to draw students' attention to it. It is best to avoid asking students to identify the incorrect response, as in the following example:

Which of the following is **NOT** an indication that a skin lesion is a Stage IV pressure ulcer?

a. Blistering*
b. Sinus tracts
c. Tissue necrosis
d. Undermining

---

*Correct answer.

The structure of this item reinforces the wrong answer and may lead to confusion when a student attempts to recall the correct information at a later time. A better way to word the item is:

Which of the following is an indication that a skin lesion is a Stage II pressure ulcer?

a. Blistering*
b. Sinus tracts
c. Tissue necrosis
d. Undermining

6. *No item should contain irrelevant clues to the correct answer.* This is a common error among inexperienced test-item writers. Students who are good test-takers can usually identify such an item and use its flaws to improve their chances of guessing the correct answer when they do not know it. Irrelevant clues include a multiple-choice stem that is grammatically inconsistent with one or more of the options, a word in the stem that is repeated in the correct option, using qualifiers such as "always" or "never" in incorrect responses, placing the correct response in a consistent position among a set of options, or consistently making true statements longer than false statements (Miller et al., 2009; Nitko & Brookhart, 2011). Such items contribute little to the validity of test results because they may not measure what students actually know, but how well they are able to guess the correct answers.

7. *No item should depend on another item for meaning or for the correct answer.* In other words, if a student answers one item incorrectly, he or she will likely answer the related item incorrectly. An example of such a relationship between two completion items follows:

1. Which insulin should be used for emergency treatment of ketoacidosis? _____
2. What is the onset of action for the insulin in Item 1?

_____

In this example, Item 2 is dependent on Item 1 for its meaning. Students who supply the wrong answer to Item 1 are unlikely to supply a correct answer to Item 2. Items should be worded in such a way as to make them independent of each other. However, a series of test items can be developed to relate to a context such as a case study, database, diagram, graph, or other interpretive material. Items that are linked to this material are called interpretive or context-dependent items, and they do not violate this general rule for writing test items because they are linked to a common stimulus, not to each other.

8. *Eliminate extraneous information unless the purpose of the item is to determine whether students can distinguish between relevant and irrelevant data.* Avoid the use of patient names in clinical scenarios; this information adds unnecessarily to reading time, it may distract from the purpose of the item, and it may introduce cultural bias (see Chapter 15). However, some items are designed to measure whether a student can evaluate the relevance of clinical data and use only pertinent information in arriving at the answer. In this case, extraneous data (but not patient names) may be included.

9. *Arrange for a critique of the items.* The best source of this critique is a colleague who teaches the same content area or at least someone who is skilled in the technical aspects of item writing. If no one is available to critique the test items, the teacher who developed them should set them aside for a few days. This will allow the teacher to review the items with a fresh perspective to identify lack of clarity or faulty technical construction.

10. *Prepare more items than the test blueprint specifies.* This will allow for replacement items for those discarded in the review process. The fortunate teacher who does not need to use many replacement items can use the remainder to begin an item bank for future tests.

PREPARING STUDENTS TO TAKE A TEST

A teacher-made test usually measures students' maximum performance rather than their typical performance. For this reason, teachers should create conditions under which students will be able to demonstrate their best possible performance. These conditions include adequate preparation of students to take the test (Miller et al., 2009; Nitko & Brookhart, 2011). Although this is the last point on the test-construction checklist (Exhibit 3.1), the teacher should begin preparing students to take the test at the time the test is scheduled. Adequate preparation includes information, skills, and attitudes that will facilitate students' maximum performance on the test.

Information Needs

Students need information about the test to plan for effective preparation. They need sufficient time to prepare for a test, and the date and time of a test should be announced well in advance. Although many teachers believe that unannounced or "pop" tests motivate students to study more, there is no evidence to support this position. In fact, surprise (unscheduled) tests can be considered punitive or threatening and, as such, represent an unethical use of testing (Nitko & Brookhart, 2011). Adult learners with multiple responsibilities may need to make adjustments to their work and family responsibilities to have adequate study time, and generous notice of a planned test date will allow them to set their priorities.

In addition, students need to know about the conditions under which they are to be tested, such as how much time will be allotted, whether they will have access to resources such as textbooks, how many items will be included, the types of item formats that will be used, and if they need special tools or supplies to take the test, such as calculators, pencils, or black-ink pens (Miller et al., 2009). They also should know what items and resources they will not be able to use during the test. For example, the teacher may direct students not to bring cell phones, personal digital assistants, chiming watches, watches with calculators, backpacks, brief-cases, or any books or papers to the testing site. Some teachers do not allow students to wear caps or hats with brims to discourage cheating. In fact, such requirements may be good practice for prelicensure students who must observe similar restrictions for the NCLEX.

Of course, students also should know what content will be covered on the test, how many items will be devoted to each content area, the cognitive level at which they will be expected to perform, and the types of items to expect. As previously discussed, giving students a copy of the test blueprint and discussing it with them is an effective way for teachers to convey this information. Students should also have sufficient opportunity to practice the type of performance that will be tested. For example, if students will be expected to solve medication dose calculation problems without the use of a calculator, they should practice this type of calculation in class exercises or out-of-class assignments. Students also need to know if spelling, grammar, punctuation, or organization will be considered in scoring open-ended items so that they can prepare accordingly. Finally, teachers should tell students how their test results will be used, including the weight assigned to the test score in grading (Miller et al., 2009; Nitko & Brookhart, 2011).

Another way that teachers can assist students in studying for a test is to have students prepare and use a "cheat sheet." Although this term can be expected to have negative connotations for most teachers, cheat sheets commonly are used in nursing practice in the form of memory aids or triggers such as procedure checklists, pocket guides, and reminder sheets. When legitimized for use in studying and test-taking, cheat sheets capitalize on the belief that although dishonest behavior must be discouraged, the skills associated with cheating can be powerful learning tools.

When students intend to cheat on a test, they usually try to guess potential test items and prepare cheat sheets with the correct answers to those anticipated items. Using this skill for a more honest purpose, the teacher can encourage all of the students to anticipate potential test items. In a test-preparation context, the teacher requires the students to develop a written cheat sheet that summarizes, prioritizes, condenses, and organizes content that they think is important and wish to remember during the test. The teacher may set parameters such as the length of the cheat sheet—for example, one side of one sheet of 8½ × 11-inch paper. The students bring their cheat sheets on the day of the test and may use them during the test; they submit their cheat sheets along with their test papers. Students who do not submit cheat sheets may be penalized by deducting points from their test scores or may not be permitted to take the test at all.

Some students may not even consult their cheat sheets during the test, but they still derive benefit from the preparation that goes into developing them. The teacher also may review the cheat sheets with students whose test scores are low to identify weaknesses in thinking that may have contributed to their errors. When used for this purpose, the cheat sheet becomes a powerful diagnostic and feedback tool.

Test-Taking Skills

Because of an increasingly diverse population of learners in every educational setting, including growing numbers of students for whom English is a second language and whose testing experiences may be different from the teacher's expectations, teachers should determine if their students have adequate test-taking skills for the type of test to be given. If the students lack adequate test-taking skills, their test scores may be lower than their actual abilities. Skill in taking tests sometimes is called *testwiseness*. To be more precise, testwiseness is the ability to use test-taking skills, clues from poorly written test items, and test-taking experience to achieve a test score that is higher than the student's true knowledge would predict. Common errors made by item writers do allow some students to substitute testwiseness for knowledge. But, in general, all students should develop adequate test-taking skills so that they are not at a disadvantage when their scores are compared with those of more testwise individuals (Nitko & Brookhart, 2011). Adequate test-taking skills include the following abilities (Miller et al., 2009):

1. Reading and listening to directions and following them accurately
2. Reading test items carefully
3. Recording answers to test items accurately and neatly
4. Avoiding physical and mental fatigue by paced study and adequate rest before the test rather than late-night cram sessions supplemented by stimulants
5. Using test time wisely and working at a pace that allows for careful reflection but also permits responding to all items that the student is likely to answer correctly
6. Bypassing difficult items and returning to them later

7. Making informed guesses rather than omitting answers
8. Outlining and organizing responses to essay items before beginning to write
9. Checking answers to test items for clerical errors and changing answers if a better response is indicated

Many teachers advise students not to change their answers to test items, believing that the first response usually is the correct answer and that changing responses will not increase a student's score. Research findings, however, do not support this position. Studies of answer-changing and its effect on test performance have revealed that most students do change their answers to about 4% of test items and that approximately two thirds of answer changes become correct responses. As item difficulty increases, however, this payoff diminishes; consequently, more knowledgeable students benefit more than less knowledgeable students from changing answers (Nitko & Brookhart, 2011).

Students should be encouraged to change their first response to any item when they have a good reason for making the change. For example, a student who has a clearer understanding of an item after re-reading it, who later recalls additional information needed to answer the item, or who receives a clue to the correct answer from another item should not hesitate to change the first answer. Improvement in test scores should not be expected, however, when students change answers without a clear rationale for making the change.

Test Anxiety

Finally, teachers should prepare students to approach a test with helpful attitudes. Although anxiety is a common response to situations in which performance is evaluated, high levels of anxiety are likely to interfere with maximum performance (Miller et al., 2009).

Whether some students can be characterized as test-anxious is a matter of frequent debate. Test anxiety can be viewed in several ways. Students who are motivated to do well often experience increased emotional tension in response to a test. Their perceptions of the testing situation affect their thoughts during test preparation and test-taking. Students who perceive a test as a challenge usually have thoughts that are task-directed. They can focus on completing the task and easily manage any tension that is associated with it. Some students perceive tests as threats because they have poor test-taking skills, inadequate knowledge, or both. These students often have task-irrelevant thoughts about testing. They focus on what could happen if they fail a test, and their feelings of helplessness cause them to desire to escape the situation (Nitko & Brookhart, 2011).

Test anxiety can be characterized as a trait with three components: physical, emotional, and cognitive. Test-anxiety research suggests an interaction among these components: negative thoughts and perceptions about testing can create negative feelings, which interfere with performance (Poorman, Mastorovich, & Molcan, 2007). The physical component, or autonomic reactivity, involves unpleasant feelings and reactions such as perspiration, increased heart rate, headaches, and gastrointestinal symptoms, although not all test-anxious individuals have physical reactions. The emotional component involves mood and feelings (e.g., nervousness, uneasiness, fear, dread, panic) associated with testing situations.

The cognitive component refers to thoughts or concerns related to performance and its consequences, occurring before or during a test. Essentially, the cognitive component involves worry about possible negative outcomes: "catastrophic fantasies" about what might happen if the student fails, and "competitive worry" that other students are doing better (Poorman et al., 2007). Cognitive indications of test anxiety include impaired ability to concentrate and easy distractibility during the test, difficulty recalling information ("going blank"), misreading or misunderstanding directions or test items, and feeling pressured to be perfect. Additionally, individuals with true test anxiety often have a history of poor performance on tests and other evaluative situations, particularly high-stakes tests. For example, these individuals may repeatedly fail a driver's license examination or achieve good scores on quizzes or unit tests but fail final examinations (Poorman et al., 2007)

The combination of negative feelings and thoughts often results in behaviors that interfere with students' ability to prepare adequately for a test. One of the most dangerous behaviors is avoidance—procrastinating rather than beginning preparation early, and engaging in activities that seem to be related to preparing for the test but really are just distractions. For example, students often report that they studied for many hours and still failed a test, but a record of their activities would reveal that much of that time was spent highlighting material in the textbook or "preparing to study"—organizing their notes, doing household chores with the intention of minimizing interruptions, and so on. Negative thinking creates anxiety, which students try to avoid by avoiding the studying that they believe is causing the discomfort (Poorman et al., 2007).

Students whose test anxiety interferes with their performance often benefit from treatment that addresses the feeling or emotional component of anxiety and the negative thinking or worry aspect as well as training to improve their general test-taking skills. For example, the test-anxious student may learn techniques for stopping negative thoughts during study periods and testing situations, and behavioral techniques such as progressive relaxation and visual imagery (Poorman et al., 2007). A more comprehensive discussion of the diagnosis and treatment of test anxiety is beyond the scope of this textbook. However, teachers may be able to identify students whose performance suggests that test anxiety may be a factor, and to refer those students for treatment.

Students need to view tests and other assessment procedures as opportunities to demonstrate what they know and what they can do. To foster this attitude, the teacher should express confidence in the students' abilities to prepare for and perform well on an upcoming test. It may be helpful for the teacher to ask the students what would help them to feel more relaxed and less anxious before and during a test. Conducting a review session, giving practice items similar to those that will be used on the test, and not talking or interrupting students during a test are examples of strategies that are likely to reduce students' anxiety to manageable levels (Miller et al., 2009; Nitko & Brookhart, 2011).

SUMMARY

Teachers who leave little time for adequate preparation often produce tests that contain poorly chosen and poorly written test items. Sufficient planning for test construction before the item-writing phase begins, followed by a careful critique of the completed test by other teachers, is likely to produce a test that will yield more valid results.

All decisions involved in planning a test should be based on a teacher's knowledge of the purpose of the test and relevant characteristics of the population of learners to be tested. The purpose for the test involves why it is to be given, what it is supposed to measure, and how the test scores will be used. A teacher's knowledge of the population that will be tested will be useful in selecting the item formats to be used, determining the length of the test and the testing time required, and selecting the appropriate scoring procedures. The students' English-language literacy, visual acuity, and previous testing experience are examples of factors that might influence these decisions.

The length of the test is an important factor that is related to its purpose, the abilities of the students, the item formats that will be used, the amount of testing time available, and the desired reliability of the test scores. The desired difficulty of the test and its ability to differentiate among various levels of performance are affected by the purpose of the test and the way in which the scores will be interpreted and used.

A test with a variety of item formats usually provides students with more opportunity to demonstrate their competence than a test with only one item format. Test items may be classified as selected-response or constructed-response types, depending on the task required of the learner. All item formats have advantages and limitations. Teachers should select item formats based on a variety of factors, such as the objectives, specific skill to be measured, and the ability level of the students. Many objectives are better measured with certain item formats.

Decisions about what scoring procedure or procedures to use are somewhat dependent on the choice of item formats. Student responses to some item formats must be hand-scored, whether they are recorded directly on the test itself or on a separate answer sheet or in a booklet. The teacher should decide whether the time and resources available for scoring a test suggest that hand-scoring or machine-scoring would be preferable.

The best way to ensure measurement validity of a teacher-constructed test is to develop a test blueprint, also known as a test plan or a table of specifications, before building the test itself. The elements of a test blueprint include (a) a list of the major topics or instructional objectives that the test will cover, (b) the level of complexity of the task to be assessed, and (c) the emphasis each topic will have, indicated by number or percentage of items or points. The test blueprint serves several important functions. It is a useful tool for guiding the work of the item writer so that sufficient items are developed at the appropriate level to test important content areas and objectives. The blueprint also should be used to inform students about the nature of the test and how they should prepare for it.

After developing the test blueprint, the teacher writes the test items that correspond to it. Regardless of the selected item formats, the teacher should follow some general rules that contribute to the development of high-quality test items. Those rules were discussed in the chapter.

Because teacher-made tests typically measure students' maximum performance rather than their typical performance, teachers should create conditions under which students will be able to demonstrate their best possible performance. These conditions include adequate preparation of the students to take the test. Adequate preparation includes information, skills, and attitudes that will facilitate students' maximum performance on the test.

REFERENCES

American Educational Research Association, American Psychological Association, & National Council on Measurement in Education. (1999). *Standards for educational and psychological testing*. Washington, DC: American Educational Research Association.

Bloom, B. S., Englehart, M. D., Furst, E. J., Hill, W. H., & Krathwohl, D. R. (1956). *Taxonomy of educational objectives: The classification of educational goals. Handbook I: Cognitive domain*. White Plains, NY: Longman.

Bosher, S. D. (2009). Removing language as a barrier to success on multiple-choice exams. In S. D. Bosher & M. D. Pharris (Eds.), *Transforming nursing education: The culturally inclusive environment* (pp. 259–284). New York, NY: Springer Publishing.

Bosher, S., & Bowles, M. (2008). The effects of linguistic modification on ESL students' comprehension of nursing course test items. *Nursing Education Perspectives, 29,* 165–172.

Miller, M. D., Linn, R. L., & Gronlund, N. E. (2009). *Measurement and assessment in teaching* (10th ed.). Upper Saddle River, NJ: Prentice Hall.

National Council of State Boards of Nursing. (2010). *2010 NCLEX-RN® detailed test plan.* Retrieved from https://www.ncsbn.org/2010_NCLEX_RN_TestPlan.pdf

Nitko, A. J., & Brookhart, S. M. (2011). *Educational assessment of students* (6th ed.). Upper Saddle River, NJ: Pearson Education.

Poorman, S. G., Mastorovich, M. L., & Molcan, K. L. (2007). *A good thinking approach to the NCLEX and other nursing exams* (2nd ed.). Pittsburgh, PA: STAT Nursing Consultants.

Waltz, C. F., Strickland, O. L., & Lenz, E. R. (2005). *Measurement in nursing and health research* (3rd ed.). New York, NY: Springer Publishing.

FOUR

True–False and

Matching

There are different ways of classifying types of test items. One way is to group items according to how they are scored—objectively or subjectively. An example of an objectively scored item is multiple choice: there is one correct or best answer. By choosing that answer, students receive a particular score, such as one point. Essay items are subjectively scored: the teacher judges the quality of the response based on criteria or a rubric for scoring. Another way is to group them by the type of response required of the test-taker. Selected-response items require the test-taker to select the correct or best answer from options provided by the teacher. Examples of these items include true–false, matching exercises, multiple-choice, and multiple-response. Constructed-response items ask the test-taker to supply an answer rather than choose from options already provided. Constructed-response items include completion and essay (short and extended). For each of the item formats presented in this book, a number of principles should be considered when writing them. Although important principles are described, the lists presented are not intended to be inclusive; other sources on test construction might include additional helpful suggestions for writing test items.

In addition to test items, other assessment strategies are written assignments, case method and case studies, discussions, simulations, presentations, and projects. These strategies and others, including methods for evaluating clinical performance, are discussed in later chapters of the book.

TRUE–FALSE

A true–false item consists of a statement that the student judges as either true or false. In some items, students also correct false statements or supply a rationale as to why the statement is true or false. True–false items are most effective for recall of facts and specific information but also may be used to test the student's comprehension of an important principle or concept. They are not intended for assessing complex thinking and understanding (Musial, Nieminen, Thomas, & Burke, 2009). Each item represents a declarative sentence stating a fact or principle and asks the learner to decide whether it is true or false, right or wrong, correct or incorrect. Some authors refer to this type of test item as alternate response, allowing for these varied response formats. For affective outcomes, agree–disagree might be used, asking the learner to agree or disagree with a value-based statement.

There are different opinions as to the value of true–false items. Although some authors express concern over the low level of testing, focusing on recall of facts, and the opportunity for guessing, others indicate that true–false items provide an efficient means of examining student acquisition of knowledge in a course. With true–false items, students can respond to a large number of items in a short time. For that reason, true–false items are useful to include on a test, and they also provide a way of testing a wide range of content. These items are easy to write and to score (Nitko & Brookhart, 2011).

Although true–false items are relatively easy to construct, the teacher should avoid using them to test meaningless information. Designed to examine student recall and comprehension of *important* facts and principles, true–false items should not be used to evaluate memorization of irrelevant information. Prior to constructing these items, the teacher should ask: Is the content assessed by the true–false item important when considering the course outcomes? Does the content represent knowledge taught in the class or through other methods of instruction? Do the students need an understanding of the content to progress through the course and for their further learning?

The main limitation to true–false items is guessing. Because one of the two responses has to be correct, the probability that a student will answer the item correctly is 50%. However, the issue with guessing is not as much of a problem as it seems. With no knowledge of the facts being tested, on a 10-point quiz, the student would only be expected to answer 5 of the items or 50% correctly. Nitko and Brookhart (2011) suggested that few students in a course respond to test items with blind or completely random guessing. Most students have some knowledge of the subject even if they need to guess an answer. It also is difficult to obtain an adequate score on a test by using random guessing only. Although students have a 50/50 chance of guessing a correct answer on one true–false item, the probability of guessing correctly on a test with many items is small. For example, if a test has 10 true–false items, a student who guesses blindly on all of those items has less than 6 chances out of 100 of having 80% or more of the items correct.

Writing True–False Items

The following discussion includes some important principles for the teacher to consider when constructing true–false items.

   1. *The true–false item should test recall of important facts and information.* The teacher should avoid constructing items that test trivia and meaningless information. The content should be worth knowing and be important in relation to the course outcomes.

   2. *The statement should be true or false without qualification*—unconditionally true or false. The teacher should be able to defend the answer without conditions.

   3. *Avoid words such as "usually," "sometimes," "often," and similar terms.* Miller, Linn, and Gronlund (2009) indicated that these words typically occur in true statements, giving the student clues as to the correct response. Along the same lines, avoid words such as "never," "always," "all," and "none," which often signal a false response.

   4. *Avoid terms that indicate an infinite degree or amount* such as "large." They can be interpreted differently by students.

   5. *Each item should include one idea to be tested* rather than multiple ones. When there are different propositions to be tested, each should be designed as a single true–false item.

   6. *Items should be worded precisely and clearly.* The teacher should avoid long statements with different qualifiers and focus the sentence instead on the main idea to be tested. Long statements take time for reading and do not contribute to testing student knowledge of an important fact or principle.

   7. *Avoid the use of negatives*, particularly double negatives. They are confusing to read and may interfere with student ability to understand the statement. For instance, the item "It is not normal for a 2-year-old to demonstrate hand-preference" (true) would be stated more clearly as, "It is normal for a 2-year-old to demonstrate hand-preference" (false). Brookhart (2011) indicated that if "not" must be used in the item, it should be highlighted.

   8. *With a series of true–false items, statements should be similar in length.* The teacher may be inclined to write longer true sentences than false ones in an attempt to state the concept clearly and precisely.

   9. *Use an equal number, or close to it, of true and false items* on a test (Miller et al., 2009; Waugh & Gronlund, 2013). Some experts recommend including slightly more false than true statements because false statements tend to differentiate better between most and least knowledgeable students. Higher discrimination power improves the reliability of test scores (Nitko & Brookhart, 2011, p. 162).

   10. *Check that the true–false items are not ordered in a noticeable pattern on the test.* For example, the teacher should avoid arranging the items in a pattern in which the answers would be TFTF or FTTFTT.

11. *Decide how to score true–false items prior to administering them to students.* In some variations of true–false items, students correct false statements; for this type, the teacher should award 2 points, 1 for identifying the statement as false and 1 for correcting it. With items of this type, the teacher should not reveal the point value of each item because this would cue students that 2-point items are false.

Sample items follow:

For each of the following statements, select T if the statement is true and F if the statement is false:

T̲   F   Type I diabetes was formerly called insulin-dependent diabetes. (T)

T̲   F   Hypothyroidism is manifested by lethargy and fatigue. (T)

T   F̲   The most common congenital heart defect in children is Tetralogy of Fallot. (F)

Variations of True–False Items

There are many variations of true–false items that may be used for testing. One variation is to ask the students to correct false statements. Students may identify the words that make a statement false and insert words to make it true. In changing the false statement to a true one, students may write in their own corrections or choose words from a list supplied by the teacher. One other modification of true–false items is to have students include a rationale for their responses, regardless of the statement being true or false. This provides a means of testing their understanding of the content.

For all of these variations, the directions should be clear and specific. Some examples follow:

If the statement is true, select T and do no more. If the statement is false, select F and underline the word or phrase that makes it false.

T   F   Tetany occurs with increased levels of calcium.

Because this statement is false, the student should select F and underline the word "increased":

T   F̲   Tetany occurs with <u>increased</u> levels of calcium. (F)

If the statement is true, select T and do no more. If the statement is false, select F, underline the word or phrase that makes it false, and write in the blank the word or phrase that would make it true.

T   F   Canned soups are high in potassium.

T   F   Fresh fruits and vegetables are low in sodium.

_____

In the first example, because the statement is false, the student should select F, underline "potassium," and write "sodium" in the blank to make the statement true. In the second example, because the statement is true, the student should only select T:

T   F̲   Canned soups are high in potassium. (F) Sodium

T̲   F   Fresh fruits and vegetables are low in sodium. (T)

_____

If the statement is true, select T and do no more. If the statement is false, select F and select the *correct* answer from the list that follows the item.

T   F   Bradycardia is a heart rate less than 80 beats per minute.
          40, 50, 60, 100

Because the statement is false, the student should select both F and 60:

T   F̲   Bradycardia is a heart rate less than 80 beats per minute.
          (F) 40, 50, 60̲, 100

If the statement is true, select T and explain why it is true. If the statement is false, select F and explain why it is false.

T̲   F   One purpose of Kegel exercises is to strengthen the pubococ-
          cygeal muscles. (T)

_____
_____

One other variation of true–false items is called multiple true–false. This is a cross between a multiple-choice and a true–false item. Multiple true–false items have an incomplete statement followed by several phrases that complete it; learners indicate which of the phrases form true or false statements. This type of item clusters true–false statements under one stem. However, rather than selecting one answer as in a multiple-choice item, students decide whether each alternative is true or false (Nitko & Brookhart, 2011). Directions for answering these items should be clear, and the phrases should be numbered consecutively because they represent individual true–false items. As with any true–false item, the phrases that complete the statement should be unequivocally true or false.

Sample items follow:

The incomplete statements below are followed by several phrases. Each of the phrases completes the statement and makes it true or false.

If the completed statement is true, select T. If the completed statement is false, select F.

A patient with a below-the-knee amputation should:

T   F   1. Avoid walking until fitted with a prosthesis. (F)
T   F   2. Keep the residual limb elevated at all times. (F)
T   F   3. Exercise the arms against resistance. (T)
T   F   4. Not sit for prolonged periods of time. (T)

Bloom's taxonomy of the cognitive domain includes the:

T   F   5. Application level. (T)
T   F   6. Knowledge level. (T)
T   F   7. Calculation level. (F)
T   F   8. Recommended actions level. (F)
T   F   9. Analysis level. (T)
T   F   10. Manipulation level. (F)
T   F   11. Synthesis level. (T)

MATCHING EXERCISES

Matching exercises consist of two parallel columns in which students match terms, phrases, sentences, or numbers from one column to the other. In a matching exercise students identify the one-to-one correspondence between the columns. One column includes a list of premises (for which the match is sought); the other column (from which the selection is made) is referred to as responses (Miller et al., 2009). The basis for matching responses to premises should be stated explicitly in the directions with the exercise. The student identifies pairs based on the principle specified in these directions. With some matching exercises, differences between the premises and responses are not apparent, such as matching a list of laboratory studies with their normal ranges, and the columns could be interchanged. In other exercises, however, the premises include descriptive phrases or sentences to which the student matches shorter responses.

Matching exercises lend themselves to testing categories, classifications, groupings, definitions, and other related facts. They are most appropriate for measuring facts based on simple associations (Miller et al., 2009). One advantage of a matching exercise is its ability to test a number of facts that can be grouped together rather than designing a series of individual items. For instance, the teacher can develop one matching exercise on medications and related side effects rather than a series of individual items on each medication. A disadvantage of matching exercises, however, is the focus on recall of facts and specific information, although in some courses this reflects an important outcome of learning.

Writing Matching Exercises

Matching exercises are intended for categories, classifications, and information that can be grouped in some way. An effective matching exercise requires the use of homogeneous material with responses that are plausible for the premises. Responses that are not plausible for some premises provide clues to the correct match. Principles for writing matching exercises include:

1. *Develop a matching exercise around homogeneous content.* All of the premises and responses to be matched should relate to that content, for example, all laboratory tests and values, all terms and definitions, and all types of health insurance and characteristics. This is the most important principle in writing a matching exercise (Miller et al., 2009).

2. *Include an unequal number of premises and responses* to avoid giving a clue to the final match. Typically there are more responses than premises, but the number of responses may be limited by the maximum number of answer options per item allowed on a scannable answer sheet. In that case, the teacher may need to write more premises than responses.

3. *Use short lists of premises and responses.* This makes it easier for the teacher to identify ones from the same content area, and it saves students reading time. With a long list of items to be matched, it is difficult to review the choices and pair them with the premises. It also prohibits recording the answers on a scannable form. Miller et al. (2009) recommended using four to seven items in each column. A longer list might be used for some exercises, but no more than 10 items should be included in either column (p. 190).

4. *For matching exercises with a large number of responses, the teacher should develop two separate matching exercises.* Otherwise students spend too much time reading through the options.

5. *Directions for the matching exercises should be clear and state explicitly the basis for matching the premises and responses.* This is an important principle in developing these items. Even if the basis for matching seems self-evident, the directions should include the rationale for matching the columns.

6. *Directions should specify whether each response may be used once, more than once, or not at all.* Matching items can be developed in which students match one response to one premise, with at least one "extra" response remaining to avoid giving a clue to the final match. Items also can be written in which students can use the responses more than once or not at all. The directions should be unambiguous about the selection of responses.

7. *Place the longer premises on the left and shorter responses on the right.* This enables the students to read the longer statement first, then search on the right for the correct response, which often is a single word or a few words.

8. *The order in which the premises and responses are listed should be alphabetical, numerical, or in some other logical order.* Alphabetical order and listing numbers in sequence eliminate clues from the arrangement of the responses (Miller et al., 2009). If the lists have another logical order, however, such as dates and sequential steps of a procedure, then they should be organized in that order. Numbers, quantities, and similar types of items should be arranged in decreasing or increasing order.

9. *The entire matching exercise should be typed on the same page and not divided across pages.* This prevents students from missing possible responses that are on the next page and their turning pages back and forth to read both premises and responses at one time. It also may decrease the time required for students to take the test (Miller et al., 2009).

Sample matching items are found in Exhibits 4.1 and 4.2.

❑Exhibit 4.1

Sample Matching Item

Directions: For each definition in Column A, select the proper term in Column B. Use each letter only once or not at all.

Column A (Premises)	Column B (Responses)
_b_ 1. Attaching a particular response to a specific stimulus	a. Cognitive styles
_f_ 2. Believing that one can respond effectively in a situation	b. Conditioning
_g_ 3. Changing gradually behavioral patterns	c. Empowerment
_d_ 4. Observing a behavior and its consequences and attempting to behave similarly	d. Modeling
_a_ 5. Varying ways in which individuals process information	e. Self-care
	f. Self-efficacy
	g. Shaping

☐Exhibit 4.2

Sample Matching Item

Directions: For each type of insulin in Column A, identify its peak action in Column B. Responses in Column B may be used once, more than once, or not at all.

Column A	Column B
_c_ 1. Regular	a. Long acting
_b_ 2. NPH	b. Intermediate acting
_a_ 3. Glargine	c. Short acting
_a_ 4. Detemir	

SUMMARY

This chapter described how to construct two types of test items: true–false and matching exercises, including variations of them. A true–false item consists of a statement that the student judges as either true or false. In some forms, students correct a false statement or supply a rationale as to why the statement is true or false. True–false items are most effective for recall of facts and specific information but also may be used to test the student's comprehension of an important principle or concept.

Matching exercises consist of two parallel columns in which students match terms, phrases, sentences, or numbers from one column to the other. One column includes a list of premises and the other column, from which the selection is made, contains the responses. The student identifies pairs based on the principle specified in the directions. Matching exercises lend themselves to testing categories, classifications, groupings, definitions, and other related facts. As with true–false items, they are most appropriate for testing recall of specific information.

REFERENCES

Brookhart, S. M. (2011). *Grading and learning: Practices that support student achievement.* Bloomington, IN: Solution Tree Press.

Miller, M. D., Linn, R. L., & Gronlund, N. E. (2009). *Measurement and assessment in teaching* (10th ed.). Upper Saddle River, NJ: Prentice Hall.

Musial, D., Nieminen, G., Thomas, J., & Burke, K. (2009). *Foundations of educational measurement.* Boston, MA: McGraw-Hill Higher Education.

Nitko, A. J., & Brookhart, S. M. (2011). *Educational assessment of students* (6th ed.). Upper Saddle River, NJ: Pearson Education.

Waugh, C. K., & Gronlund, N. E. (2013). *Assessment of student achievement* (10th ed.). Upper Saddle River, NJ: Pearson Education.

FIVE ❑

Multiple-Choice and

Multiple-Response

This chapter focuses on two other kinds of selected-response items: multiple-choice and multiple-response. Multiple-choice items, which have one correct answer, are used widely in nursing and in other fields. This test-item format includes a question or incomplete statement, followed by a list of options that answer the question or complete the statement. Multiple-response items are designed similarly, although more than one answer may be correct. Both of these test-item formats may be used for assessing learning at the recall, comprehension, application, and analysis levels, making them adaptable for a wide range of content and learning outcomes.

MULTIPLE-CHOICE ITEMS

Multiple-choice items can be used for assessing many types of learning outcomes. Some of these include:

- Knowledge of facts, specific information, and principles
- Definitions of terms
- Understanding of content
- Application of concepts, principles, and theories in clinical and other situations
- Analysis of data and clinical situations
- Comparison and selection of varied interventions
- Judgments and decisions about actions to take in clinical and other situations

Multiple-choice items are particularly useful in nursing to assess application- and analysis-level outcomes. With multiple-choice items, the teacher can introduce *new* information requiring application of concepts and theories or analytical thinking to respond to the questions. Experience with multiple-choice testing provides essential practice for students who will later encounter this type of item on licensure, certification, and other commercially prepared examinations. Multiple-choice items also allow the teacher to sample the course content more easily than with items such as essay questions, which require more time for responding. In addition, multiple-choice tests can be electronically scored and analyzed.

Although there are many advantages to multiple-choice testing, there are also certain disadvantages. First, these items are difficult to construct, particularly at the higher cognitive levels. Developing items to test memorization of facts is much easier than designing ones to measure use of knowledge in a new situation and skill in analysis. As such, many multiple-choice items are written at the lower cognitive levels, focusing only on recall and comprehension. Second, teachers often have difficulty developing plausible distractors. These distractors—also spelled distracters—are the incorrect alternatives that seem plausible for test-takers who have not adequately learned the content. If a distractor is not plausible, it provides an unintended clue to the test-taker that it is not the correct response. Third, it is often difficult to identify only one correct answer. For these reasons, multiple-choice items are time-consuming to construct.

Some critics of multiple-choice testing suggest that essay and similar types of questions to which students develop a response provide a truer measure of learning than items in which students choose from available options. However, multiple-choice items written at the application and analysis levels require *use* of concepts and theories and analytical thinking to make a selection from the available options. For items at those levels, test-takers need to compare options and make a judgment about the correct or best response.

Writing Multiple-Choice Items

There are three parts to a multiple-choice item, each with its own set of principles for development: (a) stem, (b) answer, and (c) distractors. Table 5.1 indicates each of these parts.

The stem is the lead-in phrase in the form of a question or an incomplete statement that relies on the alternatives for completion. Following the stem is a list of alternatives or options for the learner to consider and choose from. These alternatives are of two types: the answer, also called the keyed response, which is the correct or best response to answer the question or complete the statement, and distractors, which are the incorrect alternatives. The purpose of the distractors, as the word implies, is to

☐Table 5.1

PARTS OF MULTIPLE-CHOICE ITEM	
An early and common sign of pregnancy is:	**STEM in form of incomplete statement**
OPTIONS OR ALTERNATIVES	
a. amenorrhea.	*Answer*
b. morning sickness.	*Distractor*
c. spotting.	*Distractor*
d. tenderness of the breasts.	*Distractor*
In which of the following groups does Raynaud's disease occur most frequently?	**STEM in form of question**
OPTIONS OR ALTERNATIVES	
a. Men between 20–40 years old	*Distractor*
b. Men between 50–70 years old	*Distractor*
c. Women between 20–40 years old	*Answer*
d. Women between 50–70 years old	*Distractor*

distract students who are unsure of the correct answer. Suggestions for writing each of these parts are considered separately because they have different principles for construction.

Stem

The stem is the question or incomplete statement to which the alternatives relate. Whether the stem is written in question form or as an incomplete statement, the most important quality is its clarity. The test-taker should be able to read the stem and know what to look for in the alternatives without having to read through them. Thus, after reading the stem the learner should understand the intent of the item, what type of response the teacher expects (Nitko & Brookhart, 2011). One other important consideration in writing the stem is to ensure that it presents a problem or situation that relates to the learning outcome being assessed. Guidelines for writing the stem are:

   1. *The stem should present clearly and explicitly the problem to be solved.* The student should not have to read the alternatives to understand the question or the intent of the incomplete statement. The stem should provide sufficient information for answering the question or completing the statement. An example of this principle follows:

Cataracts:

a. are painful.
b. may accompany coronary artery disease.
c. occur with aging.*
d. result in tunnel vision.

The stem of this question does not clearly present the problem associated with cataracts that the alternatives address. As such, it does not guide the learner in reviewing the alternatives. In addition, the options are dissimilar, which is possible because of the lack of clarity in the stem; alternatives should be similar. One possible revision of this stem is:

The causes of cataracts include:

a. aging.*
b. arteriosclerosis.
c. hemorrhage.
d. iritis.

After writing the item, the teacher should cover the alternatives and read the stem alone. Does it explain the problem and direct the learner to the alternatives? Is it complete? Could it stand alone as a short-answer item? In writing the stem, always include the nature of the response, such as, "Which of the following *interventions, signs and symptoms, treatments, data*," and so forth. A stem that simply asks "Which of the following?" does not provide clear instructions as to what to look for in the options.

2. *Although the stem should be clear and explicit, it should not contain extraneous information unless the item is developed for the purpose of identifying significant versus insignificant data.* Otherwise, the stem should be brief, including only necessary information. Long stems that include irrelevant information take additional time for reading. This point can be illustrated as follows, using the previous cataract item:

You are caring for an elderly man who lives alone but has frequent visits from his daughter. He has congestive heart failure and some shortness of breath. Your patient was told recently that he has cataracts. The causes of cataracts include:

a. aging.*
b. arteriosclerosis.
c. hemorrhage.
d. iritis.

---

*Correct answer.

In this stem, the background information about the patient is irrelevant to the problem addressed. If subsequent items were to be written about the patient's other problems, related nursing interventions, the home setting, and so forth, then this background information might be presented as a scenario in a context-dependent item set (see Chapter 7).

Stems also should not be humorous; laughing during the test can distract students who are concentrating. If one of the distractors is humorous, it will be recognized as implausible and eliminated as an option, increasing the chance of guessing the correct answer from among the remaining alternatives. Humorous content may be confusing to test-takers who are nonnative English speakers (Bosher, 2009, p. 268).

3. *Avoid inserting information in the stem for instructional purposes.* In the example that follows, the definition of cataract has no relevance to the content tested, that is, the causes of cataracts. The goal of testing is to evaluate outcomes of learning, not to teach new information, as in this example:

Cataracts are an opacity of the lens or capsule of the eye leading to blurred and eventual loss of vision. The causes of cataracts include:

a. aging.*
b. arteriosclerosis.
c. hemorrhage.
d. iritis.

4. *If words need to be repeated in each alternative to complete the statement, shift them to the stem.* This is illustrated as follows:

An early and common sign of pregnancy:

a. *is* amenorrhea.*
b. *is* morning sickness.
c. *is* spotting.
d. *is* tenderness of the breasts.

The word "is" may be moved to the stem:

An early and common sign of pregnancy *is*:

a. amenorrhea.*
b. morning sickness.
c. spotting.
d. tenderness of the breasts.

Similarly, a word or phrase repeated in each alternative does not test students' knowledge of it and should be included in the stem. An example follows:

Clinical manifestations of Parkinson's disease include:

a. decreased perspiration, tremors at rest, and *muscle rigidity.**
b. increased salivation, *muscle rigidity*, and diplopia.
c. *muscle rigidity*, decreased salivation, and nystagmus.
d. tremors during activity, *muscle rigidity*, and increased perspiration.

This item does not test knowledge of muscle rigidity occurring with Parkinson's disease because it is included with each alternative. The stem could be revised as follows:

Clinical manifestations of Parkinson's disease include *muscle rigidity* and which of the following signs and symptoms?

a. Decreased salivation and nystagmus
b. Increased salivation and diplopia
c. Tremors at rest and decreased perspiration*
d. Tremors during activity and increased perspiration

5. *Do not include key words in the stem that would clue the student to the correct answer.* This point may be demonstrated in the earlier question on cataracts.

You are caring for an *elderly* patient who was told recently that he has cataracts. The causes of cataracts include:

a. *aging.**
b. arteriosclerosis.
c. hemorrhage.
d. iritis.

In this item, informing the student that the patient is elderly provides a clue to the correct response.

6. *Avoid the use of negatively stated stems, including words such as "no," "not," and "except."* Negatively stated stems are sometimes unclear; in addition, they require a change in thought pattern from selections that represent correct and best responses to ones reflecting incorrect and least likely responses. Most stems may be stated positively, asking for the correct or best response rather than the exception. If there is no acceptable alternative to a negatively stated stem, consider rewriting the item in a different format, such as true–false, completion or multiple response. Nitko and Brookhart (2011) recommended that if a negatively phrased item must be used, the negative word should be in the stem or an alternative but not both of them and should be <u>underlined</u> or placed in CAPITAL LETTERS.

7. *The stem and alternatives that follow should be consistent grammatically.* If the stem is an incomplete statement, each option should complete it grammatically; if not, clues may be provided as to the correct or incorrect responses. It is also important to check carefully that a consistent verb form is used with the alternatives. An example follows:

> Your patient is undergoing a right carotid endarterectomy. Prior to surgery, which information would be most important to collect as a baseline for the early recovery period? Her ability to:
>
> a. follow movements with her eyes
> b. move all four extremities*
> c. rotating her head from side to side
> d. swallow and gag

Option "c" provides a grammatical clue by not completing the statement "Her ability to." The item may be revised easily:

> Your patient is undergoing a right carotid endarterectomy. Prior to surgery, which information would be most important to collect as a baseline for the early recovery period? Her ability to:
>
> a. follow movements with her eyes
> b. move all four extremities*
> c. rotate her head from side to side
> d. swallow and gag

8. *Avoid ending stems with "a" or "an"* because these often provide grammatical clues as to the option to select. It is usually easy to rephrase the stem to eliminate the "a" or "an." For instance,

> Narrowing of the aortic valve in children occurs with *an*:
>
> a. aortic stenosis.*
> b. atrial septal defect.
> c. coarctation of the aorta.
> d. patent ductus arteriosus.

Ending this stem with "an" eliminates alternatives "c" and "d" because of an obvious lack of an grammatical agreement. The stem could be rewritten by deleting the "an":

> Narrowing of the aortic valve in children occurs with:
>
> a. aortic stenosis.*
> b. atrial septal defect.
> c. coarctation of the aorta.
> d. patent ductus arteriosus.

Ending the stem with "a or an" or "a/an" is not a satisfactory alternative because these formats require test-takers to re-read each alternative with "a" first and then "an," thereby increasing reading time unnecessarily.

9. *If the stem is a statement completed by the alternatives, begin each alternative with a lower-case letter and place a period after it because it forms a sentence with the stem.* At the end of the stem, use a comma or colon as appropriate. Use uppercase letters to begin alternatives that do not form a sentence with the stem. If the stem is a question, place a question mark at the end of the stem.

10. *Each multiple-choice item should be independent of the others.* The answer to one item should not be dependent on a correct response to another item, and the test-taker should not have to read another item to correctly interpret the item at hand. In the following example, the meaning of the second-item stem cannot be understood without referring to the stem of the first item:

> **1.** You are the community health nurse developing a teaching plan for a 45-year-old man who was treated in the Emergency Department for an asthma attack. Which action should be implemented *FIRST*?
> a. Assess other related health problems
> b. Determine his level of understanding of asthma*
> c. Review with him treatments for his asthma
> d. Teach him actions of his medications
>
> **2.** On your second home visit, the patient is short of breath. Which of these statements indicates a need for further instruction?
> a. "I checked my peak flow because I'm not feeling good."
> b. "I have been turning on the air conditioner at times like this."
> c. "I tried my Advair because my chest was feeling heavy."*
> d. "I used my nebulizer mist treatment for my wheezing."

A better format would be to develop a series of multiple-choice items that relate to a patient scenario, clinical situation, or common data set (context-dependent item set), with directions that indicate the items that pertain to the given context. This item format is discussed in Chapter 7.

11. *Write the stem so that the alternatives are placed at the end of the incomplete statement.* An incomplete statement with a blank in the middle, which the options then complete, interrupts the reading and may be confusing for the students to read and follow (Nitko & Brookhart, 2011). For example:

The nurse should check the _____ for a patient receiving warfarin.

a. activated clotting time
b. complete blood cell count
c. International Normalized Ratio*
d. partial thromboplastin time

This item would be easier to read for students if the alternatives were placed at the end of the statement:

For a patient receiving warfarin, the nurse should check the:

a. activated clotting time.
b. complete blood cell count.
c. International Normalized Ratio.*
d. partial thromboplastin time.

Alternatives

Following the stem in a multiple-choice item is a list of alternatives or options, which include (a) the correct or best answer and (b) distractors. There are varying recommendations as to the number of alternatives to include, ranging from 3 to 5. The more options—as long as they are plausible—the more discriminating the item. Five options reduce the chance of guessing the correct answer to 1 in 5 (Miller, Linn, & Gronlund, 2009). Unfortunately, it usually is difficult to develop four plausible distractors to accompany the correct answer when five options are included. For this reason, four options typically are used, allowing for one correct or best answer and three plausible distractors. Many standardized tests use four alternatives. In writing multiple-choice items, however, if one of the distractors is not plausible, it is better to use a 3-option item (Rodriguez, 2005; Tarrant & Ware, 2012). General principles for writing the alternatives follow:

1. *The alternatives should be similar in length, detail, and complexity.* It is important to check the number of words included in each option for consistency in length. Frequently the correct answer is the longest because the teacher attempts to write it clearly and specifically. Nitko and Brookhart (2011) suggested that the testwise student may realize that the longest response is the correct answer without having the requisite knowledge to make this choice. In that case, the teacher should either shorten the correct response or add similar qualifiers to the distractors so that they are similar in length as well as in detail and complexity.

Although there is no established number of words by which the alternatives may differ from each other without providing clues, one strategy is to count the words in each option and attempt to vary them by no more than a few words. This will ensure that the options are consistent in length. In the sample item, the correct answer is longer than the distractors, which might provide a clue for selecting it.

> You are assessing a 14-year-old girl who appears emaciated. Her mother describes the following changes: resistance to eating and 20-lb. weight loss over the last 6 weeks. It is most likely that the patient resists eating for which of the following reasons?
>
> a. Complains of recurring nausea
> b. Describes herself as "fat all over" and fearful of gaining weight*
> c. Has other gastrointestinal problems
> d. Seeks her mother's attention

The correct answer can be shortened to: Is fearful of gaining weight.

2. *In addition to consistency in length, detail, and complexity, the options should have the same number of parts.* The answer in the previous question is not only longer than the other options but also includes two parts, providing another clue. In the example that follows, including two causes in option "a" provides a clue to the answer. Revising that option to only "aging" avoids this.

> Causes of cataracts include:
>
> a. aging and steroid therapy.*
> b. arteriosclerosis.
> c. hemorrhage.
> d. iritis.

3. *The alternatives should be consistent grammatically.* The answer and distractors should be similar in structure and terminology. Without this consistency in format, the test-taker may be clued to the correct response or know to eliminate some of the options without being familiar with the content. In the sample item below, the student may be clued to the correct answer "a" because it differs grammatically from the others:

> You are making a home visit with a new mother who is breastfeeding. She tells you that her nipples are cracked and painful. Which of the following instructions should be given to the mother?
>
> a. Put the entire areola in the baby's mouth during feeding.*
> b. The baby should be fed less frequently until the nipples are healed.
> c. There is less chance of cracking if the nipples are washed daily with soap.
> d. Wiping off the lotion on the nipples before feeding the baby may help.

4. *The alternatives should sample the same domain, for instance, all symptoms, all diagnostic tests, all nursing interventions, varying treatments,* *and so forth.* A study by Ascalon, Meyers, Davis, and Smits (2007) examined the effects on item difficulty of different ways of writing the item stem and homogeneity of the alternatives. They found no differences in item difficulty when the stem was written as a statement versus a question. However, when alternatives of a multiple-choice item were similar, it increased the item difficulty. It is likely that when responses are dissimilar from the correct response, learners can easily eliminate them as options. In the example that follows, option "b" is not a nursing diagnosis, which may clue the student to omit it as a possibility.

> You are working in the Emergency Department, and your patient is having difficulty breathing. His respiratory rate is 40, heart rate 140, and oxygen saturation 90%. He also complains of a headache. Which of the following nursing diagnoses is of greatest priority?
>
> a. Activity intolerance
> b. Chronic obstructive pulmonary disease
> c. Impaired gas exchange*
> d. Pain

5. *Avoid including opposite responses among the options.* This is often a clue to choose between the opposites and not consider the others. A sample item follows:

> The nurse should determine the correct placement of a nasogastric tube by:
>
> a. asking the patient to swallow.
> b. aspirating gastric fluid from the tube.
> c. confirming the placement with an X-ray.*
> d. confirming the placement with capnography.

In this example, the correct response is opposite one of the distractors, which clues the student to select one of these alternatives. In addition, options "c" and "d" begin with "confirming," which may provide a visual clue to choose between them. McDonald (2007) suggested that when two sets of opposites are used in the alternatives, there is less opportunity for guessing. Using this principle, the first distractor in the example could be reworded to form a second pair of opposites:

> The nurse should determine the correct placement of a nasogastric tube by:
>
> a. aspirating air from the tube.
> b. aspirating gastric fluid from the tube.
> c. confirming the placement with an X-ray.*
> d. confirming the placement with capnography.

6. *Arrange the options in a logical or meaningful order.* The order can be alphabetical, numerical, or chronological (Nitko & Brookhart, 2011). Arranging the options in this way tends to randomly distribute the position of the correct response rather than the answer occurring most often in the same location, for example, "b" or "c," throughout the test. It also helps students locate the correct response more easily when they have an answer in mind.

7. *Options with numbers, quantities, and other numerical values should be listed sequentially, either increasing or decreasing in value, and the values should not overlap.* When alternatives overlap, a portion of a distractor may be correct, resulting in more than one correct answer. These problems are apparent in the sample item that follows:

The normal range for potassium in adults is:

a. 2.5–4.5 mEq/L.
b. 0.5–3.5 mEq/L.
c. 3.5–5.2 mEq/L.*
d. 1.5–4.5 mEq/L.

The values in these options overlap, and the alternatives would be easier to review if they were arranged sequentially from decreasing to increasing values. Laboratory and other values should be labeled appropriately, such as hemoglobin 14.0 g/dL. A revision of the prior item follows:

The normal range for potassium in adults is:

a. 0.5–1.5 mEq/L.
b. 2.0–3.2 mEq/L.
c. 3.5–5.2 mEq/L.*
d. 8.5–10.3 mEq/L.

8. *Each option should be placed on a separate line for ease of student reading.* If answers are recorded on a separate answer sheet, the teacher should review the format of the sheet ahead of time so that responses are identified as "a" through "d" or 1 through 4 as appropriate. Usually items are numbered and responses are lettered to prevent clerical errors when students use a separate answer sheet.

9. Use the option of "call for assistance" sparingly. Options that relate to getting assistance such as "notify the physician" or "call the supervisor" should be used sparingly because it is not known how they act as distractors in multiple-choice items. McDonald (2007) suggested that students do not readily choose an option such as "call the physician" and therefore it may not be a good distractor. When it is the correct or best answer, the students would need to weigh that decision against the other options. However, some teacher-made tests may overuse this option as the correct answer, conditioning students to select it without considering the other alternatives.

Correct answer. In a multiple-choice item there is one answer to be selected from among the alternatives. In some instances the best rather than the correct answer is to be chosen. Considering that judgments are needed to arrive at decisions about patient care, items can ask for the best or most appropriate response from those listed. Best answers are valuable for more complex and higher level learning such as with items written at the application and analysis levels. Even though best-answer items require a judgment to select the best option, there can be only one answer, and there should be consistency in the literature and among experts as to that response. A colleague can review the items, without knowing the answers in advance, to ensure that they are correct.

Listed below are suggestions for writing the correct answer. These suggestions are guided by the principle that the students should not be able to identify the correct response and eliminate distractors because of the way the stem or alternatives are written.

1. *Review the alternatives carefully to ensure that there is only one correct response.* For example:

Symptoms of increased intracranial pressure include:

a. blurred vision.*
b. decreased blood pressure.
c. disorientation.*
d. increased pulse.

In this sample item, both "a" and "c" are correct; a possible revision follows:

Symptoms of increased intracranial pressure include:

a. blurred vision and decreased blood pressure.
b. decreased blood pressure and increased pulse.
c. disorientation and blurred vision.*
d. increased pulse and disorientation.

2. *Review carefully terminology included in the stem to avoid giving a clue to the correct answer.* Key words in the stem, if also used in the correct response, may clue the student to select it. In the following example, "sudden weight loss" is in both the stem and the answer:

An elderly patient with *sudden weight loss*, thirst, and confusion is seen in the clinic. Which of the following signs would be indicative of dehydration?

a. Below normal temperature
b. Decreased urine-specific gravity
c. Increased blood pressure
d. *Sudden weight loss**

The question could be revised by omitting "sudden weight loss" in the stem.

An elderly patient with dry skin, thirst, and confusion is seen in the clinic. Which of the following signs would also be indicative of dehydration?

a. Below normal temperature
b. Decreased urine-specific gravity
c. Increased blood pressure
d. *Sudden weight loss**

3. *The correct answer should be randomly assigned to a position among the alternatives to avoid favoring a particular response choice.* Some teachers may inadvertently assign the correct answer to the same option (e.g., "c") or, over a series of items, a pattern may develop from the placement of the correct answers (e.g., "a, b, c, d, a, b, c, d"). As indicated earlier in the discussion of how to write the options, this potential clue can be avoided by listing the alternatives in a logical or meaningful order such as alphabetical, numerical, or chronological. However, the teacher also should double check the position of the correct answers on a test to confirm that they are more or less randomly distributed.

4. *The answers should not reflect the opinion of the teacher but instead should be the ones with which experts agree or are the most probable responses.* The answers should be consistent with the literature and not be answers chosen arbitrarily by the teacher. Alternatively, a specific authority may be referenced in the stem (e.g., "According to the Centers for Disease Control and Prevention").

Distractors. Distractors are the incorrect but plausible options offered. Distractors should appeal to learners who lack the knowledge for responding to the question without confusing those who do know the content. If the option is obviously wrong, then there is no reason to include it as an alternative. Because the intent of the distractors is to appeal to learners who have not mastered the content, at least some of the students should choose each option, or the distractors should be revised for the next administration of the test.

Each alternative should be appropriate for completing the stem. Hastily written distractors may be clearly incorrect, may differ in substance and format from the others, and may be inappropriate for the stem, providing clues as to how to respond. They also may result in a test item that does not measure the students' learning.

When writing a multiple-choice item, it is sometimes difficult to identify enough plausible distractors to have the same number of options for each item on the test. However, rather than using a filler that is obviously incorrect or would not be seriously considered by the students, the teacher should use fewer options on that item. Nitko and Brookhart (2011) indicated that there is no rationale for using the same number of alternatives for each item on a test. The goal is to develop plausible and functional alternatives, ones that attract at least some of the students, rather than filler alternatives that no one chooses. Thus, for some items there may be only three alternatives, even though the majority of questions on that test use four. The goal, however, is to develop three plausible distractors so that most items have at least four responses from which to choose.

In writing distractors, it is helpful to think about common errors that students make, phrases that "sound correct," misperceptions students have about the content, and familiar responses not appropriate for the specific problem in the stem. Another way of developing distractors is to identify, before writing any of the options, the content area or domain to which all the responses must belong, for example, all nursing interventions. If the stem asks about nursing measures for a patient with acute pneumonia, the distractors might be interventions for a patient with asthma that would not be appropriate for someone with pneumonia.

Terms used in the stem also give ideas for developing distractors. For example, if the stem asks about measures to avoid increasing anxiety in a patient who is delusional, the distractors may be interventions for a delusional patient that might inadvertently increase or have no effect on anxiety, or interventions useful for decreasing anxiety but not appropriate for a patient with a delusional disorder. Another strategy for developing distractors is to identify the category to which all alternative responses must belong. For a stem that asks about side effects of erythromycin, plausible distractors may be drawn from side effects of antibiotics as a group. Suggestions for writing distractors include:

1. *The distractors should be consistent grammatically and should be similar in length, detail, and complexity with each other and the correct answer.* Examples were provided earlier in the chapter. The distractors should be written with the same specificity as the correct response. If the correct response is "quadratus plantae," distractors that are more general such as "motor" may be a clue not to choose that option.

2. *The distractors should sample the same content area as the correct answer.* When types of options vary, they may clue the student as to the correct response or to eliminate a particular distractor. In the following example, options "a," "b," and "c" pertain to factors in the workplace. Because option "d" relates to diet, it may clue the student to omit it. A better alternative for "d" would be another factor to assess in the work setting such as how tiring the job is.

> In planning teaching for a patient with a hiatal hernia, which of these factors should be assessed?
>
> a. Amount of lifting done at work*
> b. Number of breaks allowed
> c. Stress of the job
> d. Use of high-sodium foods

3. *Avoid using "all of the above" and "none of the above" in a multiple-choice item.* As distractors these contrast with the direction of selecting one correct or best response. With "all of the above" as a distractor, students aware of one incorrect response are clued to eliminate "all of the above" as an option. Similarly, knowledge of one correct alternative clues students to omit "none of the above" as an option. Often teachers resort to "all of the above" when unable to develop a fourth option, although it is better to rephrase the stem or to modify the options to provide fewer plausible alternatives. Popham (2012), based on a review of the research, indicated that three well selected choices are almost as good as 4 or 5.

"None of the above" option is appropriate for multiple-choice items on which students perform calculations. By using "none of the above," the teacher avoids giving clues to students when their incorrect answer is not listed with the options. In the following example the student would need to know the correct answer to identify that it is not among the alternatives:

> You are working in a pediatrician's office, and a mother calls and asks you how many drops of acetaminophen to give to her infant. The order is for 40 mg every 12 hours, but the container she has at home is 80 mg/0.8 mL. You should tell the mother to give:
>
> a. 1 dropperful
> b. 1 teaspoon
> c. 1.5 mL in a 3-mL syringe
> d. None of the above*

4. *Omit terms such as "always," "never," "sometimes," "occasionally," and similar ones from the distractors.* These general terms often provide clues as to the correctness of the option. Terms such as *always* and *never* suggest that the alternatives are incorrect because rarely does a situation occur always or never, particularly in patient care.

5. *Avoid using distractors that are essentially the same.* In the following example, alternatives "a" and "c" are essentially the same. If "rest" is eliminated as an option, the students are clued to omit both of these. In addition, the correct response in this item is more general than the others and is not specific to this particular student's health problems.

> A student comes to see the school nurse complaining of a severe headache and stiff neck. Which of the following actions would be most appropriate?
>
> a. Ask the student to rest in the clinic for a few hours
> b. Collect additional data before deciding on interventions*
> c. Have a family member take the student home to rest
> d. Prepare to take the student to the emergency room

The item could be revised as follows:

> A student comes to see the school nurse complaining of a severe headache and stiff neck. Which of the following actions would be most appropriate?
>
> a. Ask the student to rest in the clinic for a few hours
> b. Check the student's health record for identified health problems*
> c. Prepare to take the student to the emergency room
> d. Send the student back to class after medicating for pain

Variation of Multiple-Choice Item

A multiple-choice item can be combined with short-answer or essay. In this format, after answering a multiple-choice item, students develop a rationale for why their answer is correct and the distractors are incorrect. The teacher should award 1 point for correctly identifying the answer and other points for providing an acceptable rationale. For example:

> Your patient is ordered 60 mg of Roxanol™ (morphine sulfate 20 mg/mL) every 4 hours for severe pain. Which of the following actions should be taken?
>
> a. Dilute in 500 cc normal saline
> b. Give the morphine as ordered
> c. Have the pharmacist review the order
> d. Call the physician about the dose*

In the space below, provide a rationale for why your answer is the best one and why the other options are not appropriate.

_____

_____

MULTIPLE-RESPONSE

In these item formats several alternatives may be correct, and students choose either all of the correct alternatives or the best combination of alternatives. Multiple-response items are included on the NCLEX® Examination as one type of item format (National Council of State Boards of Nursing, 2010). On the NCLEX and other types of computerized tests, students select all of the options that apply by checking the box that precedes each option, as in the following example:

The preliminary diagnosis for your patient, a 20-year-old college student, is meningitis. Which signs and symptoms should you anticipate finding? Select all that apply:

☐ 1. Abdominal tenderness
☑ 2. Fever
☐ 3. Lack of pain with sudden head movements
☑ 4. Nausea and vomiting
☑ 5. Nuchal rigidity
☑ 6. Sensitivity to light
☐ 7. Sudden bruising in neck area

The principles for writing multiple-response items are the same as for writing multiple-choice. Suggestions for writing these items include the following:

1. *The combination of alternatives should be plausible.* Options should be logically combined rather than grouped randomly.

2. *The alternatives should be used a similar number of times in the combinations.* If one of the alternatives is in every combination, it is obviously correct; this information should be added to the stem as described earlier in the chapter. Similarly, limited use of an option may provide a clue to the correct combination of responses. After grouping responses, each letter should be counted to be sure that it is used a similar number of times across combinations of responses and that no letter is included in every combination.

3. *The responses should be listed in a logical order, for instance, alphabetically or sequentially, for ease in reviewing.* Alternatives are easier to review if shorter combinations are listed before longer ones.

A sample item follows:

Causes of cataracts include:

1. aging.
2. arteriosclerosis.
3. hemorrhage.
4. iritis.
5. steroid therapy.
    a. 1, 2
    b. 1, 5*
    c. 2, 4
    d. 1, 3, 4
    e. 2, 3, 5

SUMMARY

This chapter described the development of multiple-choice and multiple-response items. Multiple-choice items, with one correct or best answer, are used widely in nursing and other fields. This test-item format includes a question or incomplete statement followed by a list of options that answer the question or complete the statement. Multiple-response items are designed similarly although more than one answer may be correct, or students may be asked to select one answer with the best combination of alternatives. All of these item formats may be used for evaluating learning at the recall, comprehension, application, and analysis levels, making them adaptable for a wide range of content and learning outcomes.

Multiple-choice items are important for testing the application of nursing knowledge in simulated clinical situations and analytical thinking. Because of their versatility, they may be integrated easily within most testing situations.

There are three parts in a multiple-choice item, each with its own set of principles for development: (a) stem, (b) answer, and (c) distractors. The stem is the lead-in phrase in the form of a question or an incomplete statement that relies on the alternatives for completion. Following the stem is a list of alternatives, options for the learner to consider and choose from. These alternatives are of two types: the answer, which is the correct or best option to answer the question or complete the statement, and distractors, which are the incorrect yet plausible alternatives. Suggestions for writing each of these parts were presented in the chapter and were accompanied by sample items.

The ability to write multiple-choice items is an important skill for the teacher to develop. This is a situation in which "practice makes perfect." After writing an item, the teacher should have colleagues read it and make suggestions for revision. The teacher should also try out questions with students and maintain an electronic file of items for use in constructing tests. Although time-consuming to develop, multiple-choice items are an important means for assessing learning in nursing.

REFERENCES

Ascalon, M. E., Meyers, L. S., Davis, B. W., & Smits, N. (2007). Distractor similarity and item-stem structure: Effects on item difficulty. *Applied Measurement in Education, 20,* 153–170.

Bosher, S. D. (2009). Removing language as a barrier to success on multiple-choice nursing exams. In S. D. Bosher & M. D. Pharris (Eds.), *Transforming nursing education: The culturally inclusive environment* (pp. 259–284). New York, NY: Springer Publishing.

McDonald, M. E. (2007). *The nurse educator's guide to assessing learning outcomes.* Boston, MA: Jones and Bartlett.

Miller, M. D., Linn, R. L., & Gronlund, N. E. (2009). *Measurement and assessment in teaching* (10th ed.). Upper Saddle River, NJ: Prentice Hall.

National Council of State Boards of Nursing. (2010). *2010 NCLEX-RN® detailed test plan.* Chicago, IL: Author.

Nitko, A. J., & Brookhart, S. M. (2011). *Educational assessment of students* (6th ed.). Upper Saddle River, NJ: Pearson Education.

Popham, W. J. (2012). *Selected-response tests: Building and bettering* (Vol. 12). Boston, MA: Pearson.

Rodriguez, M. C. (2005). Three options are optimal for multiple-choice items: A meta-analysis of 80 years of research. *Educational Measurement: Issues and Practice, 24*(2), 3–13.

Tarrant, M., & Ware, J. (2012). A framework for improving the quality of multiple-choice assessment. *Nurse Educator, 37,* 98–104.

SIX

Short-Answer

(Fill-in-the-Blank) and Essay

Short-answer and essay are examples of constructed response items. With these items, the test-taker supplies an answer rather than selecting from options already provided. Because students supply the answers, this type of item reduces the chance of guessing.

Short-answer items can be answered by a word, phrase, or number. There are two types of short-answer items: question and completion. One format presents a question that students answer in a few words or phrases. With the other format, completion or fill-in-the-blank, students are given an incomplete sentence that they complete by inserting a word or words in the blank space. In an essay item, the student develops a more extended response to a question or statement. Essay tests and written assignments use writing as the means of expressing ideas, although with essay items the focus of assessment is the content of the answer rather than the writing ability. Short-answer and essay items are described in this chapter.

SHORT-ANSWER

Short-answer items can be answered by a word, phrase, or number. The two types of short-answer items—question and completion—also referred to as fill-in-the-blank, are essentially the same except for format.

With the question format, students answer a question in a few words or phrases. Calculations may be included for the teacher to review the process that the student used to arrive at an answer. The questions may stand alone and have no relationship to one another, or comprise a series of questions in a similar content area.

Completion items consist of a statement with a key word or words missing; students fill in the blank to complete it. Other types of completion items ask students to perform a calculation and record the answer, or to order a list of responses.

Completion items are appropriate for recall of facts and specific information and for calculations. To complete the statement, the student recalls missing facts, such as a word or short phrase, or records the solution to a calculation problem. Although completion items appear easy to construct, they should be designed in such a way that only one answer is possible. If students provide other correct answers, the teacher needs to accept them.

Fill-in-the-blank and ordered response items are two of the alternate item formats used on the NCLEX®. Fill-in-the-blank items ask candidates to perform a calculation and type in the answer. All answers are scored as right or wrong. With ordered response items, candidates answer a question by rank ordering options or placing a list of responses in the proper order (National Council of State Boards of Nursing, 2012). For example, students might be given a list of the phases of wound healing or of Erikson's stages of development and asked to put them in the order they occur. On a computerized test, such as the NCLEX, candidates can click an option and drag it or highlight an option and use the arrow keys to arrange the options in the correct order. However, this same format can be used on a paper-and-pencil test with students writing the order on their test booklets or teacher-made answer sheets, or indicating it on a machine-scannable answer sheet.

Short-answer items are useful for measuring student ability to interpret data, use formulas correctly, complete calculations, and solve mathematical-type problems. Items may ask students to label a diagram, name anatomical parts, identify various instruments, and label other types of drawings, photographs, and the like. Nitko and Brookhart (2011) described another type of short-answer format, association variety, which provides a list of terms or pictures for which students recall relevant labels, numbers, or symbols (p. 151). For example, students might be given a list of medical terms and be asked to recall their abbreviations.

Writing Short-Answer Items

Suggestions for developing short-answer items are as follows:

1. *Questions and statements should not be taken verbatim from textbooks, other readings, and lecture notes.* These materials may be used as a basis for designing short-answer items, but taking exact wording from them may result in testing only recall of meaningless facts out of context. Such items

measure memorization of content and may or may not be accompanied by the student's comprehension of it.

2. *Phrase the item so that a unique word, series of words, or number must be supplied to complete it.* Only one correct answer should be possible to complete the statement.

3. *Write questions that are specific and can be answered in a few words, phrases, or short sentences.* The question, "What is insulin?" does not provide sufficient direction as to how to respond; asking instead "What is the peak action time of NPH insulin?" results in a more specific answer.

4. *Before writing the item, think of the correct answer first and then write a question or statement for that answer.* Although the goal is to develop an item with only one correct response, students may identify other correct answers. For this reason, it is necessary to develop a scoring sheet with all possible correct answers, and re-score student responses as needed if students provide additional correct answers that the teacher did not anticipate.

5. *Fill-in-the-blank items requiring calculations and solving mathematical-type problems should include in the statement the type of answer and degree of specificity desired,* for instance, convert pounds to kilograms, rounding your answer to one decimal point.

6. *For a statement with a key word or words missing, place the blank at or near the end of the statement.* This makes it easier for students to complete. It also is important to watch for grammatical clues in the statement, such as "a" versus "an" and singular versus plural, prior to the blank, which might give clues to the intended response. If more than one blank is included in the statement, they should be of equal lengths. Use of more than 2 blanks should be avoided because there may be insufficient information remaining to permit students to grasp the nature of the task they are to perform.

7. *When students need to write longer answers, provide for sufficient space or use a separate answer sheet.* In some situations, longer responses might indicate that the item is actually an essay item, and the teacher then should follow principles for constructing and evaluating essay items.

8. *Even though a blank space is placed at the end of the statement, the teacher may direct the student to record one-word answers in blanks arranged in a column to the left or right of the items, thereby facilitating scoring.* For example,

_____ 1. *Streptococcus pneumoniae* and *Staphylococcus aureus* are examples of _____ bacteria.

Following are some examples of question and completion (or fill-in-the-blank) formats of short-answer items:

What congenital cardiac defect results in communication between the pulmonary artery and the aorta? _____

Two types of metered-dose inhalers used for the treatment of bronchial asthma are:

_____

_____

List three methods for measuring handwashing compliance of staff in an acute care setting.

1. _____
2. _____
3. _____

You are caring for a patient who weighs 128 lb. She is ordered 20 mcg/kg of an intravenous (IV) medication. What is the correct dose in micrograms?

Answer: _____

ESSAY ITEM

In an essay test, students construct responses to items based on their understanding of the content. With this type of test item, varied answers may be possible depending on the concepts selected by the student for discussion and the way in which they are presented. Essay items provide an opportunity for students to select content to discuss, present ideas in their own words, and develop an original and creative response to an item. Essay items are useful for assessing complex learning outcomes and higher levels of learning. Higher level responses, however, are more difficult to evaluate and score than answers reflecting recall of facts.

Although some essay items are developed around recall of facts and specific information, they are more appropriate for higher levels of learning. Miller, Linn, and Gronlund (2009) recommended that essay items be used primarily for learning outcomes that cannot be measured adequately through selected-response items. Essay items are effective for assessing students' ability to apply concepts, analyze theories, evaluate situations and ideas, and develop creative solutions to problems, using multiple sources of information. In a study by Barnett and Francis (2012), students who had quizzes with essay items that required higher level thinking performed better on multiple-choice and essay items on their tests in the course compared to students whose quizzes had items that required only recall of facts.

Although essay items use writing as the medium for expression, the intent is to assess student understanding of specific content rather than judge writing ability in and of itself. Other types of assignments are better suited to evaluating the ability of students to write effectively; these are described in later chapters. Low-level essay items are similar to short-answer items and require precise responses. An example of a low-level essay is "Describe three signs of increased intracranial pressure in children under 2 years old." Broader and higher level essay items, however, do not limit responses in this way and differ clearly from short-answer items, such as "Defend the statement 'access to health care is a right.'" Essay items may be written to assess a wide range of learning outcomes. These include:

- Comparing, such as comparing the side effects of two different medications
- Outlining steps to take and protocols to follow
- Explaining and summarizing in one's own words a situation or statement
- Discussing topics
- Applying concepts and principles to a clinical scenario and explaining their relevancy to it
- Analyzing patient data and clinical situations through use of relevant concepts and theories
- Critiquing different interventions and nursing management
- Developing plans and proposals drawing on multiple sources of information
- Analyzing nursing and health care trends
- Arriving at decisions about issues and actions to take, accompanied by a rationale
- Analyzing ethical issues, possible decisions, and their consequences
- Developing arguments for and against a particular position or decision

As with other types of test items, the objective or outcome to be assessed provides the framework for developing the essay item. From the learning outcome, the teacher develops a clear and specific item to elicit information about student achievement. If the outcome to be assessed focuses on application of concepts to clinical practice, then the essay item should examine ability to apply knowledge to a clinical situation. The item should be stated clearly so that the students know what they should write about. If it is ambiguous, the students will perceive the need to write all they know about a topic.

Issues With Essay Tests

Although essay items are valuable for examining the ability to select, organize, and present ideas and they provide an opportunity for creativity and originality in responding, they are limited by low reliability and other issues associated with their scoring. The teacher should have an understanding of these issues because they may influence the decision to use essay items. Strategies are provided later in the chapter for addressing some of these issues.

Limited Ability to Sample Content

By their nature essay items do not provide an efficient means of sampling course content as compared to objective items. Often only a few essay items can be included on a test, considering the time it takes for students to formulate their thoughts and prepare an open-ended response, particularly when the items are intended for assessing higher levels of learning. As a result, it is difficult to assess all of the different content areas in a nursing course using essay items.

When the learning outcomes are memorization and recall of facts, essay items should not be used because there are more efficient means of measuring such outcomes. Instead, essay items should be developed for assessing students' ability to organize and express ideas and explain their interrelationships (Nitko & Brookhart, 2011). Essay items are best used for responses requiring originality.

Unreliability in Scoring

The major limitation of essay items is the lack of consistency in evaluating responses. Scoring answers is a complex process, and studies have shown that essay responses are scored differently by different teachers (Miller et al., 2009). Some teachers are more lenient or critical than others regardless of the criteria established for scoring. Even with preset criteria, teachers may evaluate answers differently, and scores may vary when the same teacher reads the paper again. Miller et al. (2009) suggested that frequently the reasons for unreliability in scoring are the failure of the faculty member to identify the specific outcomes being assessed with the essay item and lack of a well-defined rubric for scoring (p. 242).

Factors such as misspelled words and incorrect grammar may affect scoring beyond the criteria to which they relate. In scoring the student's response, it is important to focus on the substantive content and not be influenced by how the response is written. Factors such as writing style, spelling, and grammar should be ignored in the evaluation or scored separately (Nitko & Brookhart, 2011; Waugh & Gronlund, 2013).

The unreliability with scoring, though, depends on the type of essay item. When the essay item is highly focused and structured, such as "List three side effects of bronchodilators," there is greater reliability in scoring. Of course, these lower level items also could be classified as short-answer. Less restrictive essay items allowing for freedom and creativity in responding have lower rater reliability than more restricted ones. Items asking students to analyze, defend, judge, evaluate, critique, and develop products are less reliable in terms of scoring the response. There are steps the teacher can take, though, to improve reliability, such as defining the content to be included in a "correct" answer and using a scoring rubric. These are presented later in the chapter.

Carryover Effects

Another issue in evaluating essay items is a carryover effect in which the teacher develops an impression of the quality of the answer from one item and carries it over to the next response. If the student answers one item well, the teacher may be influenced to score subsequent responses at a similarly high level; the same situation may occur with a poor response. For this reason, it is best to read all students' responses to one item before evaluating the next one. Miller et al. (2009) suggested that reading all the answers to one item at a time improves scoring accuracy by keeping the teacher focused on the standards of each item. It also avoids carrying over an impression of the quality of the student's answer to one item onto the scoring of the next response.

The same problem can occur with tests as a whole as well as written assignments. The teacher's impression of the student can carry over from one test to the next or from one paper to the next. When scoring essay tests and grading papers, the teacher should not know whose paper it is.

Halo Effect

There may be a tendency in evaluating essay items to be influenced by a general impression of the student or feelings about the student, either positive or negative, that create a halo effect when judging the quality of the answers. For instance, the teacher may hold favorable opinions about the student from class or clinical practice and believe that this learner has made significant improvement in the course, which in turn might influence the scoring of responses. For this reason, essay tests should be scored anonymously by asking students to identify themselves by an assigned or selected number rather than by their names. Names can be matched with numbers after scoring is completed.

Effect of Writing Ability

It is difficult to evaluate student responses based on content alone even with clear and specific scoring guidelines. The teacher's judgment often is influenced by sentence structure, grammar, spelling, punctuation, and overall writing ability. Some students write well enough to cover up their lack of knowledge of the content; longer answers may be scored higher regardless of the content. The teacher, therefore, needs to evaluate the *content* of the learner's response and not be influenced by the writing style. When writing also is evaluated, it should be scored separately (Miller et al., 2009).

Rater Drift

Essay tests read early in a scoring session may be scored higher than those read near the end because of teacher fatigue and time constraints. Nitko and Brookhart (2011) described the problem of "rater drift," the tendency of the teacher to gradually stray from the scoring criteria. Over time the teacher may not pay attention to the specific criteria or may apply them differently to each response. In scoring essay items the teacher needs to check that the rubric and standards for grading are implemented equally for each student. Teachers should read papers in random order and read each response twice before computing a score. After scoring the responses to a question, the teacher should rearrange the papers to avoid being influenced by their order. It also is important to stop periodically and confirm that the responses read later are scored consistently with those read early (Nitko & Brookhart, 2011).

Time

One other issue in using essay items is the time it takes for students to answer them and for teachers to score them. In writing essay items, the teacher should estimate how long it will take to answer each item, erring on allowing too much time rather than too little. Students should be told approximately how long to spend on each item so they can pace themselves (Miller et al., 2009).

Scoring essay items also can be a pressing issue for teachers, particularly if the teacher is responsible for large numbers of students. Considering that responses should be read twice, the teacher should consider the time required for scoring responses when planning for essay tests. Scoring software is available that can scan an essay and score the response. One example of an automated essay scoring program is e-rater® used by Educational Testing Service. Programs such as e-rater score essays by identifying features that represent important aspects of writing quality and can be used to predict scores, for example, grammar, usage, style, organization, and content relevance, among others (Educational Testing Service, 2012). Nursing faculty members need to determine, however, whether such software is appropriate for use in nursing courses with their specialized content and need for higher level thinking, and whether its use is cost-effective.

Student Choice of Items

Some teachers allow students to choose a subset of essay items to answer, often because of limited time for testing and to provide options for students. For example, the teacher may include four items on the care of patients with heart disease and ask students to answer two of them. However, Miller et al. (2009) cautioned against this practice because when students choose different items to answer, they are actually taking different tests. The option to choose items to answer also may affect measurement validity.

Restricted-Response Essay Items

There are two types of essay items: restricted response and extended response. Although the notion of freedom of response is inherent in essay items, there are varying degrees of freedom in responding to the items. At one end of the continuum is the restricted-response item, in which a few sentences are required for an answer. These are short-answer essays. At the other end is the extended-response item, in which students have freedom to express their own ideas and organize them as they choose. Responses to essay items typically fall between these two extremes.

In a restricted-response item, the teacher limits the student's answer by indicating the content to be discussed and frequently the amount of discussion allowed, for instance, limiting the response to one paragraph or page. With this type of essay item, the way in which the student responds is structured by the teacher. A restricted-response item may be developed by posing a specific problem to be addressed and asking questions about that problem (Miller et al., 2009). For example, specific material, such as patient data, a description of a clinical situation, research findings, a description of issues associated with clinical practice, and extracts from the literature, to cite a few, may be included with the essay item. Students read, analyze, and interpret this accompanying material, then answer questions about it. Nitko and Brookhart (2011) referred to essay items of this type as interpretive exercises or context-dependent tasks. Examples of restricted-response items follow:

- Define patient centered care. Limit your definition to one paragraph.
- Select one environmental health problem and describe its potential effects on the community. Do not use an example presented in class. Limit your discussion to one page.

- Compare metabolic and respiratory acidosis. Include the following in your response: definitions, precipitating factors, clinical manifestations, diagnostic tests, and interventions.
- Your patient is 76 years old and 1 day postoperative following a femoral popliteal bypass graft. Name two complications the patient could experience at this time and discuss why they are potential problems. List two nursing interventions for this patient during the initial recovery period with related evidence.
- Describe five physiological changes associated with the aging process.

Extended-Response Essay Items

Extended-response essay items are less restrictive and as such provide an opportunity for students to decide how to respond: they can organize ideas in their own ways, arrive at judgments about the content, and demonstrate ability to communicate ideas effectively in writing. With these types of items, the teacher may assess students' ability to develop their own ideas and express them creatively, integrate learning from multiple sources in responding, and evaluate the ideas of others based on predetermined criteria. Because responses are not restricted by the teacher, assessment is more difficult. This difficulty, however, is balanced by the opportunity for students to express their own ideas. As such, extended-response essay items provide a means of assessing more complex learning not possible with selected-response items. The teacher may decide to allow students to respond to these items outside of class. Sample items include:

- Select an article describing a nursing research study. Critique the study, specifying the criteria used. Based on your evaluation, describe how the research findings could be used in clinical practice.
- The fall rate on your unit has increased in the last 3 months. Develop a plan for analyzing this occurrence with a rationale to support your action plan.
- Develop a plan for saving costs in the wound clinic.
- You receive a call in the allergy clinic from a mother who describes her son's problems as "having stomach pains" and "acting out in school." She asks you if these problems may be due to his allergies. How would you respond to this mother? How would you manage this call? Include a rationale for your response.
- You are caring for a child diagnosed recently with acute lymphocytic leukemia who lives with his parents and two teenage sisters. Describe how the family health-and-illness cycle would provide a framework for assessing this family and planning for the child's care.

Writing Essay Items

Essay items should be reserved for learning outcomes that cannot be assessed effectively through multiple-choice and other selected-response formats. With essays, students can demonstrate their higher level thinking, ability to integrate varied sources of information, and creativity. Suggestions for writing essay items follow.

1. *Develop essay items that require synthesis of the content.* Avoid items that students can answer by merely summarizing the readings and class discussions without thinking about the content and applying it to new situations. Assessing students' recall of facts and specific information may be accomplished more easily using other formats such as true-false and matching rather than essay.

2. *Phrase items clearly.* The item should direct learners in their responses and should not be ambiguous. Exhibit 6.1 provides sample stems for essay items based on varied types of learning outcomes. Framing the item to make it as specific as possible is accomplished more easily with restricted-response items. With extended-response items, the teacher may provide directions as to the type of response intended without limiting the student's own thinking about the answer. In the example that follows, there is minimal guidance as to how to respond; the revised version, however, directs students more clearly as to the intended response without limiting their freedom of expression and originality.

Example: Evaluate an article describing a nursing research study.

Revised Version: Select an article describing a nursing research study. Critique the study, specifying the criteria you used to evaluate it. Based on your evaluation, describe whether the research provides evidence for nursing practice and the strength of the evidence. Include a rationale supporting your decision.

3. *Prepare students for essay tests.* This can be accomplished by asking thought-provoking questions in class; engaging students in critical discussions about the content; and teaching students how to apply concepts and theories to clinical situations, compare approaches, and arrive at decisions and judgments about patients and issues. Practice in synthesizing content from different sources, presenting ideas logically, and using creativity in responding to situations will help students prepare to respond to essay items in a testing situation. This practice may come through discussions in class, in clinical practice, and online; written assignments; and small-group activities. For students lacking experience with essay tests, the teacher may use sample items for formative purposes, providing feedback to students about the adequacy of their responses.

❑Exhibit 6.1

Sample Stems for Essay Items

Comparing
Compare the side effects of...methods for...interventions for....
Describe similarities and differences between....
What do...have in common?
Group these medications...signs and symptoms....

Outlining Steps
Describe the process for...procedure for...protocol to follow for....
List steps in order for....

Explaining and Summarizing
Explain the importance of...relevance of....
Identify and discuss....
Explain the patient's responses within the framework of....
Provide a rationale for....
Discuss the most significant points of....
Summarize the relevant data.
What are the major causes of...reasons for...problems associated with...
Describe the potential effects of...possible responses to...problems that might result from....

Applying Concepts and Theories to a Situation
Analyze the situation using...theory/framework.
Using the theory of..., explain the patient's/family's responses.
Identify and discuss...using relevant concepts and theories.
Discuss actions to take in this situation using this theoretical basis.
Describe a situation that demonstrates the concept of...principle of...theory of....

Analyzing
Discuss the significance of....
Identify relevant data with supporting rationale.
Identify and describe additional data needed for decision making.
Describe possible patient problems with rationale.
What hypotheses may be formed?
Compare nursing interventions based on research findings and other evidence.
Describe multiple nursing interventions for this patient with supporting rationale.
Provide a rationale for...
Critique the nurse's responses to this patient.
Describe errors in assumptions made about...errors in reasoning....
Analyze the situation and describe alternate actions possible.
Identify all possible decisions, consequences of each, your decision, and supporting rationale.

Developing Plans and Proposals
Develop a plan for...discharge plan...teaching plan...
Develop a proposal for...protocol for...
Based on the theory of..., develop a plan for...proposal for...

Exhibit 6.1 *(continued)*

Develop a new approach for...method for...
Design multiple interventions for...

Analyzing Trends and Issues
Identify one significant trend/issue in health care and describe implications for nursing practice.
Analyze this issue and implications for...
In light of these trends, what changes would you propose?
Critique the nurse's/physician's/patient's decisions in this situation. What other approaches are possible? Why?
Analyze the ethical issue facing the nurse. Compare multiple decisions possible and consequences of each. Describe the decision you would make and why.
Identify issues for this patient/family/community and strategies for resolving them.

Stating Positions
What would you do and why?
Identify your position about...and defend it.
Develop an argument for...and against...
Develop a rationale for...
Do you support this position? Why or why not?
Do you agree or disagree with...? Include a rationale.
Specify the alternative actions possible. Which of these alternatives would be most appropriate and why? What would you do and why?

---

4. *Tell students about apportioning their time to allow sufficient time for answering each essay item.* In writing a series of essay items, consider carefully the time needed for students to answer them and inform students of the estimated time before they begin the examination. In this way students may gauge their time appropriately. Indicating the point value of each essay item also will guide students to use their time appropriately, spending more time on and writing longer responses to items that carry greater weight.

5. *Score essay items that deal with the analysis of issues according to the rationale that students develop rather than the position they take on the issue.* Students should provide a sound rationale for their position, and the evaluation should focus on the rationale rather than on the actual position.

6. *Avoid the use of optional items and student choice of items to answer.* As indicated previously, this results in different subsets of tests that may not be comparable.

7. *In the process of developing the item, write an ideal answer to it.* The teacher should do this while drafting the item to determine if it is appropriate, clearly stated, and reasonable to answer in the allotted time frame. Save this ideal answer for use later in scoring students' responses.

8. *If possible, have a colleague review the item and explain how he or she would respond to it.* Colleagues can assess the clarity of the item and whether it will elicit the intended response.

Scoring Essay Items: Holistic Versus Analytic

There are two methods of scoring essay items: holistic and analytic. The holistic method involves reading the entire answer to each item and evaluating its overall quality. With the analytic method of scoring, the teacher separately scores individual components of the answer.

Holistic Scoring

With holistic scoring, the teacher assesses and scores the essay response as a whole without judging each part separately. There are different ways of scoring essays using the holistic method.

Relative Scoring. One method of holistic scoring is to compare each student's answer with the responses of others in the group, using a relative standard. To score essay items using this system, the teacher quickly reads the answers to each item to gain a sense of how the students responded overall, then re-reads the answers and scores them. Papers may be placed in a number of piles reflecting degrees of quality with each pile of papers receiving a particular score or grade.

Model Answer. Another way is to develop a model answer for each item and then compare each student's response to that model. The model answer does not have to be written in narrative form, but can be an outline with the key points and elements that should be in the answer. Before using a model answer for scoring responses, teachers should read a few papers to confirm that students' answers are consistent with what was intended.

Holistic Scoring Rubric. A third way of implementing holistic scoring is to use a scoring rubric, which is a guide for scoring essays, papers, written assignments, and other open-ended responses of students. Rubrics also can be used for grading posters, concept maps, presentations, and projects competed by students. The rubric consists of criteria used for evaluating the quality of the student's response. With holistic scoring, the rubric includes different levels of responses, with characteristics or descriptions of each level, and the related score. The student's answer is assigned the score associated with the one description within the rubric that best reflects its quality and thus its score. The important concept in this method is that holistic scoring yields one overall score that considers the entire response to the item rather than scoring its component parts separately (Nitko & Brookhart, 2011; Popham, 2012).

Holistic rubrics are quicker to use for scoring because the teacher evaluates the overall response rather than each part of it. One disadvantage, though, is that they do not provide students with specific feedback about their answers. An example of a holistic scoring rubric for an essay item is given in Table 6.1.

Analytic Scoring

In the analytic method of scoring, the teacher identifies the content that should be included in the answer and other characteristics of an ideal response. Each of these areas is assessed and scored separately. With analytic scoring the teacher focuses on one characteristic of the response at a time (Miller et al., 2009). Often a detailed scoring plan is used that lists content to be included in the answer and other characteristics of the response to be judged. Students earn points based on how well they address each content area and the other characteristics, not their overall response.

Analytic Scoring Rubric. A scoring rubric also can be developed with points assigned for each of the content areas that should be included in

▢Table 6.1

EXAMPLE OF HOLISTIC SCORING RUBRIC FOR ESSAY ITEM ON HEALTH CARE ISSUE

SCORE	DESCRIPTION
4	Presents thorough analysis of health care issue considering its complexities. Considers multiple perspectives in analysis. Analysis reflects use of theories and research. Discussion is well organized and supports analysis.
3	Analyzes health care issue. Considers different perspectives in analysis. Analysis reflects use of theories but not research. Discussion is organized and logical.
2	Describes health care issue but does not consider its complexities or different perspectives. Basic analysis of issue with limited use of theory. Discussion accurate but limited.
1	Does not clearly describe health care issue. No alternate perspectives considered. Limited analysis with no relevant theory or literature to support ideas. Errors in answer.
0	Does not identify the health care issue. No application of theory to understand issue. Errors in answer. Off-topic.

the response and other characteristics to be evaluated. An analytic scoring rubric is useful in assessing essays and written work. First, it guides the teacher in judging the extent to which specified criteria have been met. Second, because an analytic scoring rubric provides a clear framework and scoring guide for evaluating the quality of an essay and other written assignments, it removes some of the bias that often occurs with evaluating student assignments (Shipman, Roa, Hootan, & Wang, 2012). Third, a rubric creates a standardized method for grading assignments, which is valuable when there are different faculty members in a course each grading their own students' work. Lastly, it provides feedback to students about the strengths and weaknesses of their response (Miller et al., 2009). An example of an analytic scoring rubric for the same essay item is found in Table 6.2.

⬜Table 6.2

EXAMPLE OF ANALYTIC SCORING RUBRIC FOR ESSAY ITEM ON HEALTH CARE ISSUE

SCORE	ANALYSIS OF ISSUE	MULTIPLE PERSPECTIVES	THEORY AND RESEARCH	PRESENTATION
4	Presents thorough analysis of health care issue considering its complexities	Considers multiple perspectives in analysis	Uses theories and research as basis for analysis	Discussion well organized and supports analysis.
3	Analyzes health care issue	Considers a few varying perspectives	Uses theories in analysis but no research	Discussion organized and logical
2	Describes health care issue but does not consider its complexities	Describes one perspective without considering other points of view	Reports basic analysis of issue with limited use of theory	Discussion accurate but limited
1	Does not clearly describe health care issue	Considers no alternate perspectives	Presents limited analysis with no relevant theories or literature to support ideas	Discussion has errors in content
0	Does not identify health care issue	Considers no alternate perspectives	Does not apply any theories in discussion	Discussion has errors in content. May be off-topic

Score _____

CRITERIA FOR ASSESSING ESSAY ITEMS

The criteria for assessing essay items, regardless of the method, often address three areas: (a) content, (b) organization, and (c) process. Questions that guide assessment of each of these areas are:

- *Content*: Is relevant content included? Is it accurate? Are significant concepts and theories presented? Are hypotheses, conclusions, and decisions supported? Is the answer comprehensive?
- *Organization*: Is the answer well organized? Are the ideas presented clearly? Is there a logical sequence of ideas?
- *Process*: Was the process used to arrive at conclusions, actions, approaches, and decisions logical? Were different possibilities and implications considered? Was a sound rationale developed using relevant literature and theories?

Suggestions for Scoring

1. *Identify the method of scoring to be used prior to the testing situation* and inform the students of it.
2. *Specify in advance an ideal answer.* In constructing this ideal answer, review readings, the content presented in class and online, and other instructional activities completed by students. Identify content and characteristics required in the answer and assign points to them if using the analytic method of scoring.
3. *If using a scoring rubric, discuss it with the students ahead of time* so that they are aware of how their essay responses will be judged.
4. *Read a random sample of papers* to get a sense of how the students approached the items and an idea of the overall quality of the answers.
5. *Score the answers to one item at a time.* For example, read and score all of the students' answers to the first item before proceeding to the second item. This procedure enables the teacher to compare responses to an item across students, resulting in more accurate and fairer scoring, and saves time by only needing to keep in mind one ideal answer at a time (Miller et al., 2009).
6. *Read each answer twice before scoring.* In the first reading, note omissions of major points from the ideal answer, errors in content, problems with organization, and problems with the process used for responding. Make notes about omissions, errors, and problems and record other comments on the students' paper in a format that can be modified if needed after reading the response a second time.

After reading through all the answers to the question, begin the second reading for scoring purposes.

7. *Read papers in random order.*
8. *Use the same scoring system for all papers.*
9. *Read essay answers and other written assignments anonymously.* Develop a system for implementing this in the nursing education program, for instance, by asking the students to choose a code number.
10. *Cover the scores of the previous answers* to avoid being biased about the student's ability.
11. *For important decisions or if unsure about the evaluation, have a colleague read and score the answers* to improve reliability. A sample of answers might be independently scored rather than the complete set of student tests.
12. *Adopt a policy on writing* (sentence structure, spelling, punctuation, grammar, neatness, and writing style in general) and determine whether the quality of the writing will be part of the test score. Inform students of the policy in advance of the test. If writing is assessed, then it should be scored separately, and the teacher should be cautious not to let the writing style bias the evaluation of content and other characteristics of the response.

SUMMARY

Short-answer items can be answered by a word, phrase, or number. There are two types of short-answer items: question and completion, also referred to as fill-in-the-blank. These items are appropriate for recall of facts and specific information. With short-answer items, students can be asked to interpret data, use formulas, complete calculations, and solve mathematical-type problems.

In an essay test, students construct responses to items based on their understanding of the content. With this type of test item, varied answers may be possible depending on the concepts selected by the student for discussion and the way in which they are presented. Essay items provide an opportunity for students to select content to discuss, integrate concepts from various sources, present ideas in their own words, and develop original and creative responses to items. This freedom of response makes essay items particularly useful for complex learning outcomes.

There are two types of essay items: restricted response and extended response. In a restricted-response item, the teacher limits the student's answer by indicating the content to be discussed and frequently the amount of discussion allowed, for instance, limiting the response to one paragraph or page. In an extended-response item, students have complete freedom of response, often requiring extensive writing. Although essay items use writing as the medium for expression, the intent is to assess student understanding of specific content rather than judge the writing ability in and of itself. Other types of assignments are better suited to assessing the ability of students to write effectively.

REFERENCES

Barnett, J. E., & Francis, A. L. (2012). Using higher order thinking questions to foster critical thinking: A classroom study. *Educational Psychology, 32,* 201–211.

Educational Testing Service. (2012). *How the e-rate® engine works.* Retrieved from http://www.ets.org/erater/how

Miller, M. D., Linn, R. L., & Gronlund, N. E. (2009). *Measurement and assessment in teaching* (10th ed.). Upper Saddle River, NJ: Prentice Hall.

National Council of State Boards of Nursing. (2012). *Alternate item formats frequently asked questions.* Retrieved from https://www.ncsbn.org/2334.htm#What_is_an_alternate_item_format

Nitko, A. J., & Brookhart, S. M. (2011). *Educational assessment of students* (6th ed.). Upper Saddle River, NJ: Pearson Education.

Popham, W. J. (2012). *The role of rubrics in testing and teaching* (2nd ed.). Upper Saddle River, NJ: Pearson Education.

Shipman, D., Roa, M., Hooten, J., & Wang, Z. J. (2012). Using the analytic rubric as an evaluation tool in nursing education: The positive and the negative. *Nurse Education Today, 32,* 246–249.

Waugh, C. K., & Gronlund, N. E. (2013). *Assessment of student achievement* (10th ed.). Upper Saddle River, NJ: Pearson Education.

SEVEN

Assessment of Higher

Level Learning

In preparing students to meet the needs of patients within the changing health care system, educators are faced with identifying essential content to teach in the nursing program. Mastery of this knowledge alone, however, is not enough. Students also need to develop cognitive skills for processing and analyzing information, comparing different approaches, weighing alternatives, and arriving at sound conclusions and decisions. These cognitive skills include, among others, the ability to apply concepts and theories to new situations, problem solving, critical thinking, and clinical judgment. The purpose of this chapter is to present methods for assessing these higher levels of learning in nursing.

HIGHER LEVEL LEARNING

One of the concepts presented in Chapter 1 was that learning outcomes can be organized in a cognitive hierarchy or taxonomy, with each level representing more complex learning than the previous one. Learning extends from simple recall and comprehension, which are lower level cognitive behaviors, to higher level thinking skills. Higher level cognitive skills include application, analysis, synthesis, and evaluation. With higher level thinking, students apply concepts, theories, and other forms of knowledge to new situations, use that knowledge to interpret patient needs and identify patient and other types of problems, and arrive at decisions about actions to take.

The main principle in assessing higher level learning is to develop test items and other assessment methods that require students to apply knowledge and skills in a *new* situation (Nitko & Brookhart, 2011). Only then can the teacher assess whether the students are able to use what they have learned in a different context. Considering that patients and treatments often do not match the textbook descriptions, and health status can change quickly, students need to develop their ability to think through clinical situations and arrive at the best possible decisions. By introducing novel materials into the evaluation process, the teacher can assess whether the students have developed these cognitive skills.

PROBLEM SOLVING

In the practice setting, students are continually faced with patient problems and other problems to be solved. Some of these problems relate to managing patient conditions and deciding what actions to take, whereas others involve problems associated with the nurse's role and work environment. The ability to solve patient and setting-related problems is an essential skill to be developed and evaluated. Problem solving begins with recognizing and defining the problem, gathering data to clarify it further, developing solutions, and evaluating their effectiveness. Knowledge about the problem and potential solutions influences the problem-solving process. Students faced with patient problems for which they lack understanding and a relevant knowledge base will be impeded in their thinking. This is an important point in both teaching and assessing problem solving. When students have an understanding of the problem and possible solutions, they can apply this knowledge and expertise to new situations they encounter in the clinical setting.

Past experience with similar problems, either real problems in the clinical setting or hypothetical ones used in teaching, also influences students' skill in problem solving. Experience with similar problems gives the student a perspective on what to expect in the clinical situation—typical problems the patient may experience and approaches that are usually effective for those problems. Expert nurses and beginners, such as students, approach patient problems differently (Benner, 2001). As a result of their extensive clinical experience, experts view the clinical situation as a whole and use their past experience with similar patients as a framework for approaching new problems.

Well-Structured and Ill-Structured Problems

Nitko and Brookhart (2011) defined two types of problems that students may be asked to solve: well structured and ill structured. Well-structured problems provide the information needed for problem solving; typically, they have one correct solution rather than multiple ones to consider and in general are "clearly laid out" (p. 231). These are problems and solutions that the teacher may have presented in class and then asked students about in an assessment. Well-structured problems provide practice in applying concepts and theories learned in class to hypothetical situations but do not require extensive thinking skills.

In contrast, ill-structured problems reflect real-life problems and clinical situations faced by students. Ill-structured problems are authentic (Nitko & Brookhart, 2011). With these situations, the problem may not be clear to the learner, the data may suggest a variety of problems, or there may be an incomplete data set to determine the problem. Along similar lines, the student may identify the problem but be unsure of the approaches to take; multiple solutions may also be possible. Some assessment methods for problem solving address well-structured problems, assessing understanding of typical problems and solutions. Other methods assess students' ability to analyze situations to interpret patient needs and concerns, identify possible problems given the data, identify additional data needed, compare and evaluate multiple approaches, and arrive at an informed decision as to actions to take (or not) in the situation.

Decision Making

Nurses continually make decisions about patient care—decisions about problems, solutions, other approaches that might be possible, and the best approach to use in a particular situation. Other decisions are needed for delivering care, managing the clinical environment, and carrying out other activities.

In decision making, the learner arrives at a decision after considering a number of alternatives and weighing the consequences of each. The decision reflects a choice made after considering these different possibilities. In making this choice, the student collects and analyzes information relevant to identifying the problem and making a decision, compares the decisions possible in that situation, and then decides on the best strategy or approach to use. Critical thinking helps students compare alternatives and decide what actions to take.

CRITICAL THINKING

There has been extensive literature in nursing over the last two decades about the importance of students developing the ability to think critically. The complexity of patient, family, and community needs; the amount of information the nurse needs to process in the practice setting; the types of clinical judgments required for care and supervising others in the delivery of care; and multiple ethical issues faced by the nurse require the ability to think critically. Critical thinking is reflective and reasoned thinking; by using critical thinking, the nurse decides what to do or believe in a given situation. Critical thinking is particularly important when problems are unclear and have more than one possible solution. In nursing there have been varied definitions of critical thinking over the years, and the nursing profession has not fully embraced a definition of critical thinking (Lasater, 2011). Nevertheless, an understanding of the concepts underlying critical thinking can guide the nurse educator in developing assessment strategies.

There are eight elements of reasoning to be considered in the process of critical thinking:

1. Purpose the thinking is to serve
2. Questions to be answered
3. Assumptions on which thinking is based
4. Analysis of one's own point of view and those of others
5. Data, information, and evidence on which to base reasoning
6. Key concepts and theories for use in thinking
7. Inferences and conclusions possible given the data
8. Implications and consequences of reasoning (Elder & Paul, 2010)

These elements of reasoning may be used as a framework for assessing students' thinking in nursing. Sample questions the teacher can use for assessing students' critical thinking are presented in Exhibit 7.1.

In the clinical setting, critical thinking enables the student to arrive at sound judgments about patient care. Carrying out assessment; planning care; intervening with patients, families, and communities; and evaluating the effectiveness of interventions—all these require critical thinking. In the assessment process, important cognitive skills include differentiating relevant from irrelevant data, identifying cues in the data, identifying additional data to collect prior to deciding on the problem, and specifying patient needs and problems based on these data.

Critical thinking also is reflected in the ability to compare possible interventions, considering the evidence, to arrive at a decision on the best approaches to use in a particular situation (Alfaro-LeFevre, 2013; Facione, 2011). Judgments about the quality and effectiveness of care are influenced by the learner's thinking skills. Facione and Facione (2008) indicated that even expert clinicians are never beyond the need to reflect on their clinical reasoning and to continue to build their critical thinking skills. Critical thinking is essential for all nurses to recognize emerging clinical patterns and know when and how to intervene (Berkow, Virkstis,

☐Exhibit 7.1

Sample Questions for Assessing Critical Thinking

Purpose of Thinking

Is the student's purpose (e.g., in a discussion, a research paper, an essay, a written assignment, and so forth) clear?
Can the student state the goals to be achieved as a result of the thinking?
Does the student use this purpose and these goals to stay focused?
Are the student's goals realistic and attainable?

Issue or Problem to Be Resolved

Does the student clarify the issue or problem to be resolved?
How does the student go about analyzing the issue or problem?
Does the student ask probing questions and focus on important issues and problems?
Are the questions relevant to resolving the issue or problem and unbiased?
Does the student recognize questions she or he is unable to answer and seek information independently for answering them?

Assumptions on Which Thinking Is Based

Does the student make assumptions that are clear? Reasonable? Consistent with one another?
Does the student question assumptions underlying her/his own thinking?

Analysis of Own Point of View and Those of Others

Does the student keep in mind different points of view?
Does the student realize that people approach situations, questions, issues, and problems differently?
Does the student consider multiple perspectives?
Does the student have a broad point of view about issues and problems rather than a narrow perspective?
Is the student able to recognize his or her own biases, values, and beliefs that influence thinking?
Does the student actively seek others' points of view?

Information and Evidence on Which to Base Reasoning

Does the student collect relevant data and evidence on which to base thinking?
Does the student search for information for and against his/her own position and critically analyze both sets of data?
Can the student differentiate relevant and irrelevant information for the question, issue, or problem at hand?
Does the student avoid drawing conclusions beyond the information and evidence available to support them?
Does the student present clear and accurate data and evidence on which his or her own thinking is based?

Concepts and Theories for Use in Thinking

Does the student apply relevant concepts and theories for understanding and analyzing the question, issue, or problem?

(continued)

Exhibit 7.1 *(continued)*

Is the student unbiased in presentation of ideas and thinking?
Does the student recognize implications of words used in presenting ideas?

Inferences and Conclusions

Does the student make clear and precise inferences?
Does the student clarify conclusions and make the reasoning easy to follow?
Does the student draw conclusions based on the evidence and reasons presented?
Are the conclusions consistent with one another?

Implications and Consequences of Reasoning

Does the student identify a number of significant implications of his/her own thinking?
Does the student identify different courses of action and consequences of each?
Does the student consider both positive and negative consequences?

Adapted from R. Paul & L. Elder (2011). *Using intellectual standards to assess student reasoning. Foundation for critical thinking.* Retrieved from http://www.criticalthinking.org/pages/using-intellectual-standards-to-assess-student-reasoning/602. Adapted with permission of the Foundation for Critical Thinking, 2012.

Stewart, Aronson, & Donohue, 2011). Students who demonstrate critical thinking ability:

- ask questions, are inquisitive, and willing to search for answers
- consider alternate ways of viewing information
- offer different perspectives to problems and solutions
- question current practices and express their own ideas about care
- extend their thinking beyond the readings, course and clinical activities, and other requirements
- are open-minded

These characteristics are important because they suggest behaviors that are to be developed by students as they progress through the nursing program. They also provide a framework for faculty to use when assessing whether students have developed their critical thinking abilities.

CLINICAL JUDGMENT

Tanner (2006) views clinical judgment as an interpretation of the patient's needs and problems, and decisions on actions to take, or not take, based on the patient's responses. The clinical judgment process includes four aspects: (1) noticing, (2) interpreting, (3) responding, and (4) reflecting. Tanner's model and research by Lasater (2011), which builds on this model, provide a framework for assessing students' thinking in a clinical situation or scenario. Students can be asked to describe what they would expect to find in situation, what they noticed first, and other data they need (noticing). To assess students' ability to interpret a situation, the teacher can ask them to explain specific data and what they mean, and their priorities of care (interpreting). Another series of questions can explore interventions for the patient, why students would select those interventions or not take any actions, and their rationale (responding). The teacher can ask students to reflect on their experiences with patients and discuss what they would do differently next time (reflecting). Lasater suggested that reflections written by students after their clinical experiences encourage them to think about those experiences and learn from them.

CONTEXT-DEPENDENT ITEM SETS

In assessing students' cognitive skills, the test items and other methods need to meet two criteria. They should (a) introduce *new* information not encountered by students at an earlier point in the instruction and (b) provide data on the thought process used by students to arrive at an answer, rather than the answer alone. Context-dependent item sets may be used for this purpose.

Writing Context-Dependent Item Sets

A basic principle of assessing higher level skills is that the test item or other assessment method has to introduce new or novel material for analysis. Without the introduction of new material as part of the assessment, students may rely on memorization from prior discussion or their readings about how to problem solve and arrive at decisions for the situation at hand; they may simply recall the typical problems and solutions without thinking through other possibilities themselves. In nursing education this principle is often implemented through clinical scenarios that present a novel situation for students to analyze. Nitko and Brookhart (2011) referred to these items as context-dependent item sets or interpretive exercises.

In a context-dependent item set, the teacher presents introductory material that students then analyze and answer questions about. The introductory material may be a description of a clinical situation, patient data, research findings, issues associated with clinical practice, and varied types of scenarios. The introductory material also may include diagrams, photographs, tables, figures, and excerpts from reading materials. Students read, analyze, and interpret the introductory material and then answer questions about it or complete other tasks. One advantage of a context-dependent item set is the opportunity to present new information for student analysis that is geared toward clinical practice. In addition, the introductory material provides the same context for analysis for all students.

The questions asked about the introductory material may be selected- or constructed-response items. With selected-response items such as multiple-choice, however, the teacher is not able to assess the underlying thought process used by students in arriving at the answer; their responses reflect instead the outcomes of their thinking. If the intent is also to assess the thinking process used by students, then open-ended items such as short-answer and essay should be used.

Interpretive Items on the NCLEX®

On the NCLEX, candidates may be asked to interpret tables, charts, graphics, and images, which may include multimedia, and to respond to questions about them using the standard multiple-choice format or alternate item formats (National Council of State Boards of Nursing, 2010). Alternate formats include multiple-response, fill-in-the-blank, hot-spot, chart/exhibit, and ordered response items. Multiple-response items were presented in Chapter 5 and fill-in-the-blank and ordered response were discussed in Chapter 6. In a hot-spot item, candidates are asked a question about an image; they answer the question by clicking on the image with their mouse. In chart/exhibit items, candidates are given a problem, and to answer that problem, they need to read and interpret information in a chart or an exhibit. Examples of hot-spot and chart/exhibit items are included later in the chapter in Exhibit 7.3.

Students should have experience answering these types of questions and other forms of context-dependent items as they progress through a nursing program. Items can be incorporated into quizzes and tests; can be developed for small-group analysis and discussion in class, as out-of-class assignments, and as online activities; and can be analyzed and discussed by students in postclinical conferences.

Layout

The layout of the context-dependent item set, that is, the way it is arranged on the page, is important so that it is clear to the students which questions relate to the introductory material. Exhibit 7.2 illustrates one way of arranging the material and related items on a page.

A heading should be used to indicate the items that pertain to the introductory material, for example, "Questions 1 through 3 refer to the scenario below." Nitko and Brookhart (2011) suggested that the material for interpretation be placed in the center of the page so that it is readily apparent to the students. If possible, the context and all items pertaining to it should be placed on the same page.

Strategies for Writing Context-Dependent Items

Suggestions follow for writing context-dependent item sets. The examples in this chapter are designed for paper-and-pencil testing; however, the scenarios and other types of introductory material for analysis may be presented through multimedia and other types of instructional technology.

If the intent is to assess students' skills in problem solving and critical thinking, the introductory material needs to provide sufficient information for analysis without directing the students' thinking in a particular direction. The first step is to draft the types of questions to be asked about the situation, then to develop a scenario to provide essential information for analysis. If the scenario is designed on the basis of clinical practice, students may be asked to analyze data, interpret the scenario, identify patient problems, decide on nursing interventions, evaluate outcomes of care, and examine ethical issues, among other tasks. The case method, discussed later in this chapter, uses a short clinical scenario followed by one or more open-ended questions.

The introductory material should be geared to the students' level of understanding and experience. The teacher should check the terminology used, particularly with beginning students. The situation should be of reasonable length without extending the students' reading time unnecessarily.

The questions should focus on the underlying thought process used to arrive at an answer, not on the answer alone. In some situations, however, the goal may be to assess students' ability to apply principles or procedures learned in class without any original thinking about them. In these instances, well-structured problems with one correct answer and situations that are clearly laid out for students are appropriate.

The teacher also should specify how the responses will be scored, if the responses are restricted in some way, such as by page length, and the criteria used for evaluation. Context-dependent items may be incorporated within a test, completed individually or in small groups for formative

☐Exhibit 7.2

Layout of Context-Dependent Item Sets

Questions 1 through 3 relate to the scenario below.

Scenario (and other types of introductory material) here

1. Item 1 here

2. Item 2 here

3. Item 3 here

evaluation, discussed in class for instructional purposes, completed during postclinical conferences, or done as out-of-class assignments, either graded or ungraded. If group work is evaluated for summative purposes, students should have an opportunity to evaluate each other's participation. In Chapter 14, a sample form (Exhibit 14.11) is provided for this purpose.

Item sets focusing on assessment of problem-solving ability may ask students to complete the following tasks:

- Identify the problem and alternate problems possible
- Develop questions for clarifying the problem further
- Identify assumptions made about the problem and solutions
- Identify additional data needed for interpreting the situation
- Differentiate relevant and irrelevant information in the situation
- Propose solutions, possible alternatives, advantages and disadvantages of each, and their choices
- Identify obstacles to solving a problem
- Relate information from different sources to the problem to be solved
- Evaluate the effectiveness of solutions and approaches to solving problems and the outcomes achieved

The following item set assesses students' skill in problem solving. After reading the introductory situation about the patient, students are asked to identify *all possible* problems and provide data to support them. Other questions ask students about additional data to be collected, again with a rationale for their answer

> Your 8-year-old patient had a closed head injury 4 weeks ago after falling off his bike. You visit him at home and find that he has weakness of his left leg. His mother reports that he is "getting his rest" and "sleeping a lot." The patient seems irritable during your visit. When you ask him how he is feeling, he tells you, "My head hurts where I hit it." The mother appears anxious, talking rapidly and changing position frequently.

> 1. List all possible problems in this situation. For each problem describe supporting assessment data.
> 2. What additional data are needed, if any, to decide on these problems? Provide a rationale for collecting this information.
> 3. What other assessment data would you collect at this time? Why is this information important to your decision making?

Context-dependent items may focus on actions to be taken in a situation. For this purpose, the teacher should briefly describe a critical event, then ask learners what they would do next. Because the rationale underlying the thinking is as important if not more important than the decision or outcome, students should also include an explanation of the thought process they used in their decision making. For example:

> You are a new employee in a long term care setting. At mealtime you find the patients sitting in chairs with their arms tied to the sides of the chair.
>
> 1. What would you do? Why did you choose this action?
> 2. Develop a quality improvement project for reducing the use of restraints in this setting.

If the goal is to assess students' ability to think through different decisions possible in a situation, two approaches may be used with the item set. The introductory material (a) may present a situation up to the point of a decision, then ask students to make a decision or (b) may describe a situation and decision and ask whether they agree or disagree with it. For both of these approaches, the students need to provide a rationale for their responses. Examples of these strategies follow.

> Your nurse manager on a busy surgery unit asks you to cover for her while she attends a meeting. You find out later that she left the hospital to run an errand instead of attending the meeting.
>
> 1. Identify three possible actions you could take in this situation.
> 2. Describe the possible consequences of each course of action.
> 3. What decision would you make? Why?

> A patient calls the office to see if he can receive his flu shot today. He had a cold a few days ago but is feeling better and has returned to work. The nurse instructs the patient to come in for his flu shot.
>
> 1. Do you agree or disagree with the nurse's decision?
> 2. Why or why not?

Often context-dependent item sets are developed around clinical scenarios. However, they also are valuable techniques to assess student ability to analyze issues and describe how they would resolve them, articulate different points of view and the reasoning underlying each one, evaluate evidence used to support a particular position, and draw inferences and conclusions that follow from the evidence. Students can be given articles and other material to read and analyze, presented with graphs and tables for interpretation, and given images and diagrams with questions to answer. Context-dependent items provide a way for teachers to examine how well students use information and think through situations. Examples of context-dependent item sets are found in Exhibit 7.3.

☐Exhibit 7.3

Sample Context-Dependent Item Sets and Hot-Spot and Chart/Exhibit Items

Examples of Context-Dependent Item Sets

Questions 1 to 4 relate to the situation below.

A 36-year-old patient scheduled for a breast biopsy has been crying on and off for the last 3 hours during her diagnostic testing. When the nurse attempts to talk to the woman about her feelings, the patient says, "Everything is fine. I'm just tired."

1. What is the patient experiencing in this situation?
2. What assumptions about the patient did you make?
3. What additional information would you collect from the patient and her health records before intervening?
4. Why is this information important?

Questions 1 and 2 relate to the situation below.

You are unsure about a medication for one of your patients. When you call the pharmacy to learn more about the drug, you discover that the amount ordered is twice the acceptable dose. You contact the attending physician who tells you to "give it because your patient needs that high a dose."

1. What are your different options at this time? Describe advantages and disadvantages of each.
2. How would you solve this dilemma?

Questions 1 to 3 relate to the situation below.

Your ventilated patient has his bed elevated 45°. He is being turned, but you notice he is developing a pressure ulcer. Another nurse tells you to lower the head of the bed.

1. Do you agree with that decision? Why or why not?
2. What would you do?
3. What evidence supports your decision?

Items 1 to 4 relate to the scenario below.

A 1-month-old girl is brought to the pediatrician's office for a well-baby checkup. You notice that she has not gained much weight over the last month. Her mother explains that the baby is "colicky" and "spits up a lot of her feeding." There is no evidence of projectile vomiting and other GI symptoms. The baby has a macular-type rash on her stomach, her temperature is normal, and she appears well-hydrated.

1. Describe possible problems this baby may be experiencing. What additional data would you collect next? Why?
2. What would you do in this situation? What evidence supports those interventions?
3. Specify outcomes for evaluating the effectiveness of the interventions you selected.

Exhibit 7.3 *(continued)*

4. What information presented in this situation is irrelevant to your decision making? Why?

Questions 1 and 2 relate to the scenario below.

A patient is seen in the clinic for a severe headache, nausea, and vomiting, which has lasted for 3 days. In the last hour the patient's headache has become progressively worse, and she is losing vision in her right eye.

1. What data are most important and why?
2. What are your next steps?

The following items are based on the readings you completed in preparation for this test.

Reading A: Smith et al. Effects of nurse practitioners in family-centered medical homes

Reading B: Jones et al. Using nurse practitioners in hospital-to-home transitional programs

1. From these readings, draw two conclusions supported by both studies.
2. What are differences between the model presented in Reading A and the one presented in B? Which model was most effective in improving quality of care and reducing costs? Provide a rationale.

Use this table to answer the question.

| | MEN | | WOMEN | | |
IMPORTANCE RATINGS	M	(*SD*)	M	(*SD*)	*t*
Able to call RN with questions	4.23	(.93)	4.92	(.95)	2.76[a]
Have RN teach illness, medications, treatment options	4.47	(.79)	4.40	(.90)	.568
Have RN teach health promotion	4.35	(.90)	4.00	(1.1)	2.51[a]

[a]$p < .01$.

Based on the data presented in the table, which of the following conclusions is accurate?

1. Health-promoting activities were more important to men than to women.*
2. It was more important to men to be able to call a registered nurse with questions after a visit.
3. Men valued teaching by the registered nurse more than women.
4. Teaching about health was more important to women than men.

(continued)

---

*Correct answer.

Exhibit 7.3 *(continued)*

Read the short paragraph below and analyze the credibility of this statement. Respond to items 1 and 2.

The board of directors of a nursing organization in which you are actively involved announced at the annual meeting that membership had increased 30% over the last year. The board reported that this increase was the direct result of the continuing education programs offered to nurses.

1. Analyze the credibility of this statement. Indicate which parts are credible and which are not, including your reasons.

   Credible Parts of Statement   Reasons Why Credible

   _____

   _____

   _____

2. What additional data would you obtain to understand the reasons for the membership increase?

Examples of Hot-Spot Items

On the electrocardiogram shown below, mark the area of the ST segment.

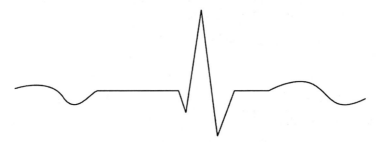

Your patient has an aortic sterosis. Mark the spot where you would place the stethoscope to best hear the murmur.

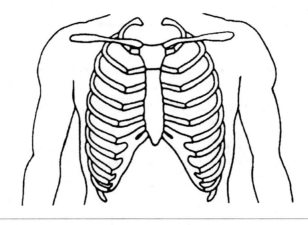

Exhibit 7.3 *(continued)*

Click on the area that represents the beginning of the contraction.

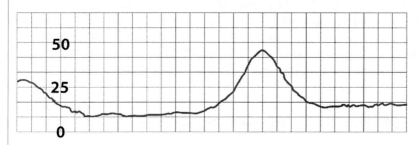

Example of Chart/Exhibit Item

You are caring for a 2-day postpartum patient with a history of lupus. She had an emergency cesarean delivery at 36 weeks gestation and during the delivery began to bleed, leading to hypovolemic shock. She received blood and fluid replacements. In morning report you are told that the patient is stable but drowsy. You check the flow sheet below.

VITAL SIGNS

DATE	TIME	TEMP	PULSE	RESP	B/P
2/1	0600				
	1000	99.4	80	28	102/52
	1400				
	1800		88		
	2200				
	0200				
2/2	0600	99.8	88	30	124/60
	1000				
	1400		100	30	
	1800				
	2200	100.2	120	32	98/56
	0200				

Which of the following information is most important to collect next?
a. Appearance of the incision site
b. Breath sounds
c. Type of vaginal discharge
d. Urinary output for the last 24 hours*

ASSESSMENT METHODS FOR HIGHER LEVEL COGNITIVE SKILLS

Although context-dependent item sets provide one means of assessing higher level cognitive skills, other methods are available for this purpose. Those alternate approaches include: case method, case study, and unfolding cases; discussion; debate; media clips; short written assignments; and varied clinical evaluation methods, which are presented in Chapter 14. Many of the assessment methods described in this section of the chapter also may be used for clinical evaluation.

Case Method, Case Study, and Unfolding Cases

With cases, students analyze a clinical scenario and answer related questions. The focus might be on interpreting patient needs and problems, identifying additional data to collect, applying concepts and theories from class and readings to the case, examining the case from different points of view, and identifying interventions. When used in these ways, cases are effective for developing problem-solving and higher level thinking skills Gaberson & Oermann, 2010; Harrison, 2012; Popil, 2011). In the case method, the cases tend to be short, providing only essential information about the scenario, in contrast to case studies, which are longer and offer more detail.

Cases work well for group analysis and discussion, either in class or online as small-group activities or in postclinical conference. In groups, students can critique each others' thinking; compare different interpretations of the problem, interventions, and decisions possible; and learn how to arrive at a group consensus. Used as a small-group activity, the case method is more easily evaluated for formative than summative purposes. Exhibit 7.4 presents examples of a case method, case study, and unfolding case.

A case study provides a hypothetical or real-life situation for students to analyze and then arrive at varied decisions. Case studies are more comprehensive than the introductory material presented with the case method (Exhibit 7.4). With case studies, students are able to provide detailed and in-depth analyses and describe the evidence on which their conclusions are based. The case study also provides a means for students to apply relevant concepts and theories from class and from their readings. A case study may be completed as an individual assignment and assessed similarly to other written assignments as long as the students provide a rationale for their decisions. The results of the case analysis may be presented orally for group critique and feedback.

One other method to use to assess higher level learning is unfolding cases, which provide a means of simulating a patient situation that

❏Exhibit 7.4

Sample Case Method, Case Study, and Unfolding Case

Case Method

A 92-year-old man is brought to the emergency department by his son. The patient seems to be dragging his right leg and has slurred speech. His blood pressure is 220/110.

1. What are possible problems this patient might be experiencing?
2. What additional data will you collect from the son, and why is this information important to confirming the problem?

Case Study

A 20-year-old woman has had abdominal pain for the last 2 weeks. Some mornings she has vomiting, but today she complains mainly of severe abdominal cramps and nausea. She has lost 8 pounds since last week and has no appetite. She reports having diarrhea for the last few days. She has no masses that you can feel although she complains of increased pain with even a slight touching of her abdominal area. Her vital signs are normal.

Her mother, who brought her to the office today, reports that the patient has always been healthy and has had no prior illnesses except for colds and an occasional flu. She lives with both parents and her younger brother, and she is a student at the local college.

1. What are possible problems that this patient might have? What data would you collect to narrow down your list of problems?
2. What laboratory tests would you expect to be ordered? Why?
3. As you talk with the patient's mother, you learn that the family was on a cruise a few weeks ago, but no one "got sick on the cruise." How might this new information influence your thinking about the patient's possible problems?
4. Considering only the data presented in the case, develop a care plan to meet the patient's current needs. Provide a rationale for each intervention in your plan.

Unfolding Case

You are making a home visit to see a 71-year-old woman who has a leg ulcer that began after she fell. The patient is coughing and wheezing; she tells you she "feels terrible."

1. What additional data would you collect in the initial assessment? Why?
2. What actions would you take during this home visit? Provide a rationale.

In 3 days you visit this patient again. She has increased shortness of breath, more fatigue, and a pale color, and she seems cyanotic around her mouth.

1. Does this new information change your impression of her problems? Why or why not?
2. List priority problems for this patient with a brief rationale.

(continued)

> **Exhibit 7.4 *(continued)***
>
> **3.** What will you report to the physician when you call?
>
> The patient recovers from that episode, and you are able to visit her one more time. At this last visit, she is still short of breath but otherwise seems improved. Using the form from your agency, write your final report on this patient.

changes over time. Rather than writing one short case, as in a case method, or a more comprehensive one with background information, as in a case study, unfolding cases describe changes in a patient's condition or a setting of care similar to what might occur with an actual patient (Exhibit 7.4). Unfolding case studies are valuable for guiding students in applying theory and classroom learning to clinical practice and developing their thinking skills. Day and others suggested that this method also enables students to identify the most salient aspects of a case, develop their clinical imagination, and begin to think like a nurse (Benner, Sutphen, Leonard, & Day, 2010; Day, 2011).

Ulrich and Glendon (2005) developed a model for writing unfolding cases, which then can be evaluated. This strategy includes at least three paragraphs for analysis and discussion by students. The case is presented in the first paragraph, followed by questions for problem solving and critical thinking. The case unfolds as the teacher presents new information about the patient or clinical situation in a second paragraph, again accompanied by higher level questions for students to answer. By introducing new data in subsequent paragraphs, the teacher presents a changing patient scenario. In Ulrich and Glendon's model, at the end of the unfolding case, students complete a reflective writing exercise to identify where further learning is needed and to share their reactions to the case. Azzarello (2008) developed a rubric for evaluating the quality of the students' analysis of an unfolding case. Students receive higher scores when they identify critical problems early in the case and request information to clarify a problem or solution.

Discussion

Discussions with students individually and in small groups are an important strategy for assessing problem solving, decision making, critical thinking, and clinical judgment skills. In a discussion, the teacher has an opportunity to ask questions about students' thinking and the rationale they used for arriving at decisions and positions on issues. Discussions may be impromptu, used for formative evaluation, or structured by the teacher to provide a context and questions to which students respond. Use of discussion for assessing cognitive skills, however, requires careful questioning with a focus on the thinking used by students to arrive at answers. In these discussions, the teacher can ask students about possible decisions, implications of options they considered and different points of view in the situation. In these discussions students can argue their thoughts and decisions persuasively (Nickitas, 2012).

The difficulty level of questions asked is significant; one should avoid a predominance of factual questions and focus instead on clarifying and higher level questions. With factual questions, students recall facts and specific information about the problem and issue being discussed. For example, factual questions are: "What is dyspnea?" and "What are subjective data?" Clarifying and explanatory questions require further thought and discussion. For instance, a clarifying question is: "Tell me the relationship between your patient's shortness of breath and her cardiac problems." For these questions, students explain their answers using their own terminology. Higher level questions, geared toward critical thinking, cannot be answered by memory alone and require an evaluation or a judgment of the situation (Gaberson & Oermann, 2010; Oermann, 2008). Examples of higher level questions are: "What are similarities and differences between the assessment and diagnoses for Mrs. S and for the patient you had last week?" and "Which pain interventions would you propose for this patient? Why did you decide on these interventions rather than the others?"

Questions for discussions should be sequenced from a low to a high level, beginning with factual questions to evaluate students' knowledge of relevant concepts and theories and their ability to apply them to the situation, problem, and issue, and progressing to questions that assess students' thinking and clinical judgments. Bloom's taxonomy can be used as a framework for developing questions for discussions focusing on higher level thinking. With this schema, low-level questions would ask for recall of facts and comprehension. Higher level questions would focus on application, analysis, synthesis, and evaluation. This taxonomy of the cognitive domain was described and examples of each level were provided in Chapter 1.

This discussion of the level of questions asked by the teacher is important because research suggests that teachers by nature do not ask higher level questions of students. Questions asked of nursing students tend to focus on recall and comprehension rather than on higher levels of thinking (Gaberson & Oermann, 2010; Hsu, 2007; Oermann, 2008; Profetto-McGrath, Smith, Day, & Yonge, 2004). If discussions are to be geared toward assessment of problem solving and higher level thinking, the teacher needs an awareness of the level of questions asked for this purpose. When a student answers a question correctly, the teacher should explore alternate possibilities and then proceed to a higher level question. The questions presented in Exhibit 7.1 for assessing critical thinking may be used to guide discussions. In a discussion, the teacher or preceptor should ask students about:

- questions, issues, and problems to be resolved
- assumptions on which their thinking is based
- their own points of view and those of others
- the information and evidence on which they are basing their thinking
- concepts and theories applicable to the question, issue, or problem being discussed
- inferences and conclusions possible
- implications and consequences of their reasoning

With a logical sequence of questions, students can analyze complex issues, examine alternate points of view, and draw generalizations across different content areas. However, these outcomes will not be achieved without carefully thought-out questions by the teacher.

Debate

Debate provides an effective mechanism for assessing students' ability to analyze problems and issues in depth, consider alternative points of view, and formulate a position. The process of analyzing the issue for the debate, considering alternative viewpoints, developing a sound position, and preparing arguments for the position taken provide opportunities for an assessment of students' critical thinking skills. Bradshaw and Lowenstein (2011) also suggested that the debate itself allows students to gain experience in speaking to a group and to develop their oral communication skills.

The focus in evaluating a debate should be on the strength of the argument developed and presented to the group. Areas to consider in evaluating debates include:

1. Clarity and comprehensiveness of the analysis of the issue
2. Rationale developed for the position taken, including use of the literature and available research
3. Consideration of alternative positions
4. Clarity of responses to the opposing side
5. Organization and development of the argument
6. Degree of persuasiveness in presenting the argument
7. Presentation skills, including keeping the audience interested and focused, presenting the information logically and clearly, and keeping within the allotted time frame

Depending on the size of the class, not all students may be able to participate in the debate, but they can all learn from it. Debates promote students' competence and learning, expand their understanding of an issue, develop their awareness of opposing views, encourage them to critically analyze issues, and help them develop persuasive arguments (Bradshaw & Lowenstein, 2011; Doody & Condon, 2012).

Multimedia

Multimedia may be used to present a scenario for assessing higher level learning. Multimedia adds to the reality of the situation as compared with presenting the scenario in print form. Any type of media may be used for this purpose. For example, images, video and audio clips, virtual reality, and many other educational and computer technologies can be used to develop real-life scenarios for students to analyze and discuss. There is a wealth of resources on the Web for presenting scenarios and other situations for teaching and assessing higher level cognitive skills. These can be integrated easily within an online learning environment, and students can work individually or in groups to analyze them.

Short Written Assignments

Evaluation of written assignments is presented in Chapter 9. For the purposes of assessing higher level thinking and other cognitive skills, however, these assignments should reflect additional principles. Assignments for this purpose should be short and require students to think critically about the topic. With term papers and other long assignments, students often summarize the literature and report on the ideas of others, rather than thinking about the topic themselves. Short written assignments, in contrast, provide an opportunity for students to express their thinking in writing and for teachers to give prompt and specific feedback to them on their reasoning.

Students should have clear directions as to what to write about and the expected length of the assignment. Assignments can be planned throughout a course and level in a nursing program so that they build on one another, helping students to develop gradually their thinking and writing skills. Beginning assignments should ask students to describe a problem or an issue and how they would solve it. In these papers and other assignments students should use multiple information resources, which are of value in preparing them for evidence-based practice (Oermann, 2006). In later assignments students can develop arguments to support their own positions about issues.

Examples of written assignments for assessing critical thinking, appropriate for either formative or summative evaluation, include short papers (one to two pages) that:

- Compare different data sets
- Compare problems and alternative interventions that could be used
- Analyze issues
- Analyze different points of view, perspectives, and positions on an issue
- Compare a student's own and others' positions on an issue or topic
- Present evidence on which their reasoning is based
- Analyze conclusions drawn, evidence to support these conclusions, and possible alternatives given the same evidence
- Present an argument to support a position

SUMMARY

This chapter provided a framework for assessing higher level learning skills among nursing students. The ability to solve patient and setting related problems is an essential ability to be developed and evaluated. The nurse continually makes decisions about problems, solutions, possible alternative approaches, and the best approach to use in a particular situation, after weighing the consequences of each. Critical thinking is reflective and reasoned thinking.

In assessing these cognitive skills, as a basic principle the teacher introduces new or novel material for analysis. Without the introduction of new material as part of the assessment, students may rely on memorization of content from prior discussion or their readings on how to problem solve and arrive at decisions for the situation at hand; they may simply recall the typical problem and solutions without thinking through alternative possibilities themselves. As a result, an essential component of this assessment is the introduction of new information not encountered by the student at an earlier point in the instruction. In nursing this is frequently accomplished by developing scenarios that present a novel situation to which students apply concepts and theories, problem solve, arrive at decisions, and engage in higher level thinking. These items are referred to as context-dependent item sets or interpretive exercises.

In a context-dependent item set, the teacher presents introductory material that students then analyze and answer questions about. The introductory material may be a description of a clinical situation, patient data, research findings, issues associated with clinical practice, and tables, among other types. Students read, analyze, and interpret this material and then answer questions about it or complete other tasks.

Other methods for assessing cognitive skills in nursing were presented in the chapter: case method and study, unfolding cases, discussions using higher level questioning, debate, multimedia, and short written assignments. In addition to these strategies, clinical evaluation methods that provide for an assessment of cognitive skills will be presented in Chapter 14.

REFERENCES

Alfaro-LeFevre, R. (2013). *Critical thinking, clinical reasoning, and clinical judgment: A practical approach* (5th ed.). St. Louis, MO: Elsevier.

Azzarello, J. (2008). Unfolding case studies: Dynamic mental models in a public health context. In N. C. Facione & P. A. Facione (Eds.), *Critical thinking and clinical reasoning in the health sciences* (pp. 75–83). Millbrae, CA: California Academic Press.

Benner, P. E. (2001). *From novice to expert: Excellence and power in clinical nursing practice.* Upper Saddle River, NJ: Prentice Hall.

Benner, P. E., Sutphen, M., Leonard, V., & Day, L. (2010). *Educating nurses: A call for radical transformation.* San Francisco, CA: Jossey-Bass.

Berkow, S., Virkstis, K., Stewart, J., Aronson, S., & Donohue, M. (2011). Assessing individual frontline nurse critical thinking. *Journal of Nursing Administration, 41,* 168–171.

Bradshaw, M. J., & Lowenstein, A. J. (2011). *Innovative teaching strategies in nursing and related health professions* (5th ed.). Sudbury, MA: Jones and Bartlett.

Day, L. (2011). Using unfolding case studies in a subject-centered classroom. *Journal of Nursing Education, 50,* 447–452.

Doody, O., & Condon, M. (2012). Increasing student involvement and learning through using debate as an assessment. *Nurse Education in Practice, 12,* 232–237.

Elder, L., & Paul, R. (2010). *The thinker's guide to analytic thinking.* Tomales, CA: Foundation for Critical Thinking.

Facione, N. C., & Facione, P. A. (2008). *Critical thinking and clinical reasoning in the health sciences: An international multidisciplinary teaching anthology.* Millbrae, CA: California Academic Press.

Facione, P. (2011). *Critical thinking: What it is and why it counts.* Retrieved from http://www.insightassessment.com/CT-Resources/Critical-Thinking-What-It-Is-and-Why-It-Counts

Gaberson, K. B., & Oermann, M. H. (2010). *Clinical teaching strategies in nursing* (3rd ed.). New York, NY: Springer Publishing.

Harrison, E. (2012). How to develop well-written case studies. *Nurse Educator, 37,* 67–70.

Hsu, L-L. (2007). Conducting clinical post-conference in clinical teaching: A qualitative study. *Journal of Clinical Nursing, 16,* 1525–1533.

Lasater, K. (2011). Clinical judgment: The last frontier for evaluation. *Nurse Education in Practice, 11,* 86–92.

National Council of State Boards of Nursing. (2010). *Frequently asked questions about NCLEX alternate item formats.* Retrieved from https://www.ncsbn.org/Alternate_Item_Formats_FAQ.pdf

Nickitas, D. M. (2012). Asking questions and appreciating inquiry: A winning strategy for the nurse educator and professional nurse learner. *Journal of Continuing Education in Nursing, 43,* 106–110.

Nitko, A. J., & Brookhart, S. M. (2011). *Educational assessment of students* (6th ed.). Upper Saddle River, NJ: Pearson Education.

Oermann, M. H. (2006). Short written assignments for clinical nursing courses. *Nurse Educator, 31,* 228–231.

Oermann, M. H. (2008). Ideas for postclinical conferences. *Teaching and Learning in Nursing, 3*, 90–93.

Paul, R., & Elder, L. (2011). *Using intellectual standards to assess student reasoning. Foundation for critical thinking.* Retrieved from http://www.criticalthinking.org/pages/using-intellectual-standards-to-assess-student-reasoning/602

Popil, I. (2011). Promotion of critical thinking by using case studies as teaching method. *Nurse Education Today, 31*, 204–207.

Profetto-McGrath, J., Smith, K. B., Day, R. A., & Yonge, O. (2004). The questioning skills of tutors and students in a context based baccalaureate nursing program. *Nurse Education Today, 24*, 363–372.

Tanner, C. A. (2006). Thinking like a nurse: A research-based model of clinical judgment. *Journal of Nursing Education, 45*, 204–211.

Ulrich, D. L., & Glendon, K. J. (2005). *Interactive group learning: Strategies for nurse educators* (2nd ed). New York, NY: Springer Publishing.

EIGHT

Test Construction and Preparation of Students for Licensure and Certification Examinations

One of the outcomes of prelicensure nursing programs is for graduates to pass an examination that measures their knowledge and competencies to engage in safe and effective nursing practice. At the entry level for professional nursing, graduates take the National Council Licensure Examination for Registered Nurses (NCLEX-RN®) or, if graduating from a practical or vocational nursing program, they take the National Council Licensure Examination for Practical Nurses (NCLEX-PN®). Certification validates knowledge and competencies for professional practice in a specialized area of nursing. As part of this process nurses may take certification examinations that assess their knowledge and skills in a nursing specialty such as critical care or pediatric nursing. Other certification examinations measure knowledge and competencies for advanced practice, for teaching, and for administrative roles. As students progress through a nursing program, they should have experience with tests that are similar to and prepare them for taking licensure and certification examinations when they graduate.

Because the focus of the NCLEX and most certification examinations is on nursing practice, the other advantage to incorporating items of these types in teacher-made tests is that it provides a way of assessing whether students can apply their theoretical learning to clinical situations. Teachers can develop items that present new and complex clinical situations for students to critically analyze. Items can focus on collecting and analyzing data, setting priorities, selecting interventions, and evaluating outcomes as related to the content taught in the course. This type of testing is a means of assessing higher and more complex levels of learning and provides essential practice before students encounter similar questions on licensure and certification examinations.

This chapter begins with an explanation of the NCLEX test plans and implications for nurse educators. Examples are provided of items written at different cognitive levels, thereby avoiding tests that focus only on recall and memorization of facts. The chapter also describes how to write questions within the framework of clinical practice or based on the nursing process and provides sample stems for use with those items. The types of items presented in the chapter are similar to those found on the NCLEX and many certification tests. By incorporating items of these types on tests in nursing courses, teachers help students acquire experience with this type of testing as they progress through the program, preparing them for taking licensure and certification examinations as graduates. The reader should keep in mind that Chapter 7 presented other ways of assessing higher level learning such as context-dependent testing, case method, and other strategies for assessing critical thinking and clinical reasoning.

NCLEX TEST PLANS

In the United States and its territories, graduates of nursing programs cannot practice as registered nurses (RNs) or as practical nurses (PNs) or vocational nurses (VNs) until they have passed a licensure examination. These examinations are developed by the National Council of State Boards of Nursing, Inc. (NCSBN) based on extensive analyses of the practice requirements of RNs and licensed practical nurses (LPNs) or vocational nurses (LVNs). Because the NCLEX examinations are high-stakes, items are piloted and tested extensively to ensure they are valid, reliable, and legally defensible, including an analysis of potential biases such as those related to ethnicity and gender (Woo & Dragan, 2012, p. 29). The licensure examination results then are used by the state boards of nursing as one of the requirements for practice in that state or territory.

NCLEX-RN EXAMINATION TEST PLAN

In developing the NCLEX-RN, the NCSBN conducts an analysis of the current practice of newly licensed RNs across clinical areas and settings. This is a continuous process allowing the licensure examination to stay current with the knowledge and competencies needed by entry level nurses. To ensure that the NCLEX-RN measures the essential competencies for safe and effective practice by a newly licensed RN, the NCSBN reviews the test plan or blueprint every 3 years (NCSBN, 2012a). For the most recent revision of the test plan, nearly 3,000 newly licensed RNs prioritized how frequently they performed 141 nursing care activities and rated the overall importance of each activity considering patient safety and the threat of complications (NCSBN). A test plan is developed from this analysis, guiding the selection of content to be tested and the percentage of items for each of the categories of the test. The NCLEX-RN Examination is based on this test plan.

Client Needs

Test items on the NCLEX-RN are categorized by client needs: (a) safe and effective care environment, (b) health promotion and maintenance, (c) psychosocial integrity, and (d) physiological integrity. Two of the categories, safe and effective care environment and physiological integrity, also have subgroups. The client needs represent the content tested on the examination. Table 8.1 lists the percentage of items on the examination from each of the categories or subcategories.

Safe and Effective Care Environment

In the Safe and Effective Care Environment category, two subcategories of content are tested on the NCLEX-RN: (a) management of care and (b) safety and infection control. In the management of care subcategory, the

Table 8.1

PERCENTAGE OF ITEMS IN NCLEX-RN EXAMINATION TEST PLAN

CLIENT NEEDS	PERCENTAGE OF ITEMS FROM EACH CATEGORY OR SUBCATEGORY
Safe and effective care environment	
Management of care	16–22
Safety and infection control	8–14
Health promotion and maintenance	6–12
Psychosocial integrity	6–12
Physiological integrity	
Basic care and comfort	6–12
Pharmacological and parenteral therapies	13–19
Reduction of risk potential	10–16
Physiological adaptation	11–17

Source: A. Wendt, L. Kenny, & L. Schultz (2010). *2010 NCLEX-RN® detailed test plan.* Chicago: National Council of State Boards of Nursing, p. 4.

questions focus on providing and directing nursing care that protects clients and health care providers. Examples of content tested in this category include advance directives, advocacy, case management, collaboration with the interdisciplinary team, concepts of management, confidentiality/information security, continuity of care, delegation, ethical practice, legal rights and responsibilities, performance improvement (quality improvement), and supervision, among others (Wendt, Kenny, & Schultz, 2010).

In the Safety and Infection Control subcategory, test items focus on prevention of accidents, emergency response planning, ergonomic principles, error prevention, handling hazardous and infectious materials, reporting of incidents and irregular occurrences, safe use of equipment, and use of restraints, among others (Wendt et al., 2010).

Health Promotion and Maintenance

The second category of client needs is Health Promotion and Maintenance. There are no subcategories of needs. Examples of content tested in this category are aging process, ante/intra/postpartum and newborn care, developmental stages and transitions, health and wellness, health promotion and screening, lifestyle choices, physical assessment techniques, and teaching and learning principles.

Psychosocial Integrity

The third category of client needs, Psychosocial Integrity, also has no subgroups. This category focuses on nursing care that promotes the emotional, mental, and social well-being of clients experiencing stressful events, and the care of patients with acute and chronic mental illness (Wendt et al., 2010). Examples of content tested include abuse, behavioral interventions, chemical and other dependencies, cultural diversity, end-of-life care, grief and loss, mental health, sensory and perceptual alterations, and therapeutic communication and environment (Wendt et al., 2010).

Physiological Integrity

The final Client Needs category, Physiological Integrity, is a significant content area tested on the NCLEX-RN. Items in this category focus on nursing care that promotes physical health and comfort, reduces risk potential, and manages health alterations. Four subcategories of content are examined by these items on the NCLEX-RN Examination:

   1. *Basic Care and Comfort*: In this area, items focus on comfort measures and assistance with activities of daily living. Related content includes assistive devices, elimination, mobility and immobility, nonpharmacological comfort interventions, nutrition and oral hydration, personal hygiene, and rest and sleep.

2. *Pharmacological and Parenteral Therapies*: Items focus on adverse effects, contraindications, side effects, and interactions; blood and blood products; calculating dosages; central venous access devices; medication administration; parenteral/intravenous therapy; pharmacological pain management; and total parenteral nutrition.

3. *Reduction of Risk Potential*: The content in this subcategory relates to measures for reducing the risk of developing complications or health problems. For example, items relate to diagnostic tests; laboratory values; potential for complications from tests, treatments, and procedures; and system-specific assessments, among others.

4. *Physiological Adaptation*: The last subcategory, physiological adaptation, includes nursing care of patients with acute, chronic, or life-threatening physical health problems. Sample content areas are alterations in body systems, fluid and electrolyte imbalances, hemodynamics, management of illness and medical emergencies, pathophysiology, and unexpected responses to therapies (Wendt et al., 2010).

Integrated Processes

Four processes are integrated throughout each of the categories of the test plan: (a) nursing process, (b) caring, (c) communication and documentation, and (d) teaching and learning. Thus there can be test items on teaching patients and the nurse's ethical and legal responsibilities in patient education as part of the Management of Care subcategory, teaching nursing assistants about the use of restraints in the Safety and Infection Control subcategory, health education for different age groups in the Health Promotion and Maintenance category, and teaching about diagnostic tests in the Reduction of Risk Potential subcategory. The other processes are integrated similarly throughout the test plan. Many of the items on the NCLEX examinations are developed around clinical situations. Those situations can involve any age group of patients in hospitals, long-term care, community health, or other types of settings.

Cognitive Levels

Bloom's taxonomy for the cognitive domain is used for developing and coding items on the NCLEX-RN Examination (Wendt et al., 2010). This taxonomy was presented in Chapter 1. Items are developed at the knowledge, comprehension, application, and analysis levels, with the majority of items at the application and higher cognitive levels (Wendt et al.). This has implications for testing in prelicensure nursing education programs. Faculty members should avoid preparing only recall and comprehension items on their tests. Although some low-level questions are essential to assess knowledge and understanding of facts and basic principles, test items also need to ask students to *use* their knowledge and think critically to arrive at an answer. Test blueprints can be developed to list not only the content and number of items in each content area but also the level of cognitive complexity at which items should be written. An example of a blueprint of this type was provided in Exhibit 3.3 in Chapter 3.

NCLEX-PN EXAMINATION TEST PLAN

The test plan for the NCLEX-PN is developed and organized similarly to the RN examination. For the 2011 test plan, PNs and VNs who were newly licensed were asked how frequently they performed 150 nursing activities and the importance of those activities (NCSBN, 2010). The activities were then used as the framework for the development of the test plan for the PN examination.

The test plan is structured around client needs and integrated processes fundamental to the practice of practical and vocational nursing. The same four client needs categories are used for the NCLEX-PN Examination with differences in some of the subcategories, related content, and percentage of items in each category and subcategory. Table 8.2 lists the percentage of items in each client need category or subcategory. Similar to the NCLEX-RN Examination, four processes are integrated throughout the test: (a) the clinical problem-solving process (nursing process), (b) caring, (c) communication and documentation, and (d) teaching and learning. Items are developed at all cognitive levels with the majority written at the application or higher levels of cognitive abilities, consistent with the NCLEX-RN test plan (NCSBN, 2011).

TYPES OF ITEMS ON THE NCLEX EXAMINATIONS

The NCLEX examinations contain the standard four-option multiple-choice items and alternate item formats. Earlier chapters described how to construct each type of item used on the NCLEX: multiple-choice (Chapter 5); and the alternate formats of multiple-response (Chapter 5), fill-in-the-blank and ordered response (Chapter 6), and hot-spot and chart or exhibit (Chapter 7). Any of these item formats on the NCLEX including multiple choice might include a table, a chart, or an image as part of the item. Items also may include sound and video. Wendt and Harmes (2009) described

⬜Table 8.2

PERCENTAGE OF ITEMS IN NCLEX-PN EXAMINATION TEST PLAN

CLIENT NEEDS	PERCENTAGE OF ITEMS FROM EACH CATEGORY OR SUBCATEGORY
Safe and effective care environment	
Coordinated care	13–19
Safety and infection control	11–17
Health promotion and maintenance	7–13
Psychosocial integrity	7–13
Physiological integrity	
Basic care and comfort	9–15
Pharmacological therapies	11–17
Reduction of risk potential	9–15
Physiological adaptation	9–15

Source: National Council of State Boards of Nursing. (2011). *2011 NCLEX-PN® detailed test plan.* Chicago: Author, p. 4.

the development of innovative items that incorporated sound and video. These items have the capacity to assess higher levels of thinking and do so more authentically than a text-based item.

The NCLEX-RN Detailed Test Plan provides valuable information about the practice activities used for developing the items and content areas assessed in each of the categories and subcategories on the examination. As described earlier, the NCSBN analyzes the current practices of newly licensed RNs and PNs/VNs across clinical specialties and settings. This analysis identifies nursing activities that are used frequently by entry-level nurses and are important to ensure patient safety. Development of the NCLEX examinations using these practice activities provides evidence of reliability and validity to support the use of the NCLEX as a measure of competent entry-level nursing practice (Wendt et al., 2010).

The NCLEX-RN Detailed Test Plan includes a list of the activity statements and related content for each category and subcategory. This information is of value in developing items for tests in a nursing program. For example, in the Safety and Infection Control subcategory, the activity statements describe the practices that RNs use to protect clients and health care personnel from health and environmental hazards. An example of one of these activity statements is: "Apply principles of infection control (e.g., hand hygiene, room assignment, isolation, aseptic/sterile technique, universal/standard precautions)" (p. 15). A sample test item also is provided with each category and subcategory. The sample item in the Safety and Infection Control subcategory assesses student understanding about infection control precautions for a patient with streptococcal pneumonia. In the NCLEX-PN Test Plan, the categories and subcategories are described with related content areas.

ADMINISTRATION OF NCLEX EXAMINATIONS

The NCLEX examinations are administered to candidates by computerized adaptive testing (CAT). The CAT model is such that each candidate's test is assembled interactively as the person is answering the questions. Each item on the NCLEX has a predetermined difficulty level. As each item is answered, the computer re-estimates the candidate's ability based on whether the answer is correct or incorrect. The computer then searches the item bank for an item with the same degree of difficulty (Wendt et al., 2010). This is an efficient means of testing, avoiding questions that do not contribute to determining a candidate's level of nursing competence.

The standard for passing the NCLEX is criterion-referenced. The standard is set by the NCSBN based on an established protocol and is used as the basis for determining if the candidate has passed or failed the examination. The NCLEX-RN can range from 75 to 265 items, with 15 of those being pretest items that are not scored. After candidates answer the minimum number of items, the testing stops when the candidate's ability is above or below the standard for passing, with 95% certainty (Wendt et al., 2010). Because the NCLEX is an adaptive test, candidates complete different numbers of items, and therefore the test takes varying amounts of time. If a candidate's ability has not been determined by the time the maximum number of items has been presented or when the time limit has been reached, the examination then stops.

All RN candidates must answer a minimum number of 75 items. The maximum number they can answer is 265 within a time limit of 6 hours (NCSBN, 2012b). On the NCLEX-PN, PN and VN candidates must answer a minimum of 85 items. The maximum number of items they can answer is 205, during the 5-hour testing period allowed (NCSBN, 2012b).

PREPARATION OF ITEMS AT VARIED COGNITIVE LEVELS

When courses have higher level outcomes, tests in those courses need to measure learning at the application and analysis levels rather than at recall and comprehension. This principle was discussed in earlier chapters. Items at higher levels of cognitive complexity are more difficult and time-consuming to develop, but they provide a way of evaluating ability to apply knowledge to new situations and to engage in analytical thinking. The majority of items on the NCLEX are written at higher levels of cognitive ability, requiring application of knowledge and analytical thinking.

Students are at a disadvantage if they encounter only recall and comprehension test items as they progress through a nursing program. Low-level items assess how well students memorize specific information, not if they can use that knowledge to analyze clinical situations and arrive at the best decisions possible for those situations. Students need experience answering questions at the application and analysis levels before they take the NCLEX. More important, if course outcomes are at higher levels of cognitive complexity, then tests and other methods need to assess learning at those levels. In graduate nursing programs, test items should be developed at higher cognitive levels to assess students' ability to problem solve and think critically and to prepare them for certification examinations they might take as graduates.

When developing a new test, a blueprint is important in planning the number of items at each cognitive level for the content areas to be assessed. By using a blueprint, teachers can avoid writing too many recall and comprehension items. For existing tests that were not developed using a blueprint, teachers can code items using Bloom's taxonomy and then decide if more higher level items should be added.

Knowledge or Recall

In developing items at varying cognitive levels, it is important to remember the learning outcome intended at each of these levels. Questions at the knowledge level deal with facts, principles, and other specific information that is memorized and then recalled to answer the item. An example of a multiple-choice item at the knowledge level follows:

> Your patient is taking pseudoephedrine for his stuffy nose. Which of the following side effects is common among patients using this medication?

> a. Diarrhea
> b. Dyspnea
> c. Hallucinations
> d. Restlessness*

Comprehension

At the comprehension level, items assess understanding of concepts and ability to explain them. These questions are written at a higher level than

---

*Correct answer.

recall, but they do not assess problem solving or use of information in a new context. An example of an item at the comprehension level is:

> An adult female patient is a new admission with the diagnosis of acute renal failure. Her total urine output for the previous 24 hours was 90 mL. A urinary output of this amount is known as _____.

Application

At the application level, students apply concepts and theories as a basis for responding to the item. At this level, test questions measure *use* of knowledge in new or unique situations. One method for developing items at this level is to prepare stems that have information that students did not encounter in their learning about the content. The stem might present patient data, diagnoses, or treatments different from the ones discussed in class or in the readings. If examples in class related to nursing care of adults, items might test ability to use those concepts when the patient is an adolescent or has multiple co-existing problems. An example of an item at the application level is:

> A mother tells you that she is worried about her 4-year-old daughter's development because her daughter seems to be "behind." You complete a developmental assessment. Which of the following behaviors suggests the need for further developmental testing?
>
> a. Cannot follow five commands in a row
> b. Has difficulty holding a crayon between thumb and forefinger*
> c. Is unable to balance on each foot for 6 seconds
> d. Keeps making mistakes when asked about the day of the week

Analysis

Questions at the analysis level are the most difficult to construct. They require analysis of a clinical or other situation to identify critical elements and relationships among them. Items should provide a new situation for students to analyze, not one encountered previously for which the student might recall the analysis. Many of these items require learners to solve a problem and make a decision about priorities or the best approach to take among the options. Or, items might ask students to identify the most immediate course of action to meet patient needs or manage the clinical situation.

The difference between application and analysis items is not always readily apparent. Analysis items, though, should ask students to identify relevant data, critical elements, component parts, and their interrelationships. In analysis level items students should distinguish between significant and nonsignificant information and select the best approach or priority among those cited in the alternatives. An example of an item written at the analysis level is:

> You receive a report on the following patients at the beginning of your evening shift at 3 p.m. Which patient should you assess first?
> a. An 82-year-old with pneumonia who seems confused at times*
> b. A 76-year-old patient with cancer with 300 mL remaining of an intravenous infusion
> c. A 40-year-old who had an emergency appendectomy 8 hours ago
> d. An 18-year-old with chest tubes for treatment of a pneumothorax following an accident

PREPARATION OF ITEMS WITHIN FRAMEWORK OF CLINICAL PRACTICE OR NURSING PROCESS

One of the processes integrated into the NCLEX test plans is the nursing process. This is also a framework taught in many nursing programs. If not presented as the nursing process, most clinical courses address, in some form, assessment, data analysis, problems or diagnoses, interventions, and evaluation. These areas provide another useful framework for developing test questions. Items can examine assessment of patients with varied needs and health problems, analysis of data, identification of problems, selection of evidence-based interventions and treatments, and evaluation of the outcomes of care.

Current practices suggest that many test items focus on scientific rationale, principles underlying patient care, and selection of interventions. Fewer items are developed on collecting and analyzing data, determining patient problems, setting priorities and realistic goals of care, and evaluating the effectiveness of interventions and outcomes. Developing items based on clinical scenarios in the stems provides an opportunity to examine these outcomes of learning. These items also facilitate testing at a higher cognitive level because they are written in relation to specific clinical scenarios in the stems, requiring students to apply their knowledge to the clinical situation.

The process for developing items within the framework of clinical practice or the nursing process begins with identifying the total number of items to be written. This includes specifying the number of items on each phase of the nursing process or more generally on assessment, problem identification, and so forth. On some tests, greater weight may be given to certain areas, for example, assessment, if these were emphasized in the instruction. As part of this planning, the teacher also maps out the clinical scenario to be developed in the stem as related to the course content. For instance, the teacher may develop a scenario on a young adult with sickle cell disease being seen in the emergency department and plan for two assessment items on pain, an item on a high-risk medication, and one item on evaluating the quality of the nurse's communication with the patient. A similar process may be used with other content areas for which this type of testing is intended. Items may stand alone, or a series of items may be developed related to one clinical scenario. In the latter format the teacher has an option of adding data to the situation and creating an unfolding case, which was discussed in Chapter 7.

Examples of stems that can be used to develop these items are provided in Exhibit 8.1. Teachers can select a stem and add content from their own course, providing an easy way of writing items within the framework of clinical practice or the nursing process. Sample items follow.

Assessment

An 8-year-old boy is brought to the emergency room by his mother after falling off his bike and hitting his head. Which of the following data is most important to collect in the initial assessment?

a. Blood pressure
b. Level of consciousness
c. Pupillary response
d. Respiratory status*

Analysis

The nurse practitioner is admitting a patient who complains of fatigue and myalgia, and has a rash across the bridge of the nose and cheeks. The practitioner finds a few ulcers in the patient's mouth. Prior laboratory tests included a positive C-reactive protein. These findings support a likely diagnosis of:

a. fibromyalgia.
b. rheumatoid arthritis.
c. scleroderma.
d. systemic lupus erythematosus.*

❏Exhibit 8.1

Examples of Stems for Clinical Practice and Nursing Process Items

Assessment

The nurse should collect which of the following data?

Which of the following information should be collected as a priority in the assessment?

Which data should be collected first?

Which questions should the nurse ask [the patient, the family, others] in the assessment?

Your patient develops [symptoms]. What data should the nurse collect now?

What additional data are needed to establish the patient's problems?

Which resources should be used to collect the data?

Which of the following information is a priority to report in a SBAR (Situation-Background-Assessment-Recommendation) communication to the [physician, nurse, other provider]?

Analysis

These data support the [diagnosis, problem] of_____

Which [diagnosis, problem] is most appropriate for this patient?

The priority nursing diagnosis is _____

The priority problem of this [patient, family, community] is _____

A patient with [a diagnosis of, symptoms of] is at risk for developing which of the following complications?

Planning

Which outcomes are most important for a patient with a [problem of]?

What are the priority outcomes for a patient receiving [treatment]?

Which nursing measures should be included in the plan of care for a patient with [problem, surgery, treatment, diagnostic test]?

Which of the following nursing interventions would be most effective for a patient with [diagnosis of, problem of, symptoms of]?

The nurse is teaching a patient who is [years old]. Which teaching strategy would be most appropriate?

Which intervention is most likely to be effective in managing [symptoms of]?

Implementation

Which of the following actions should be implemented immediately?

Nursing interventions for this patient include:

Following this [procedure, surgery, treatment, test], which nursing measures should be implemented?

Which of these nursing interventions is a priority for a patient with [problem]?

(continued)

Exhibit 8.1 *(continued)*

What evidence supports [nursing intervention]?

A patient with [a diagnosis of] complains of [symptoms]. What should the nurse do first?

Which explanation should the nurse use when teaching a patient [with a diagnosis of, prior to procedure, surgery, treatment, test]?

Which of the following instructions should be given to the [patient, family, caregiver, nurse] at discharge?

Which of the following situations [incidents] should be reported immediately?

Evaluation

Which of these responses indicates that the [intervention, medication, treatment] is effective?

A patient is taking [medication] for [diagnosis, problem]. Which of these data indicate a side effect of the medication?

Which response by the patient indicates improvement?

Which of the following observations indicates that the [patient, caregiver] knows how to [perform the procedure, give the treatment, follow the protocol]?

Which statement by the [patient, caregiver] indicates the need for further teaching?

Planning

Your patient is being discharged after a sickle cell crisis. Which of the following measures should be included in your teaching plan for this patient? Select all that apply.

- ☐ 1. Avoid warm temperatures inside and outdoors.
- ☐ 2. Do not use nonsteroidal anti-inflammatory drugs for pain.
- ☑ 3. Drink at least 8 glasses of water a day.
- ☑ 4. Eat plenty of grains, fruits, and green leafy vegetables.
- ☑ 5. Get a vaccination for pneumonia.
- ☐ 6. Keep cold packs handy for joint pain.

Implementation

Your patient is in active labor with contractions every 3 minutes lasting about 1 minute. She appears to have a seizure. Which of the following interventions is the top priority?

a. Assess her breathing pattern*
b. Attach an external fetal monitor
c. Call the physician
d. Prepare for a cesarean delivery

Evaluation

A male adult patient was discharged following a below-the-knee amputation. You are making the first home health visit after his discharge. Which of the following statements by the patient indicates that he needs further instruction?

   a. "I know to take my temperature if I get chills again like in the hospital."
   b. "I won't exert myself around the house until I see the doctor."
   c. "The nurse said to take more insulin when I start to eat more."*
   d. "The social worker mentioned a support group. Maybe I should call about it."

PREPARATION OF STUDENTS FOR THE NCLEX EXAMINATIONS

A number of studies have been done over the years to identify predictors of success on the NCLEX-RN. Some factors related to performance on the NCLEX-RN are: SAT and ACT scores (Grossbach & Kuncel, 2011); scores on exit or prelicensure readiness examinations (Frith, Sewell, & Clark, 2006; Lauchner, Newman, & Britt, 2008; McGahee, Gramling, & Reid, 2010; Morrison, Adamson, Nibert, & Hsia, 2004); grades in nursing courses and graduation grade point average (Grossbach & Kuncel, 2011; Landry, Davis, Alameida, Prive, & Renwanz-Boyle, 2010; McGahee et al., 2010; Stuenkel, 2006; Tipton et al., 2008); and grades in science courses (Abbott, Schwartz, Hercinger, Miller, & Foyt, 2008; McGahee et al., 2010). Academic achievement, in terms of nursing course grades and overall grade point average, has been found across studies as predictive of student performance on the NCLEX-RN. In a meta-analysis of 31 independent samples with 7,159 participants, admissions test scores (SAT and ACT) and grades earned in nursing programs, especially grades in the second year, were the best predictors of performance on the NCLEX (Grossbach & Kuncel, 2011).

A second area of the literature on the NCLEX-RN focuses on methods of preparing students to pass the examination. One development in this area has been the use of standardized examinations designed to predict student performance on the NCLEX-RN. A number of companies publish standardized tests that are intended to measure students' readiness for the NCLEX. By analyzing the results of standardized tests for NCLEX readiness, faculty members and students can work together to design individual plans for remediation so that students will be more likely to experience first-time success on the licensure examination. Carr (2011) described how her school of nursing reversed a downward trend in the number of students passing the NCLEX. Faculty identified areas of weakness in the curriculum, revised courses, changed the standardized exit examination they were using, implemented a mid-curriculum assessment, and developed remedial courses and learning activities for students who had low achievement on standardized examinations. This comprehensive approach was successful.

Other approaches such as self-assessment of content areas needing improvement, instruction for content mastery, test-taking tips, managing test anxiety, cooperative study groups, courses that guide formal NCLEX-RN preparation, and careful planning for the day of testing have been used by nursing faculty to assist students in preparing for the NCLEX examinations (Anderson, 2007; Frith et al., 2006; Herrman & Johnson, 2009; March & Ambrose, 2010; Poorman, Mastorovich, & Molcan, 2007; Thomas & Baker, 2011). Experience with test items that are similar to the NCLEX prepares students for the types of items they will encounter on the licensing examination. In addition to these item formats, students also need experience in taking practice tests.

SUMMARY

The chapter summarized the NCLEX test plans and their implications for nurse educators. One of the principles emphasized was the need to prepare items at different cognitive levels as indicated by the outcomes of the course. Items at the recall level assess how well students memorized facts and specific information; they do not, however, provide an indication of whether students can use that information in practice or can engage in analytical or higher level thinking. To assess those higher level outcomes, items must be written at the application or analysis levels or evaluated by methods other than tests. It is worthwhile for faculty members to develop a test blueprint that specifies the number of items to be developed at each cognitive level for content areas in the course. By using a blueprint, teachers can avoid writing too many recall and comprehension items on an examination.

As students progress through a nursing program, they develop knowledge and skills to assess patients, analyze data, identify patient needs and problems, set priorities for care, select appropriate interventions, and evaluate the outcomes of care. Testing within the framework of clinical practice or the nursing process provides an opportunity to assess those learning outcomes. Items may be written about data to collect in the particular clinical scenario, possible problems, approaches to use, priorities of care, decisions to be made, varying judgments possible in a scenario, and other questions that examine students' thinking and clinical judgment as related to the situation described in the stem of the item. This format of testing also provides experience for students in answering the types of items encountered on licensure and certification examinations.

REFERENCES

Abbott, A., Schwartz, M., Hercinger, M., Miller, C., & Foyt, M. (2008). Student issues. Predictors of success on National Council Licensure Examination for Registered Nurses for accelerated baccalaureate nursing graduates. *Nurse Educator, 33,* 5–6.

Anderson, R. (2007). Individualized student advisement for preparation for the National Council Licensure Examination for Registered Nurses: A community college experience. *Nurse Educator, 32,* 117–121.

Carr, S. M. (2011). NCLEX-RN pass rate peril: One school's journey through curriculum revision, standardized testing, and attitudinal change. *Nursing Education Perspectives, 32,* 384–388.

Frith, K. H., Sewell, J. P., & Clark, D. J. (2006). Best practices in NCLEX-RN readiness preparation for baccalaureate student success. *Computers in Nursing, 23,* 322–329.

Grossbach, A., & Kuncel, N. R. (2011). The predictive validity of nursing admission measures for performance on the National Council Licensure Examination: A meta-analysis. *Journal of Professional Nursing, 27,* 124–128.

Herrman, J. W., & Johnson, A. N. (2009). From beta-blockers to boot camp: Preparing students for the NCLEX-RN. *Nursing Education Perspectives, 30,* 384–388.

Landry, L., Davis, H., Alameida, M., Prive, A., & Renwanz-Boyle, A. (2010). Predictors of NCLEX-RN success across 3 prelicensure program types. *Nurse Educator, 35,* 259–263.

Lauchner, K. A., Newman, M., & Britt, R. B. (2008). Predicting licensure success with a computerized comprehensive nursing exam: The HESI Exit Exam. *CIN: Computers, Informatics, Nursing, 26*(5 Suppl), 4S–9S.

March, K. S., & Ambrose, J. M. (2010). Rx for NCLEX-RN success: Reflections on development of an effective preparation process for senior baccalaureate students. *Nursing Education Perspectives, 31,* 230–232.

McGahee, T. W., Gramling, L., & Reid, T. F. (2010). NCLEX-RN® success: Are there predictors. *Southern Online Journal of Nursing Research, 10,* 208–221.

Morrison, S., Adamson, C., Nibert, A., & Hsia, S. (2004). HESI exams: An overview of reliability and validity. *CIN: Computers, Informatics, Nursing, 22,* 220–226.

National Council of State Boards of Nursing. (2010). *Report of findings from the 2009 LPN/VN practice analysis: Linking the NCLEX-PN® examination to practice.* Chicago, IL: Author.

National Council of State Boards of Nursing. (2011). *2011 NCLEX-PN® detailed test plan.* Chicago, IL: Author.

National Council of State Boards of Nursing. (2012a). *2011 RN Practice analysis: Linking the NCLEX-RN® examination to practice.* Chicago, IL: Author.

National Council of State Boards of Nursing. (2012b). *2012 NCLEX® Examination Candidate Bulletin.* Retrieved from https://www.ncsbn.org/2012_NCLEX_Candidate_Bulletin.pdf

Poorman, S. G., Mastorovich, M. L., & Molcan, K. L. (2007). *A good thinking approach to the NCLEX® and other nursing exams* (2nd ed.). Pittsburgh, PA: STAT Nursing Consultants.

Stuenkel, D. (2006). At-risk students: Do theory grades + standardized examinations = success? *Nurse Educator, 31,* 207–212.

Thomas, M. H., & Baker, S. S. (2011). NCLEX-RN success: Evidence-based strategies. *Nurse Educator, 36,* 246–249.

Tipton, P., Pulliam, M., Beckworth, C., Illich, P., Griffin, R., & Tibbitt, A. (2008). Predictors of associate degree nursing students' success students. *Southern Online Journal of Nursing Research, 8*(1). Retrieved October 5, 2008.

Wendt, A., & Harmes, J. C. (2009). Developing and evaluating innovative items for the NCLEX. Part 2, item characteristics and cognitive processing. *Nurse Educator, 34,* 109–113.

Wendt, A., Kenny, L., & Schultz, L. (2010). *2010 NCLEX-RN® detailed test plan. Item writer/ item reviewer/nurse educator version.* Chicago, IL: National Council of State Boards of Nursing.

Woo, A., & Dragan, M. (2012). Ensuring validity of NCLEX® with differential item functioning analysis. *Journal of Nursing Regulation,* 2(4), 29–31.

NINE

Assessment of
Written Assignments

In most nursing courses, students complete some type of written assignment. With these assignments students can develop their critical thinking skills, gain experience with different types of writing, and achieve other outcomes specific to a course. Written assignments with feedback from the teacher help students develop their writing ability, which is an important outcome in any nursing program from the beginning level through graduate study. This chapter focuses on developing and assessing written assignments for nursing courses.

PURPOSES OF WRITTEN ASSIGNMENTS

Written assignments are a major instructional and assessment method in nursing courses. They can be used to achieve many learning outcomes, but need to be carefully selected and designed considering the instructional goals. With written assignments students can: (a) critique and synthesize the literature and report on their findings; (b) search for, critique, and integrate evidence for nursing practice; (c) analyze concepts and theories and apply them to clinical situations; (d) improve their problem-solving and higher level thinking skills; (e) gain experience in formulating their ideas and communicating them in a clear and coherent way to others; and (f) develop writing skills. Many of the written assignments in clinical courses assist students in thinking through their plan of care and identifying areas in which they need further instruction. Some assignments, such as keeping journals, also encourage students to examine their own feelings, beliefs, and values and to reflect on their learning in a course.

Not all written assignments achieve each of these purposes, and the teacher plans the assignment based on the intended goals of learning.

Assignments should meet *specific* objectives of a course and should not be included only for the purpose of having a written assignment as a course requirement. Instead, they should be carefully selected to help students improve their writing skills and achieve course outcomes.

Because writing is a developmental process that improves with practice, writing assignments should build on one another throughout a course and throughout the entire nursing program. A sequence of papers across courses encourages the improvement of writing more effectively than having students complete a different type of paper in each course. This planning also eliminates excessive repetition of assignments in the program. Along the same lines, faculty members should decide the number of written assignments needed by students to achieve the outcomes of a course or clinical practice experience. In some clinical nursing courses, students complete the same assignments repeatedly throughout a course, leading to their frustration with the "paperwork" in the course. How many times do students need to submit a written assessment of a patient? Written assignments are time-consuming for students to prepare and teachers to read and respond to. Thus, such assignments should be carefully selected to meet course goals and should benefit the students in terms of their learning.

Writing in the Discipline and Writing-to-Learn Activities

Writing assignments in a nursing course in which students receive feedback on their writing guide students in learning how to write clearly for varied audiences. The ability to communicate ideas in writing is an essential outcome of a nursing program at all educational levels (American Association of Colleges of Nursing, 2006, 2008, 2011). The dissemination of new ideas and innovations, outcomes of clinical projects, and findings of research studies requires skill in writing. This skill can be developed through formal papers in a nursing course, such as term papers, in which students receive feedback on their writing; this is often referred to as writing in the discipline (The Writing across the Curriculum [WAC] Clearinghouse, 2011a). Assignments are typically completed over a period of time, and both the content and writing skill are assessed. Formal papers also provide an opportunity to learn a reference style such as the *Publication Manual of the American Psychological Association* (APA) although this is only one aspect of the assessment (APA, 2010). The goal with written assignments such as formal papers is to learn to write effectively and communicate ideas clearly, not only how to use APA or other writing style.

Formal papers can be divided into smaller writing assignments and sequenced progressively through a course. This makes completion of the paper more manageable for students, allows the teacher to assess and provide feedback on each part of the paper, and encourages students to use that feedback for revisions as they are preparing the longer paper. Luthy, Peterson, Lassetter, and Callister (2009) also suggested that smaller assignments that build on one another are less daunting for students. For example, students might be asked to prepare a paper on a potential safety issue in the clinical setting using the National Patient Safety Goals. The first assignment might be the description of the clinical setting and patient population, issue they identified with supporting data, and relevant safety goal. The second assignment might be a literature review related to the safety goal such as the need to communicate important test results to the right person on time, why this is important, and initiatives to improve staff communication. The third assignment might be a description of the initiative they selected for implementation on their unit, their rationale based on the literature and their analysis of the clinical setting, and a plan for implementation and evaluation of outcomes. With each of these written assignments, the teacher can provide feedback, followed by student revision of both the content and writing.

Other types of writing assignments in a nursing course such as journals and in-class writing activities guide students in reflecting on their experiences or learning course content but do not promote development of writing ability. These are considered writing-to-learn activities: they are typically short and informal, and may be impromptu (Oermann, in press; WAC Clearinghouse, 2011b). For example, if students are unclear about content presented in class, they can be asked to write down their questions or summarize in their own words key concepts from class. The outcome of writing-to-learn activities is *learning*, not improving writing skill. The assessment would be formative with feedback on the content, not writing, in contrast to writing in the discipline papers (Oermann, in press).

Drafts and Rewrites

Formal papers enable the teacher to assess students' ability to present, organize, and express ideas effectively in writing. Through these written assignments, students develop an understanding of the content they are writing about, and they learn how to communicate their ideas in writing. To improve their writing abilities, though, students need to complete drafts of papers on which they receive feedback from the teacher.

Drafts and rewrites of papers are essential if the goal is to develop skill in writing (Oermann, 2010). Teachers should critique papers for quality of the content; organization; process of developing ideas and arguments; and writing style such as clarity of expression, sentence structure, punctuation, grammar, spelling, length of the paper, and accuracy and format of the references (Oermann & Hays, 2011). This critique should be accompanied by feedback on how to improve writing. Students need specific suggestions about revisions, not general statements such as *"writing is unclear."* Instead, the teacher should identify the problem with the writing and give suggestions as to how to improve it, for example, *"Introductory sentence does not relate to the content in the paragraph. Replace it with a sentence that incorporates the three nursing measures you discuss in the paragraph."* Drafts combined with feedback from the teacher are intended to improve students' writing skills. Because they are used for this purpose, they should not be graded.

Providing feedback on writing is time-consuming for teachers. Another method that can be used is for students to critique each other's writing in small groups or pairs. Peers can provide valuable feedback on content, organization, how the ideas are developed, and whether the writing is clear. Although they may not identify errors in grammar and sentence structure, they often can find problems with errors in content and clarity of writing. Students can post on a wiki or an online discussion board sections of their papers or questions about writing; peers and the teacher can provide feedback and answer the questions, which can benefit the group as a whole (Collier, 2010; McMillan & Raines, 2010). Peers also can assess writing in small-group activities in the classroom, online, and in postclinical conference if the writing assignment deals with clinical practice. Small-group critique provides a basis for subsequent revisions.

TYPES OF WRITTEN ASSIGNMENTS

Many types of writing assignments are appropriate for assessment in nursing education. Some of these assignments provide information on how well students have learned the content but do not necessarily improve their writing skill. For example, structured assignments that involve short sentences and phrases, such as nursing care plans and write ups of assessments and physical examinations, do not foster development of writing skills nor do they provide sufficient data for assessing writing.

Other assignments such as formal papers can be used for assessing students' understanding as well as writing ability. Therefore, not all written assignments provide data for assessing writing skill, and again the teacher needs to be clear about the outcomes to be evaluated with the assignment. Many written assignments can be used in nursing courses. These include:

- Term paper
- Research paper and development of research protocol
- Literature reviews and systematic reviews

- Evidence-based practice paper in which students critique and synthesize the evidence and report on its use in clinical practice
- Paper analyzing concepts and theories and their application to clinical practice
- Paper comparing different interventions with their underlying evidence base
- Paper on how the class content compares with what the students read in their textbook and in other sources, and how it applies to patient care
- Critical analysis papers in which students analyze issues, compare different options, and develop arguments for a position
- Case study analysis with written rationale
- Journals and reflective writing assignments

For clinical courses, written assignments that accompany the clinical practicum are valuable for encouraging critical thinking and development of clinical judgment. They also provide a strategy for students to analyze ethical issues in the clinical setting and reflect on their personal experiences with patients and staff. Writing assignments such as reflective journals bridge the gap between classroom learning and clinical practice, encourage students to think about practice decisions and evaluate choices, promote self awareness and professional growth, and provide valuable feedback for faculty in identifying students having difficulty with clinical judgment and other learning needs (Langley & Brown, 2010; Lasater, 2011; Lasater & Nielsen, 2009). Short papers in clinical courses are useful in focusing an assignment on a particular learning outcome and making it easier for teachers to give prompt feedback to students (Oermann, 2006). For example, students might write a one-page paper on an alternate intervention for a patient with a rationale for its use, or prepare a short paper on an issue encountered in clinical practice and an alternate approach that could have been used.

Written assignments for clinical learning include:

- Concept map, a graphic arrangement of key concepts related to a patient's care, which includes a written description of the meaning of the interrelationships
- Concept analysis paper in which students describe a concept, its characteristics, and how it relates to care of a simulated or an actual patient situation
- Analysis of a clinical experience, the care given by the student, and alternative approaches that could have been used
- Paper that examines how readings apply to care of patient
- Short paper related to clinical practice

- Teaching plan
- Nursing care plan
- Analysis of interactions with individuals and groups in the clinical setting
- Report of observations made in clinical settings
- Journal and other reflective writing activities
- Portfolio, a collection of projects and materials that demonstrate student learning in clinical practice

In-Class and Small-Group Writing Activities

Not all written assignments need to be prepared by students individually as out-of-class work that is assessed by the teacher. In-class writing assignments provide practice in expressing ideas and an opportunity for faculty and peers to give feedback on writing. For example, students can write their thoughts about the content presented in a face-to-face class or one presented online. They can list one or two questions about the content and give the questions to other students to answer in writing or to post in a discussion board. The teacher can pose a question about how the content could be applied in a different context, and ask students to write a response to the question. In a face-to-face class, several students can volunteer or be called on to read their responses aloud, and the teacher can collect all written responses for later analysis. In an online course, students can post their individual responses for critique by other students. An activity such as this one assists students in organizing their thoughts before responding to questions raised by the teacher and others. Another option is for students to write a few paragraphs about how the content compares with their readings: What new learning did they gain from the class that was not in their readings?

As another writing activity, the teacher can give students short case studies related to the content being learned in the course. In small groups or individually, students analyze these cases, identify possible problems, and develop plans of care, and then report in a few paragraphs the results of their analysis and rationale for their plan. They also can describe in writing how the case is similar to or differs from what they learned in class or from their readings.

These short written activities are valuable at the end of a class to summarize the new content and actively involve students in learning. With any of these activities, students can "pass their writing" to peers whose task is to critique both content and writing, adding their own thoughts about the topic and assessing the writing. The teacher also can review the written work to provide feedback.

Students can work in pairs or small groups for writing assignments. For example, a small group of students can write an editorial or a letter to the editor; develop a protocol for patient care based on the content presented in the lecture and readings for class; and review, critique, and summarize research and other evidence that relates to patient care. Students also can prepare a manuscript or work through the steps in writing for publication beginning with an outline, preparing a draft, and revising the draft for a final product. These assignments among others encourage acquisition of content and development of skill in writing; they also provide experience in group writing, learning about its benefits and pitfalls.

Writing Activities for Postclinical Conferences

In postclinical conferences, students can work in pairs or in small groups to critically analyze a clinical situation, decide on alternate interventions that might be used, and then write a short paper about their discussion. They can write about their own clinical activities and document the care they provided during that clinical experience. "Pass the writing" assignments work well in clinical conferences because they encourage peers to critically analyze the content, adding their own perspectives, and to identify how writing can be improved. These assignments also actively involve students in learning, which is important during a tiring clinical practice day. Group writing exercises are effective in postclinical conferences as long as the groups are small and the exercises are carefully focused.

ASSESSING WRITTEN ASSIGNMENTS

Papers and other types of written assignments should be assessed using predetermined criteria that address quality of content; organization of ideas; and the process of arriving at decisions and, depending on the assignment, at developing an argument. Writing style should also be considered. General criteria for this purpose, which can be adapted for most written assignments, are found in Exhibit 9.1.

Scoring rubrics work well for assessing papers. A rubric is a scoring guide used for the assessment of performance. Rubrics outline the criteria to meet in the paper, or describe the characteristics of the paper and the points allotted for its assessment. The points assigned to each criterion or characteristic in the rubric should reflect its importance in the paper. A description and examples of holistic and analytic scoring rubrics were provided in Chapter 6. Rubrics should be given to students before they begin writing so

❏Exhibit 9.1

Criteria for Assessing Papers and Other Written Assignments

Content
Content is relevant.
Content is accurate.
Significant concepts and theories are presented.
Concepts and theories are used appropriately for analysis.
Content is comprehensive.
Content reflects current research and evidence.
Hypotheses, conclusions, and decisions are supported.

Organization
Content is organized logically.
Ideas are presented in logical sequence.
Paragraph structure is appropriate.
Headings are used appropriately to indicate new content areas.

Process
Process used to arrive at approaches, decisions, judgments, and so forth is adequate.
Consequences of decisions are considered and weighed.
Sound rationale is provided based on theory and research as appropriate.
For papers analyzing issues, rationale supports position taken.
Multiple perspectives and new approaches are considered.

Writing Style
Ideas are described clearly.
Sentence structure is clear.
There are no grammatical errors.
There are no spelling errors.
Appropriate punctuation is used.
Writing does not reveal bias related to gender, sexual orientation, racial or ethnic identity, or disabilities.
Length of paper is consistent with requirements.
References are cited appropriately throughout paper.
References are cited accurately according to required format.

Source: K. B. Gaberson & M. H. Oermann (2010). *Clinical teaching strategies in nursing* (3rd ed., p. 363). New York, NY: Springer Publishing Company. Copyright 2010 by Springer Publishing Company. Reprinted with permission.

they are clear about how the paper will be assessed. In this way the rubric can be viewed as an instructional guide and assessment tool (Nitko & Brookhart, 2011). An example of a rubric for scoring papers and other written assignments, based on the general criteria outlined in Exhibit 9.1, is shown in Table 9.1.

⊔Table 9.1

SAMPLE SCORING RUBRIC FOR TERM PAPERS AND OTHER WRITTEN ASSIGNMENTS

CONTENT		
Content relevant to purpose of paper, comprehensive and in depth	Content relevant to purpose of paper	Some content not relevant to purpose of paper, lacks depth
10 9 8	7 6 5 4	3 2 1
Content accurate	Most of content accurate	Major errors in content
10 9 8	7 6 5 4	3 2 1
Sound background developed from concepts, theories, and literature	Background relevant to topic but limited development	Background not developed, limited support for ideas
20–15	14–7	6–1
Current research synthesized and integrated effectively in paper	Relevant research summarized in paper	Limited research in paper, not used to support ideas
10 9 8	7 6 5 4	3 2 1

ORGANIZATION		
Purpose of paper/thesis well developed and clearly stated	Purpose/thesis apparent but not developed sufficiently	Purpose/thesis poorly developed, not clear
5	4 3 2	1
Ideas well organized and logically presented, organization supports arguments and development of ideas	Clear organization of main points and ideas	Poorly organized, ideas not developed adequately in paper
10 9 8	7 6 5 4	3 2 1
Thorough discussion of ideas, includes multiple perspectives and new approaches	Adequate discussion of ideas, some alternate perspectives considered	Discussion not thorough, lacks detail, no alternate perspectives considered
10 9 8	7 6 5 4	3 2 1
Effective conclusion and integration of ideas in summary	Adequate conclusion, summary of main ideas	Poor conclusion, no integration of ideas
5	4 3 2	1

(continued)

Table 9.1 (continued)

WRITING STYLE AND FORMAT		
Sentence structure clear, smooth transitions, correct grammar and punctuation, no spelling errors	Adequate sentence structure and transitions; few grammar, punctuation, and spelling errors	Poor sentence structure and transitions; errors in grammar, punctuation, and spelling
10 9 8	7 6 5 4	3 2 1
Professional appearance of paper, all parts included, length consistent with requirements	Paper legible, some parts missing or too short/too long considering requirements	Unprofessional appearance, missing sections, paper too short/too long considering requirements
5	4 3 2	1
References used appropriately in paper, references current, no errors in references, correct use of APA style for references	References used appropriately in paper but limited, most references current, some citations or references with errors and/or some errors in APA style for references	Few references and limited breadth, old references (not classic), errors in references, errors in APA style for references
5	4 3 2	1

Total Points _____ (sum points for total score)

Popham (2012) recommended that faculty members evaluate the quality of rubrics they have developed for their courses. Rubrics for assessing papers should meet these criteria:

1. Significance: Are the characteristics assessed in the paper important? Are the points allotted to each characteristic or criterion appropriate in relation to others in the rubric?

2. Evaluative criteria: Are the characteristics or criteria in the rubric appropriate for the written assignment considering its purpose, length, and complexity? Is the number appropriate, that is, not too few or too many? Are the characteristics or criteria labeled clearly and succinctly?

3. Quality distinctions: Are there clear descriptions of qualitative differences for each of the rubric's characteristics or criteria, enabling teachers to use the rubric as intended and consistently across student papers?

4. Usability: Will students and other educators who need to use the rubric for scoring papers understand the meaning of each characteristic or criterion and how to score it?

Consistent with other evaluation methods, written assignments may be assessed either formatively (not graded) or summatively (graded). With formative evaluation the intent is to give feedback on the quality of the content and writing so that students can further develop their writing ability. Feedback is of value only if given promptly and with enough detail for students to understand how they can improve their writing. With some assignments, such as reflective journals, only formative evaluation may be appropriate.

Many nursing faculty members are concerned about the amount of time spent giving feedback on students' technical writing errors, such as grammatical, punctuation, and spelling errors. If teachers focus entirely on assessing the quality of content of written assignments, students will not understand how their technical writing skills affect their ability to communicate relevant and important information. There is a difference between giving feedback on the quality of technical writing skills and actually correcting errors for students. One method for avoiding the latter approach on a graded assignment is to signify technical writing errors with a particular symbol such as a checkmark, or more specifically, by identifying the type of error, such as "spelling" or "sp" and then require students to make the appropriate corrections to improve their scores. Another approach is to establish a "gateway" criterion for all graded written assignments. For example, the teacher specifies that no more than five grammatical, spelling, and punctuation errors will be accepted; if a paper contains more than the specified number, the teacher stops reading and scoring the paper and returns it to the student. The student then corrects the technical errors and resubmits the paper, possibly for a lower overall score. These methods can be incorporated into any scoring rubric that a nursing faculty member develops for written assignments, as previously discussed.

Suggestions for Assessing and Grading Written Assignments

The suggestions that follow for assessing papers and other written assignments do not apply to every written assignment used in a course, as these are general recommendations to guide teachers in this process.

1. *Relate the assignments to the learning outcomes of the course.* Papers and other written assignments should be planned to meet particular learning objectives. All too often students complete papers that may have a questionable relationship to course goals.

2. *Consider the number of written assignments to be completed by students, including drafts of papers.* How many teaching plans, concept maps, research proposals, one-page papers, and so forth are needed to meet the goals of the course? Students should not complete repetitive assignments unless they are essential to meeting course goals or personal learning needs.

3. *Avoid assignments that require only summarizing the literature and substance of class and online discussions unless this is the intended purpose of the assignment.* Otherwise students merely report on their readings, often without thinking about the content and how it relates to varied clinical situations. If a review of the literature is the intended outcome, the assignment should direct students to read these articles critically and synthesize them, not merely report on each article.

4. *Include clear directions about the purpose and format of the written assignment.* The goals of the written assignment—why students are writing the paper and how it relates to the course outcomes—should be identified clearly, and generally the more detailed the directions, the better, for both students and the teacher grading the papers. If there is a particular format to be followed, the teacher should review this with students and provide a written or electronic copy for their use in preparing the paper. Students need the criteria for grading and the scoring rubric before they begin the assignment, so it is clear how the paper will be assessed.

5. *Specify the number of drafts to be submitted, each with required due dates, and provide prompt feedback on the quality of the content and writing, including specific suggestions about revisions.* These drafts are a significant component of formal papers because the intent is to improve thinking and writing through them. Drafts in most instances are used as a means of providing feedback to students and should not be graded.

6. *Develop specific criteria for assessment and review these with the students prior to their beginning the assignment.* The criteria should relate to the quality of the content; organization of content; process of developing ideas and arguments; and elements of writing style such as clarity of expression, sentence structure, punctuation, grammar, spelling, length of the paper, and accuracy and format of the references. Table 9.2 offers a checklist that teachers can use in assessing writing structure and style. Other criteria would be specific to the outcomes to be met through the assignment. If a scoring rubric is used, it should be shared and discussed with the students before they begin the paper.

7. *For papers dealing with analysis of issues, focus the assessment and criteria on the rationale developed for the position taken rather than the actual position.* This type of assignment is particularly appropriate as a group activity in which students critique each other's work.

8. *Read all papers and written assignments anonymously.* The rationale for this is the same as with essay testing—the teacher needs to remove potential bias from the assessment process. Reading papers anonymously helps avoid the chance of a carryover effect in which the teacher develops an impression of the quality of a student's work, for example, from prior papers, tests, or clinical practice, and is then influenced by that impression when grading other assignments. By grading papers anonymously, the teacher also avoids a halo effect.

❑Table 9.2

CHECKLIST FOR WRITING STRUCTURE AND STYLE

✓ Content organized clearly
✓ Each paragraph focuses on one topic and presents details about it
✓ Clear sequence of ideas developed within and between paragraphs
✓ Clear transitions between paragraphs
✓ First sentence of paragraph introduces subject and provides transition from preceding paragraph
✓ Paragraphs are of appropriate length
✓ Sentences clearly written and convey intended meaning
✓ Sentences are of appropriate length
✓ Clear transitions between sentences within paragraphs
✓ Words express intended meaning and used correctly
✓ Subjects and verbs agree in each sentence
✓ Clear antecedents for pronouns
✓ No misplaced modifiers
✓ Excessive and unnecessary words omitted
✓ Stereotypes, impersonal writing, jargon, and abbreviated terms avoided
✓ Active voice used
✓ Grammar: Correct?
✓ Punctuation: Correct?
✓ Capitalization: Correct?
✓ Spelling: Correct?
✓ Writing keeps reader's interest
✓ References used appropriately in paper
✓ References current
✓ No errors in references
✓ Correct use of APA or other style for references

Source: Adapted from M. H. Oermann & J. C. Hays (2011). *Writing for publication in nursing* (2nd ed., p. 251). New York, NY: Springer Publishing Company. Copyright 2011 by Springer Publishing Company. Adapted with permission.

9. *Skim a random sample of papers to gain an overview of how the students approached the topic of the paper, developed their ideas, and addressed other aspects of the paper that would be graded.* In some instances the assessment criteria and scoring rubric might be modified, for example, if no students included a particular content area that was reflected in the grading criteria.

10. *Read papers in random order.* Papers read first in the group may be scored higher than those read at the end. To avoid any bias resulting from the order of the papers, it is best to read papers in a random order instead of always organizing papers in the same way (e.g., alphabetical) before reading them. The teacher also should take frequent breaks from grading papers to keep focused on the criteria for evaluation and avoid fatigue, which could influence scoring papers near the end.

11. *Read each paper twice before scoring.* In the first reading, the teacher can note omissions of and errors in content, problems with organization and development of ideas, issues with the process used for developing the paper, and writing style concerns. Comments and suggestions can be recorded on sticky notes or in pencil in case they need to be modified once the paper is read in its entirety. If papers are submitted electronically, the teacher can insert comments and suggestions in the paper using the "track changes" or "comments" tools, or by using different-colored highlighting, making it easy to identify the remarks.

12. *If unsure about the assessment of a paper, have a colleague also read and evaluate the paper.* The second reader should review the paper anonymously, without knowledge of the grade given by the original teacher, and without information about the reason for the additional review. Scores can be averaged, or the teacher might decide to read the paper again depending on the situation. An additional reader also might be used if the grade on the paper will determine whether the student passes the course and progresses in the program. In decisions such as these, it is helpful to obtain a "second opinion" about the quality of the paper.

13. *Consider incorporating student self-critique, peer critique, and group writing exercises within the sequence of writing assignments.* These experiences help students improve ability to assess their own writing: they can "step back" and reflect on their papers, identify where their ideas may not be communicated clearly, and decide on revisions. Students should be encouraged to ask peers to review and critique their work, similar to asking colleagues to review manuscripts and reports. Group-writing activities prepare students for working collaboratively to produce a product, which is similar to nursing practice in real clinical settings and to writing a manuscript as a group.

14. *Prepare students for written assignments by incorporating learning activities in the course, completed in and out of class.* These activities provide practice in organizing and expressing ideas in writing.

SUMMARY

Through formal papers, students develop an understanding of the content they are writing about and improve their ability to communicate their ideas in writing. With this type of written assignment, students can analyze and integrate the literature and report on their findings, analyze theories and how they apply to nursing practice, improve their thinking skills, and learn how to write more effectively. To improve their writing abilities, though, students need to complete drafts and rewrites on which they get prompt feedback from the teacher on both content and writing.

There are many types of papers and written assignments that students can complete individually or in small groups in a nursing course. Written assignments should be assessed using predetermined criteria that address quality of content, organization of ideas, the process of arriving at decisions and developing arguments, and writing style. General criteria for evaluating papers, an example of a scoring rubric, and suggestions for assessing and grading written assignments were provided in the chapter.

REFERENCES

American Association of Colleges of Nursing. (2006). *The essentials of doctoral education for advanced nursing practice.* Washington, DC: Author.

American Association of Colleges of Nursing. (2008). *The essentials of baccalaureate education for professional nursing practice.* Washington, DC: Author.

American Association of Colleges of Nursing. (2011). *The essentials of master's education in nursing.* Washington, DC: Author.

American Psychological Association. (2010). *Publication manual of the American Psychological Association* (6th ed.). Washington DC: Author.

Collier, J. (2010). Wiki technology in the classroom: Building collaboration skills. *Journal of Nursing Education, 49,* 718.

Gaberson, K. B., & Oermann, M. H. (2010). *Clinical teaching strategies in nursing* (3rd ed.). New York, NY: Springer Publishing.

Langley, M., & Brown, S. (2010). Perceptions of the use of reflective learning journals in online graduate nursing education. *Nursing Education Perspectives, 31,* 12–17.

Lasater, K. (2011). Clinical judgment: The last frontier for evaluation. *Nurse Education in Practice, 11,* 86–92.

Lasater, K., & Nielsen, A. (2009). Reflective journaling for development of clinical judgment. *Journal of Nursing Education, 48,* 40–44.

Luthy, K. E., Peterson, N. E., Lassetter, J. H., & Callister, L. C. (2009). Successfully incorporating writing across the curriculum with advanced writing in nursing. *Journal of Nursing Education, 48,* 54–59.

McMillan, L., & Raines, K. (2010). Headed in the 'write' direction: Nursing student publication and health promotion in the community. *Journal of Nursing Education, 49,* 418–421.

Nitko, A. J., & Brookhart, S. M. (2011). *Educational assessment of students* (6th ed.). Upper Saddle River, NJ: Pearson.

Oermann, M. H. (2006). Short written assignments for clinical nursing courses. *Nurse Educator, 31,* 228–231.

Oermann, M. H. (2010). Writing for publication in nursing: What every nurse educator needs to know. In L. Caputi (Ed.), *Teaching nursing: The art and science* (2nd ed., pp. 146–166). Glen Ellyn, IL: College of DuPage.

Oermann, M. H., & Hays, J. (2011). *Writing for publication in nursing* (2nd ed.). New York, NY: Springer Publishing.

Oermann, M. H. (in press). Enhancing writing in online education. In K. H. Frith & D. Clark (Eds.), *Distance education in nursing* (3rd ed.). New York, NY: Springer Publishing.

Popham, W. J. (2012). *The role of rubrics in testing and teaching* (2nd ed.). Upper Saddle River, NJ: Pearson.

The Writing across the Curriculum Clearinghouse. (2011a). What is writing in the disciplines? Retrieved from http://wac.colostate.edu/intro/pop2e.cfm

The Writing across the Curriculum Clearinghouse. (2011b). What is writing to learn? Retrieved from http://wac.colostate.edu/intro/pop2d.cfm

PART III

Elements of Test Construction,

Administration, and Analysis

TEN

Assembling and

Administering Tests

In addition to the preparation of a test blueprint and the skillful construction of test items that correspond to it, the final appearance of the test and the way in which it is administered can affect the validity of the test results. A haphazard arrangement of test items, directions that are confusing, and typographical and other errors on the test may contribute to measurement error. By following certain design rules, teachers can avoid such errors when assembling a test. Administering a test usually is the simplest phase of the testing process. There are some common problems associated with test administration, however, that also may affect the reliability of the resulting test scores and consequently the validity of inferences made about those scores. Careful planning can help the teacher avoid or minimize such difficulties. This chapter discusses the process of assembling the test and administering it to students.

TEST DESIGN RULES

Allow Enough Time

As discussed in Chapter 3, preparing a high-quality test requires time for the design phases as well as for the item-writing phase. Assembling the test is not simply a clerical or technical task; the teacher should make all decisions about the arrangement of test elements and the final appearance of the test even if someone else types or reproduces the test. The teacher must allow enough time for this phase to avoid errors that could affect the students' test scores.

Arrange Test Items in a Logical Sequence

Various methods for arranging items on the test have been recommended, including by order of difficulty and according to the sequence in which the content was taught. However, if the test contains items of two or more formats, the teacher should first group items of the same format together. Because each item format requires different tasks of the student, this type of arrangement makes it easier for students to maintain the mental set required to answer each type of item, and prevents errors caused by frequent changing of tasks. Keeping items of the same format together also requires fewer sets of directions and facilitates scoring if a scannable answer sheet is not used (Miller, Linn, & Gronlund, 2009). Miller et al. (2009) recommended arranging sections of item types in the following order, from simplest to most complex:

1. True–false items
2. Matching exercises
3. Short-answer or completion items
4. Multiple-choice items
5. Context-dependent or interpretive exercises
6. Restricted-response essay items
7. Extended-response essay items (p. 341)

Constructing a test with all of the above-listed item types is not recommended, even for a test with a large sample of items administered to a highly skilled group of learners. The longer the test, the more item formats can be included, but complex formats require more reading and processing time for the student, so they should be combined with only one or two other types.

Next, within each item format, items may be arranged according to the order in which the content was taught, which may assist students in recalling information more easily. Finally, combining the item format and content-sequence grouping, teachers should arrange items in order of increasing difficulty. Even well-prepared students are likely to be somewhat anxious at the beginning of a test, and encountering difficult items may increase their anxiety and interfere with their optimum performance. Beginning with easier items may build the students' confidence and allow them to answer these items quickly and reserve more time for difficult items. By having confidence in their ability to answer the beginning items correctly, students may have less anxiety about the remainder of the test (Gronlund, 2006; Miller et al., 2009).

Write Directions

The teacher cannot assume that the students know the basis on which they are to select or provide answers or how and where to record their answers to test items. Depending on the level of students and their familiarity with the type of items and assessment procedures, it is not reasonable to expect that the assessment will be self-explanatory. This is especially true with students who are non-native English speakers or for those whose primary and secondary education occurred in countries where objectively scored item formats are less common.

The test should begin with a set of clear general directions. These general directions should include instructions on:

- How and where to record responses
- What type of writing implement to use
- Whether or not students may write on the test booklet
- The amount of time allowed
- The number of pages and items on the exam
- The types and point values of items
- Whether students may ask questions during the test
- What to do after finishing the exam (Gronlund, 2006; Miller et al., 2009; Nitko & Brookhart, 2011)

Students may need to know some of these instructions while they are preparing for the test, such as whether their answers to items requiring them to supply the names of medications must be spelled accurately to be scored as correct.

Each section consisting of a particular item format should begin with specific instructions. For multiple-choice items, the student needs to know whether to select the *correct* or *best* response. Directions for completion and essay items should state whether spelling, grammar, punctuation, and organization will be considered in scoring, and the length of the desired response. For computation items, directions should specify the degree of precision required, the unit of measure, whether to show the calculation work, and what method of computation to use if there is more than one option (Miller et al., 2009). Matching exercise directions should clearly specify the basis on which the match is to be made (Gronlund, 2006). An example is: "For each definition in Column A, select the proper term in Column B. Use each letter in Column B only once or not at all."

Use a Cover Page

The general test directions may be printed on a cover page (Exhibit 10.1). A cover page also serves to keep the test items hidden from view during the distribution of the exam so that the first students to receive the test will not have more time to complete it than students who receive their copies

☐Exhibit 10.1

Example of a Cover Page With General Directions

Exam Number _____

BEHAVIORAL HEALTH NURSING FINAL EXAM

Directions

1. This test comprises 12 pages. Please check your test booklet to make sure you have the correct number of pages in the proper sequence.

2. Parts I and II contain 86 multiple-choice and matching items. You may write on the test booklet but **you must record your answers to these items on your answer sheet.** This part of the test will be machine-scored; read carefully and follow the instructions below:

   a. Use a #2 pencil.

   b. Notice that the items on the answer sheet are numbered **DOWN** the page in each column.

   c. Choose the **ONE BEST** response to each item. Items with multiple answer marks will be counted as incorrect. Fill in the circle completely; if you change your answer, erase your first answer thoroughly.

   d. Print your name (last name, first name) in the blocks provided, then completely fill in the corresponding circle in each column. If you wish to have your score posted, fill in an identification number of up to 9 digits (**DO NOT** use your Social Security Number) and fill in the corresponding circle in each column.

   e. Above your name, write your test booklet number.

3. Part III consists of two essay items. Directions for this section are found on page 12. Write your answers to these items on the lined paper provided. You may use pen or pencil. On each page of your answers, write your **TEST BOOKLET NUMBER. DO NOT** write your name on these pages.

4. If you have a question during the test, do not leave your seat—raise your hand and a proctor will come to you.

5. You have until 11:00 a.m. to complete this test.

---

later. If the directions on the cover page indicate the number of pages and items, the students can quickly check their test booklets for completeness and correct sequence of pages. The teacher can then replace defective test booklets before students begin answering items.

When a separate answer sheet is used, the cover page may be numbered to help maintain test security; students are directed to record this number in a particular place on the answer sheet. With this system, the teacher can track any missing test booklets after the test is done. Additionally, if the teacher asks students to record responses to short-answer or essay items directly on the test booklet, those answers can be scored anonymously; the score from the answer sheet then can be added to the score from the supply-type items for a total test score that is associated with each student's name.

Avoid Crowding

Test items are difficult to read when they are crowded together on the page; learning-disabled students and non-native English speakers may find crowding particularly trying. Techniques that allow students to read efficiently and to prevent errors in recording their responses include leaving sufficient white space within and between items and indenting certain elements. Teachers should allow enough blank space between and around items so that each item is distinct from the others. If not, the students might inadvertently read a line from a preceding or following item and think it belongs to the item they are answering. Tightly packing words on a page may minimize the amount of paper used for testing, but facilitating maximum student performance on a test is worth a small additional expense for a few more sheets of paper (Miller et al., 2009).

Optimum spacing varies for each item format. The response options for a multiple-choice item should not be printed in tandem fashion, as the following example illustrates:

1. Which method of anesthesia involves injection of an agent into a nerve bundle that supplies the operative site? A. General; B. Local; C. Regional; D. Spinal; E. Topical

The options are much easier to read if listed in a single column below the stem (Miller et al., 2009), as in this example:

1. Which method of anesthesia involves injection of an agent into a nerve bundle that supplies the operative site?

   A. General
   B. Local
   C. Regional
   D. Spinal
   E. Topical

Notice in this example that the second line of the stem is indented to the same position as the first line and that the responses are slightly indented. This spacing makes the item number and its content easier to read.

Keep Related Material Together

The stem of a multiple-choice item and all related responses should appear on the same page. Both columns of a matching exercise should also be printed side by side and on one page, including the related directions; using short lists of premises and responses makes this arrangement easier. With context-dependent and interpretive exercises, the introductory material and all related items should be contained on the same page, if possible. This facilitates reading the material and related questions (Gronlund, 2006; Miller et al., 2009).

Facilitate Scoring

If the test will be scored by hand, the layout of the test or the answer sheet should facilitate easy scoring. A separate answer sheet can be constructed to permit rapid scoring by comparing student responses to an answer key. If the students record their answers directly on the test booklet, the test items should be arranged with scoring in mind. For example, a series of true–false items should be organized with columns of Ts and Fs, preferably at the left margin (Gronlund, 2006; Miller et al., 2009) so that students need only circle their responses, as in the following example:

> T   F   1. A stethoscope is required to perform auscultation.
> T   F   2. Physical exam techniques should be performed in the order of least to most intrusive.
> T   F   3. When using percussion, it is easier to detect a change from dullness to resonance.

Circling a letter rather than writing or printing it will prevent misinterpretation of the students' handwriting. With completion items, printing blank spaces for the answers in tandem, as in the following example, makes scoring difficult:

> 1. List three responsibilities of the circulating nurse during induction of general anesthesia.
>
> _____   _____   _____

Instead, the blanks should be arranged in a column along one side of the page, preferably on the left, as in this example:

> 1. _____   1–3. List three responsibilities of the
> 2. _____   circulating nurse during induction of
> 3. _____   general anesthesia.

Arrange the Correct Answers in a Random Pattern

Many teachers have a tendency to favor certain response positions for the correct or keyed answer to objective test items, for example, to assign the correct response to the A or D position of a multiple-choice item. Some teachers arrange test items so that the correct answers form a pattern that makes scoring easy (e.g., T-F-T-F or A-B-C-D). Students who detect a pattern of correct answers (e.g., the correct answer never appears in the same position two or more consecutive times) may use this information to obtain higher test scores than their knowledge would warrant (Gronlund, 2006).

Many item analysis software programs calculate the number of times the keyed response occurs in each position. While reviewing these reports, teachers may determine if the correct answer positions occur in approximately equal numbers, keeping in mind that multiple-choice, true–false, and matching items may have differing numbers of response options. While these reports would not be available until after the test is administered and scored, they could alert teachers to use a different technique to more evenly distribute the correct answer position if the test (in its entirety or with minor item revisions) is used again. The teacher also can tally the number of Ts and Fs, or As, Bs, Cs, and Ds on the answer key by hand. For true–false items, if either true or false statements are found to predominate, some items may be rewritten to make the distribution more equal (although it is recommended by some experts to include more false than true items).

Gronlund (2006) recommended that the position of the correct response in multiple-choice items be randomly assigned. One method for obtaining a random order is to place all responses to multiple-choice items and all premises and responses in a matching exercise in alphabetical order by the first letter in each, as described below.

Arrange Options in Logical or Numerical Order

The response alternatives for multiple-choice items and the premises and responses of a matching exercise should be arranged according to a logical or meaningful order, such as alphabetical or chronological order, or in order of size or degree. This type of arrangement reduces reading time and helps students who know the correct answer to search though the options to find it. This strategy also tends to randomly distribute the correct answer position as discussed above, especially on lengthy tests. When the options are numbers, they should always be in numerical order, preferably ascending (Gronlund, 2006). This principle can be seen in the example shown in Exhibit 10.2.

❏Exhibit 10.2

Arrangement of Options: Not Ordered Versus Ordered Numerically

Options Not Ordered	*Options in Numerical Order*
Your patient is ordered guiaifenesin 300 mg four times daily. It comes 200 mg/5 mL. How many milliliters should you give per dose?	Your patient is ordered guaifenesin 300 mg four times daily. It comes 200 mg/5 mL. How many milliliters should you give per dose?
a. 5.0 mL	a. 2.5 mL
b. 2.5 mL.	b. 5.0 mL
c. 10 mL	c. 7.5 mL*
d. 7.5 mL*	d. 10 mL

Number the Items Consecutively Throughout the Test

Although test items should be grouped according to format, they should be numbered consecutively throughout the test. That is, the teacher should not start each new item format section with item number 1 but continue numbering items in continuous sequence. This numbering system helps students to find items they may have skipped and to avoid making errors when recording their answers, especially when using a separate answer sheet.

Proofread

The goal throughout the preparation and use of assessments is to obtain valid evidence that students have met learning goals. Although validity is a major focus of the planning for a test (e.g., through use of a test blueprint), careful assembly and administration of the test will assure that it will function as intended (Miller et al., 2009).

The test items and directions should be free of spelling, punctuation, grammatical, and typing errors. Such defects are a source of measurement error and can cause confusion and distraction, particularly among students who are anxious (Haladyna, 2004). Typographical and similar errors are a problem for any student but more so for non-native English speakers or those who have learning disabilities. Often the test designer does not recognize his or her own errors; another teacher who knows the content may be asked to proofread a copy of the test before it is duplicated. The spell-check or grammar-check features of a word processing program may not recognize punctuation errors or words that are spelled correctly but used in the wrong context, and they may not always detect structural errors such as giving two test items the same number or two responses the same letter.

---

*Correct answer.

Prepare an Answer Key

Whether the test will be machine-scored or hand-scored, the teacher should prepare and verify an answer key in advance to facilitate efficient scoring and to provide a final check on the accuracy of the test items. Scannable answer sheets also can be used for hand-scoring; an answer key can be produced by punching holes to indicate the correct answers. The teacher also should prepare ideal responses to essay items, identify intended responses to completion items, and prepare scoring rubrics if the analytical scoring method is used.

REPRODUCING THE TEST

Assure Legibility

Legibility is an important consideration when printing and duplicating the test; poor-quality copies may interfere with optimum student performance. A font that includes only upper-case letters is difficult to read; upper- and lower-case lettering is recommended. The master or original copy should be letter-quality, produced with a laser or other high-quality printer so that it can be clearly reproduced. For best results, the test should be photocopied or printed on a machine that has sufficient toner to produce crisp, dark print without any stray lines or artifacts.

Print on One Side of the Page

The test should be reproduced on only one side of each sheet of paper. Printing on both sides of each page could cause students to skip items unintentionally or make errors when recording their scores on a separate answer sheet. It also creates distractions from excessive page-turning during the test. If the test is to be hand-scored and students record their answers on the test rather than on a separate answer sheet, printing only on one side makes it easier to score.

Reproduce Enough Copies

The teacher should duplicate more test copies than the number of students to allow for extra copies for proctors or to replace defective copies that may have been inadvertently distributed to students. Displaying test items on a screen from a projector, or writing them on the chalkboard or interactive whiteboard, may save costs or the teacher's preparation time, but these procedures may cause problems for students with learning or visual disabilities. When students do not have their own copies of a test for whatever reason, they cannot control the pace at which they answer items or return to a previous item. Dictating test items is not recommended except when the objective is to test knowledge of correct spelling; in addition to creating problems for students with hearing impairments, this method wastes time that students could otherwise spend in thinking about and responding to the items. In addition, there is no record of how the items were worded, which could present a problem if a student later questions how an answer was scored.

Maintain Test Security

Teachers have a serious responsibility to maintain the security of tests by protecting them from unauthorized access. Carelessness on the part of the teacher can enable dishonest students to gain access to test materials and use them to obtain higher scores than they deserve. This contributes to measurement error, and it is unfair to honest students who are well-prepared for the test. It is up to the teacher to make arrangements to secure the test while it is being prepared, reproduced, stored, administered, and scored.

Test materials should be stored in locked areas accessible only to authorized personnel. Computer files that contain test items should be protected with passwords, encryption, or similar security devices. Only regular employees should handle test materials; student employees should not be asked to type, print, or reproduce tests. While test items are being typed, they should be protected from the view of others by turning the monitor off if an unauthorized individual enters the area. Printed drafts of tests should be destroyed by shredding pages rather than discarding them in trash or recycling receptacles.

One suggestion for preventing cheating during test administration to large groups is to prepare alternative forms of the test. This can be done by presenting the same questions but in a different order on each form. For calculation items the teacher can modify values within the same question on different forms; in that way the responses will not be identical. Faculty members can prepare alternative forms of the test for students to complete online. Software is also available that allows for random sequencing of items on an online exam. The problem with this technique is that a random sequence may not be consistent with principles for ordering items on a test. It also may result in alternative forms of a test that are not equivalent.

Similarly, the order of responses to multiple-choice and matching items might be scrambled to produce an alternative form of the test. However, the psychometric properties of alternative forms produced in these ways might be sufficiently different as to result in different scores, especially when the positions of items with unequal difficulty are switched. If there is little or no evidence for the true equivalence of these alternative forms, it is best not to use this approach. Other ways to prevent cheating are discussed in the next section of this chapter.

TEST ADMINISTRATION

Environmental Conditions

The environmental conditions of test administration can be a source of measurement error if they interfere with the students' performance. If possible, the teacher should select a room that limits potential distractions during the test. For example, if windows must be open for ventilation during warm weather, the students may be distracted by lawn mowing or construction noise; requesting a room on another side of the building for testing may prevent the problem. Placing a sign such as "Testing— Quiet Please" on the door of the classroom may reduce noise in the hallway (Miller et al., 2009).

For online courses, it is critical to determine prior to the test administration that students have the computer capabilities and Internet access to take the exam for the time period allotted. Students with dial-up modems may experience "timing out," which means being disconnected from the Internet by their Internet Service Providers after a set period of time or what appears to be inactivity on the part of the user. When that occurs, the students cannot transmit their completed exams, and course management systems may not permit them to access another copy. A more extensive discussion of effective approaches to online testing can be found in Chapter 11.

Distributing the Test Materials

Careful organization allows the teacher to distribute test materials and give instructions to the students efficiently. With large groups of students, several proctors may be needed to assist with this process. If a separate answer sheet is used, it usually can be distributed first, followed by the test booklets. During distribution of the test booklets, the teacher should instruct students not to turn over the test booklet and begin the test until told to do so. At this point, the students should check their test booklets for completeness, and the proctors should replace defective booklets. The teacher then should read the general directions aloud while the students read along. Hearing the directions may help non-native English speakers, students with learning disabilities, and students whose anxiety may interfere with their comprehension of the written instructions. Once the teacher answers any general questions about the test procedures, the students can begin the test.

However, do not take any more time than necessary before allowing students to begin the test. Extended remarks and instructions may interfere with students' mental set for the test, increase students' anxiety, and possibly create hostility toward the teacher (Miller et al., 2009).

Answering Questions During the Test

Some students may find it necessary to ask questions of the teacher during a test, but responding to these questions is always somewhat disturbing to other students. Also, by responding to student questions during a test, a proctor may inadvertently give hints to the correct answer, which would put that student at an advantage while not making the same information available to other students (Miller et al., 2009). However, it is not appropriate to refuse to allow questions during a test. One of the teacher's responsibilities to administer a test professionally is to provide "reasonable opportunities for individuals to ask questions about the assessment procedures or directions prior to and at appropriate times during administration" (National Council on Measurement in Education, 1995, p. 6). If a student asks a question that the proctor cannot answer, the student may be instructed to record the question on a separate piece of paper identified with the student's name; questions can be collected with the other test materials. Then if a student identifies a flaw in a test item, the teacher can take the necessary action after the test is completed rather than interrupt the test to announce corrections. Chapter 12 includes a discussion of how to adjust test scores if an item is found to be fatally flawed.

While answering student questions during the test, distraction can be kept to a minimum by telling students to raise their hands if they have questions rather than leaving their seats to approach the teacher; a proctor then goes to the student's seat. Proctors should answer questions as quietly and briefly as possible. In answering questions, proctors certainly should address errors in the test copy and ambiguity in directions but should avoid giving clues to the correct answers. When writing items, teachers should work to eliminate cultural bias and terms that would be unfamiliar to non-native English speakers. This is discussed further in Chapter 15.

Preventing Cheating

Cheating is widely believed to be common on college campuses in the United States. Nitko and Brookhart (2011) suggested that when teachers know their students, interact with them about their learning, and give meaningful assignments, they create an environment in which cheating is less likely to occur.

Cheating is defined as any activity whose purpose is to gain a higher score on a test or other academic assignment than a student is likely to earn on the basis of achievement. Traditional forms of cheating on a test include but are not limited to the following:

- Acquiring test materials in advance of the test or sharing materials with others
- Arranging for a substitute to take a test
- Preparing and using unauthorized notes or other resources during the test
- Exchanging information with others or copying answers from another student during the test
- Copying test items or retaining test materials to share with others who may take the test later

In addition to the low-technology forms of cheating on a test such as writing on body parts, clothing (e.g., the underside of the bill of a cap, the inside of a sleeve or waistband), or belongings (e.g., backpack, jewelry, facial tissue) and copying answers from others, technological advances have created many new, more sophisticated methods. For example, students with cell phones (especially smartphones) can "beam" information to other students or solicit help from them via text messaging, instant messaging, email, and camera. Cell phones and other "smart" devices are easily concealed by students under desk tops or in baggy clothing. The widespread use of Bluetooth technology makes this practice even easier. Students with iPods can listen to pre-recorded content related to the domain being tested—a sort of auditory cheat sheet. Teachers who allow students to use hand-held devices during a test to access tools helpful in solving problems (e.g., calculators for solving medication dosage calculation problems) must be especially vigilant. The faculty member should fully understand the functions of such devices to curb such practices as pre-programming and multiple screens that can be minimized (Hulsart & McCarthy, 2009).

With adequate test security and good proctoring during the test, the teacher usually can prevent these opportunities for cheating. Students who do act honestly resent those who cheat, especially if dishonest students are rewarded with high test scores. Honest students also resent faculty members who do not recognize and deal effectively with cheating.

Because of the widespread and growing use of technological aids to cheating, teachers should consider instituting standard procedures to be followed during all tests, especially if testing large groups of students. Included in these procedures may be conditions such as the following:

- No personal belongings may be brought into the testing room other than a writing implement. Backpacks; books; papers; cell phones, pagers, and other hand-held devices; purses; briefcases; tissues; candy or cough drops; beverage bottles or cups; "lucky charms"; and so forth, must be left outside the classroom.
- Outerwear such as coats, jackets, and caps with a bill or brim may not be worn.
- Sunglasses or visors may not be worn.
- Earplugs or earbuds may not be worn. If students wish to use earplugs to block environmental noise during tests, they should inform the teacher in advance, and the teacher may supply inexpensive, disposable ones.
- The teacher may provide a supply of scratch paper to be used during the test and submitted with other test materials before students leave the testing room.
- The teacher may provide a supply of tissues and extra writing implements to be used if needed during the test.
- Bathroom breaks during the test may be prohibited or limited, depending on the testing time allowed. Students may need to be accompanied to rest rooms by proctors, who may search rest rooms for hidden devices and print resources before students are permitted to use them.
- Students will occupy every other seat in a row, directly behind students in the row in front of them.
- Students must keep test materials on the desk or table in full view of the proctors and not spread out over a large area. If a student must leave the testing room for any reason, all test materials should be turned face-down during the student's absence.
- If the use of calculators is permitted during exams, the faculty may purchase the necessary quantity of an inexpensive model with limited functionality to be distributed and collected with the test materials.
- Students may not leave their seats without permission until they have completed the test and are submitting their test materials.

While some of these measures may appear extreme, many of them are variations of the test conditions under which graduates of the nursing education program will take the National Council Licensure Examination or certification examinations. Students may benefit from becoming accustomed to taking tests under these conditions. Teachers should decide which, if any, of these suggestions are appropriate for use in their particular circumstances.

Although a number of methods for preventing cheating during a test have been proposed, the single most effective method is careful proctoring. There should be enough proctors to supervise students adequately during exams; for most groups of students, at least two proctors are suggested so that one is available to leave the room with a student in case of emergency without leaving the remaining students unsupervised. When proctoring a test, it is important to be serious about the task and devote full attention to it rather than grading papers, checking email and other messages, or reading. If more than one proctor is available, they should locate themselves at different places in the room to observe students from different vantage points. Proctors should avoid walking around the room unless in response to a student's raised hand; such walking can be distracting, especially to students with test anxiety.

A particularly troubling situation for teachers is how to deal with a student's behavior that suggests cheating during a test. Prior to administering the test, the teacher must know the policies of the nursing program and college or university regarding cheating on an examination or another assessment. If a teacher is certain that a student is cheating, the teacher should quietly collect the test and answer sheet and ask the student to leave the room. However, if it is possible that the teacher's interpretation of the behavior is incorrect, it may be best not to confront the student at that time. In addition to preventing a potentially innocent student from completing the test, confiscating test materials and ordering a student to leave will create a distraction to other students that may affect the accuracy of all the students' test scores. A better response is to continue to observe the student, making eye contact if possible to make the student aware of the teacher's attention. If the student was attempting to cheat, this approach usually effectively stops the behavior. If the behavior continues, the teacher should attempt to verify this observation with another proctor, and if both agree, the student may be asked to leave the room.

While many testing experts would argue that the appropriate penalty for cheating on a test is a score of zero for that test, Nitko and Brookhart (2011) referred to this approach as "the deadly zero" (p. 333). Depending on the number of components that contribute to the course grade and the relative weight of each, a test score of zero as a consequence of cheating may result in a failing grade for the course. (See Chapter 17 for a more comprehensive discussion of grading components.) However, simply deducting a pre-determined number of points from the test score suggests that the low score represents the offending student's true level of achievement, which is not the case. Nitko and Brookhart discussed several strategies for computing a course grade when one component was missing (an assignment that was not submitted); in one of the strategies, the teacher assigns the highest possible failing score according to the grading scale in use instead of a zero, which tends to have a less devastating effect on the course grade. Although their recommendations were made in the context of a missing assignment, the same principles might be applied to the question of an appropriate sanction for cheating on a test. Whatever strategy teachers choose as a sanction for cheating on a test, they are using grades to control students' behavior by lowering a score that is meant to indicate achievement "for behavior that is unrelated to achievement" (Nitko & Brookhart, 2011, p. 333). The sanction for cheating on a test should be specified in an academic honesty policy that is consistent with that of the parent institution, and students should be informed of the policy before it is enforced.

If the teacher learns that a copy of a test is circulating in advance of the scheduled date of administration, the teacher should attempt to obtain verifiable evidence that some students have seen it. In this case, the teacher needs to prepare another test or develop an alternative way of assessing student learning. As described in this book, there are many assessment strategies applicable for measuring learning outcomes in nursing.

Online Testing

As more courses and programs are offered through distance education, teachers are faced with how to prevent cheating on an assessment when they cannot directly observe the students. Various approaches can be used, ranging from administering the tests in a proctored computer testing center to high-technology solutions such as remote proctoring. A more extensive discussion of this topic can be found in Chapter 11.

Collecting Test Materials

For traditional on-site tests, when students are finished with the test and are preparing to leave the room, the resulting confusion and noise can disturb students who are still working. The teacher should plan for efficient collection of test materials to minimize such distractions and to maintain test security. It is important to be certain that no test materials leave the room with the students. Therefore, teachers should take care to verify that the students turn in their test booklets, answer sheets, scratch paper, and any other test materials. With a large group of students, one proctor may be assigned the task of collecting test materials from each student; this proctor should check the test booklet and answer sheet to assure that the directions for marking answers were followed, that the student's name (or number) is recorded as directed, and that the student has not omitted any items. Any such errors can then be corrected before the student leaves the room, and test security will not be compromised.

If students are still working near the end of the allotted testing time, the remaining amount of time should be announced, and they should be encouraged to finish as quickly as possible. When the time is up, all students must stop, and the teacher or proctor must collect the rest of the tests. Students who have not finished the test at that point cannot have additional time unless they have qualified learning disabilities. In those cases, the testing time may be extended if the student's learning disability has been confirmed according to college or university policies. This decision should be made in advance of the test and the necessary arrangements made. Extended testing time is not an appropriate remedy for every learning disability, however. It should be provided only when specifically prescribed based on a psychoeducational evaluation of a student's abilities and needs. Chapter 15 includes additional discussion of accommodations for students with disabilities.

Collaborative Testing

Collaborative testing, an assessment method in which pairs or small groups of students work together during summative assessments, is gaining support from both teachers and students at all educational levels. There are a number of methods of collaborative testing, but most involve students taking the same test twice: once individually, and then after submitting their answer sheets, the second time in small groups to discuss the test items and then retake the test. In most cases, pairs or small groups are randomly assigned at the time of the test. The manner of re-testing varies; in some methods, the dyads or small groups discuss the test items but submit separate answer sheets, resulting in individual scores. In this procedure, students are not required to answer on the basis of group consensus or vote on the answer to each item, but instead record their own answers after the discussion. Teachers may record the sum or mean scores of the two individual tests. In other methods, the pairs or groups discuss the test items until they reach consensus on the answers, and one answer sheet is submitted for the pair or group. Each student's total score for the two tests is then determined by the sum or mean of the individual and the group scores.

Studies of collaborative testing in chiropractic and nursing education programs have demonstrated better performance in the collaborative testing groups and student preference for collaborative testing. In both research and anecdotal reports, students have consistently reported positive perceptions of collaborative testing, including decreased test anxiety, improved thinking skills, and increased motivation. By encouraging students to participate as active learners, collaborative testing may support positive attitudes about the importance of course content, enhance depth of learning, and improve higher-level thinking skills (Meseke, Nafziger, & Meseke, 2010; Sandahl, 2010). However, reported effects of collaborative testing on longer-term knowledge retention have not been consistent, and results may vary according to the cognitive level being measured by the test, with students performing better on collaborative tests with relatively low-level items. One explanation offered for students' dislike of higher cognitive level items on collaborative tests is the difficulty of reaching consensus about the correct answers, and students' individual answers on the re-test did not always correlate with the answer recommended by the group after discussion. Students also have reported that lower-level items did not enhance their critical thinking skills because the group was able to reach consensus quickly without much discussion (Meseke et al., 2010; Sandahl, 2010). Collaborative testing apparently benefits both low- and high-performing students, but low performers have shown significantly higher group test than individual test scores. Students involved with collaborative testing have reported studying no more than they would have normally but demonstrated better overall course performance as compared to students involved in traditional solo testing (Meseke et al., 2010).

Despite the reported benefits of collaborative testing, students in some studies have reported concern that their unprepared classmates may have earned higher exam scores than they deserved. It has been noted that some individuals contribute little to the collaborative efforts while reaping the benefits of the group interaction, a phenomenon known as "social loafing," "free-riding," or "freeloading." Although this behavior may disrupt group functioning, it may appear to be advantageous to low-achieving students who receive input from their peers without reciprocating. However, "parasitic" students who do not participate fully in the discussion may not learn as deeply as those who do, and even though high-achieving students may be annoyed by this behavior, it probably does them little harm because they will benefit from the discussion and group feedback. The freeloading problem is less problematic in smaller-sized groups (no more than four students) due to a level of peer pressure that promotes participation (Meseke et al., 2010).

Collaborative testing typically is used for only some of the tests in a nursing course, most often selected quizzes and unit exams. While students may benefit in a number of ways from this testing method, they still must develop sufficient skill at taking individual tests to support their success on licensure and certification examinations that they will take on completion of the nursing education program.

SUMMARY

The final appearance of a test and the way in which it is administered can affect the validity of the test results. Poor arrangement of test items, confusing or missing directions, typographical errors, and careless administration may contribute to measurement error. Careful planning can help the teacher to avoid or minimize these difficulties.

Rules for good test design include allowing sufficient time, arranging test items in a logical sequence, writing general and item-format directions, using a cover page, spacing test elements to avoid crowding, keeping related material together, arranging the correct answers in a random pattern, numbering items consecutively throughout the test, proofreading the test, and preparing an accurate answer key. In preparing to reproduce the test, the teacher should assure legibility, print the test on one side of each page, prepare enough copies for all students and proctors, and maintain the security of test materials.

Although administering a test usually is the simplest phase of the testing process, there are some common problems that may affect the reliability of the resulting scores. Teachers should arrange for favorable environmental conditions, distribute the test materials and give directions efficiently, make appropriate plans for proctoring and answering questions during the test, and collect test materials efficiently. Teachers have an important responsibility to prevent cheating before, during, and after a test. Various forms of cheating were discussed, and suggestions were given for preventing cheating on a test, including careful proctoring.

The chapter also included a brief discussion of collaborative testing. Several methods of this testing paradigm were described. Studies have reported satisfaction with collaborative testing, but some expressed concern about unprepared peers and those who contribute little to group discussion receiving higher test scores than they deserved. In general, collaborative testing appears to benefit both high- and low-achieving students, but probably should not be used for all tests whose scores will contribute to course grades.

REFERENCES

Gronlund, N. E. (2006). *Assessment of student achievement* (8th ed.). Boston, MA: Pearson Education.

Haladyna, T. M. (2004). *Developing and validating multiple-choice test items*. Mahwah, NJ: Erlbaum.

Hulsart, R., & McCarthy, V. (2009). Educators' role in promoting academic integrity. *Academy of Educational Leadership Journal, 13*(4), 49–61.

Meseke, C. A., Nafziger, R., & Meseke, J. K. (2010). Student attitudes, satisfaction, and learning in a collaborative testing environment. *Journal of Chiropractic Education, 24,* 19–29.

Miller, M. D., Linn, R. L., & Gronlund, N. E. (2009). *Measurement and assessment in teaching* (10th ed.). Upper Saddle River, NJ: Prentice Hall.

National Council on Measurement in Education. (1995). *Code of professional responsibilities in educational measurement (CPR)*. Retrieved from http://ncme.org/resource-center/code-of-professional-responsibilities-in-educational-measurement/

Nitko, A. J., & Brookhart, S. M. (2011). *Educational assessment of students* (6th ed.). Upper Saddle River, NJ: Pearson Education.

Sandahl, S. S. (2010). Collaborative testing as a learning strategy in nursing education. *Nursing Education Perspectives, 11*, 142–147.

ELEVEN

Online Testing and
Assessment of Learning

ANNA N. VIORAL AND KATHLEEN B. GABERSON

Contemporary nursing students expect educational institutions to provide flexible instructional methods that help them balance their academic, employment, family, and personal commitments (Jones & Wolf, 2010). Online education has rapidly developed as a potential solution to these demands. The growth rate of online student enrollment in all disciplines has far exceeded the growth rate of traditional course student enrollment in United States higher education (Allen & Seaman, 2007). Over 5.6 million students enrolled in at least one college-level online course during the fall 2009 academic term (Allen & Seaman, 2010). In nursing, the American Association of Colleges of Nursing reported that 173 registered nurse (RN)-to-master's degree programs and more than 400 RN-to-bachelor of science in nursing programs were offered at least partially online in 2005. These numbers are projected to increase considering student demand for convenience and access (Allen & Seaman, 2010).

The terms distance education, online education, and online learning often are treated as synonymous in the literature on this topic. For the purposes of this chapter, *distance education* refers to a structured two-way participation distinct from the traditional classroom setting (Moore & Kearsley, 2005). This type of education may not always involve technology. For example, correspondence courses occur at a distance and do not always involve a computer or technology. Conversely, *online education* refers to any form of learning or teaching that takes place via a computer network or course management system (Moore & Kearsley, 2005). Examples of various course management systems used for online education include Blackboard, Desire2Learn, and Moodle. *Online learning* or *e-learning* involves a subset of teaching and learning activities offered through webinars, interactive multimedia via the internet, video conferencing, simulations, and other interactive teaching and learning methods (Zerwekh, 2011).

This chapter discusses recommendations for assessment of learning in online courses, including testing and appraising course assignments, to determine if course goals and outcomes have been met. Assessment of online courses themselves, of teaching effectiveness in online programs, and of online nursing education programs is discussed in Chapter 18.

ASSESSMENT OF LEARNING AT THE INDIVIDUAL LEARNER LEVEL

Online assessment and evaluation principles do not differ substantially from the approaches used in the traditional classroom environment. As with traditional format courses, assessment of individual achievement in online courses should involve multiple methods such as tests, written assignments, and contributions to online discussions. Technological advances in testing and assessment have made it possible to administer tests on a computer and assess other products of student thinking even in traditional courses (Miller, Linn, & Gronlund, 2009). But courses and programs that are offered only online or in a hybrid format depend heavily or entirely on technological methods to assess the degree to which students have met expected learning targets or outcomes.

Online Testing

The choice to use online testing inevitably raises concerns about academic dishonesty. How can the course instructor be confident that students who are enrolled in the course are the ones who are taking the tests? How can teachers prevent students from consulting unauthorized sources while taking tests or sharing information about tests with students who have not yet taken them? To deter cheating and promote academic integrity, faculty members should incorporate a multilayered approach to online testing (Christe, 2003). Educators can employ low and high technology solutions to address this problem.

One example of a low technology solution includes creating an atmosphere of academic integrity in the classroom by including a discussion of academic integrity expectations in the syllabus or student handbook (Conway-Klaassen & Keil, 2010; Hart & Morgan, 2009). When teachers have positive relationships with students, interact with them regularly about their learning, and convey a sense of confidence about students' performance on tests, they create an environment in which cheating is less likely to occur (Miller et al., 2009; Nitko & Brookhart, 2011). Faculty members should develop and communicate clear policies and expectations about cheating on online tests, plagiarism, and other examples of academic dishonesty. Unfortunately, students do not always view cheating or sharing as academic dishonesty; they believe it is just collaboration (Wideman, 2011).

Another low technology option is administering a tightly timed examination (Kolitsky, 2008). This approach also may deter students from looking up answers to test items for fear of running out of time to complete the assessment (Christe, 2003). Other suggestions to minimize cheating on online examinations include randomizing the test items and response options; displaying one item at a time and not allowing students to review previous items and responses; creating and using different versions of the test for the same group of learners; and developing open-book examinations (Conway-Klaassen & Keil, 2010). However, each of these approaches has disadvantages that teachers of online courses must take into consideration before implementing them.

Randomized Sequence of Test Items and Response Options

As discussed in Chapter 10, the sequence of test items may affect student performance and therefore assessment validity. Many testing experts recommend arranging items of each format in order of difficulty, from easiest to most difficult, to minimize test anxiety and allow students to respond quickly to the easy items and spend the majority of testing time on the more difficult ones. Another recommendation is to sequence test items of each format in the order in which the content was taught, allowing students to use the content sequence as a cognitive map by which they can more easily retrieve stored information. A combination of these approaches—content sequencing with difficulty progression within each content area—may be the ideal design for a test (Nitko & Brookhart, 2011). Many testing experts also recommend varying the position of the correct answer to multiple-choice and matching items in a random way to avoid a pattern that may help test-wise but uninformed students achieve higher scores than their knowledge warrants. A simple way to obtain sufficient variation of correct answer position is to arrange the responses in alphabetical or numerical order (Gronlund, 2006; Nitko & Brookhart, 2011). Therefore, scrambling the order of test items and response options on an online test may affect the validity of interpretation of the resulting scores, and there is no known scientific evidence to recommend this practice as a way of preventing cheating on online tests.

Displaying One Item at a Time and Not Allowing Students to Review Previous Items

This tactic is appropriate for the computerized adaptive testing model in which each student's test is assembled interactively as the person is taking the test. Because the answer to one item (correct or incorrect) determines the selection of the next item, there is nothing to be gained by reviewing previous items. However, in teacher-constructed assessments for traditional or online testing, students should be permitted and encouraged to return to a previous item if they recall information that would prompt them to change their responses. While helping students develop test-taking skills to perform at the level at which they are capable, teachers should encourage students to bypass difficult items and return to them later to use the available time wisely (Nitko & Brookhart, 2011). Therefore, presenting only one item at a time and not permitting students to return to previous items may produce test scores that do not accurately reflect students' abilities.

Creating and Using Different Forms of an Examination With the Same Group of Students

As discussed in Chapter 2, alternate forms of a test are considered to be equivalent if they were developed from the same test blueprint or table of specifications, and if they produce highly correlated results. Equivalent test forms are widely used in standardized testing to assure test security, but alternate forms of teacher-constructed tests usually are not subjected to the rigorous process of obtaining empirical data to document their equivalence. Therefore, alternate forms of a test for the same group of students may produce results that are not comparable, leading to inaccurate interpretations of test scores.

Developing and Administering Open-Book Tests

Tests developed for use in traditional courses usually do not permit test-takers to consult references or other resources to arrive at correct responses, and most academic honesty codes and policies include expectations that students will not consult such resources during assessments without the teacher's permission. However, for online assessments, particularly at the graduate level, teachers may develop tests that permit or encourage students to make use of appropriate resources to select or supply correct answers. Commonly referred to as "open-book" or "take-home" tests, these assessments should gauge students' higher-order thinking abilities by requiring use of knowledge and skill in novel situations. One of the higher-order skills that may be important to assess is the ability to identify and use appropriate reference materials for problem solving, decision making, and clinical reasoning. Teachers can use test item formats such as essay and context dependent item sets (interpretive exercises) to craft novel materials for students to analyze, synthesize, and evaluate. Because these item formats typically require more time than true-false, multiple-choice, matching, and completion items, teachers should allot sufficient time for online open-book testing. Therefore, administering an open-book assessment as a tightly timed examination to deter cheating will not only produce results that do not accurately reflect students' true abilities but will likely also engender unproductive feelings of anxiety and anger among students (Nitko & Brookhart, 2011).

An additional low-technology strategy to deter cheating may be the administration of tests in a timed synchronous manner, where students' test results are not revealed until after all students have finished the examination. While synchronous online testing may be inconvenient, adequate advance knowledge of test days and times could alleviate scheduling conflicts that some students may encounter.

High technology solutions to prevent cheating on unproctored tests include browser security programs such as Respondus™ to keep students from searching the Internet while taking the examination (Hart & Morgan, 2009). However, this security feature does not prevent students from using a second computer or seeking assistance from other people during the test. For those wanting to use the best technology available to prevent academic dishonesty, faculty members could use remote proctoring to assure student identity and monitor student actions (Dunn, Meine, & McCarley, 2010). Remote proctors incorporate a web camera, biometric scanner, and microphone into a single device, which avoids students having to arrange for an approved proctor (Dunn et al., 2010, p. 4).

Students also may be required to use webcams to confirm their identities to the faculty member. Some course management systems have password-protected access and codes to prevent printing, copying, and pasting. However, these methods do not prevent students from receiving help from other students. Therefore a reasonable compromise to these dilemmas may be the use of proctored testing centers (Krsak, 2007; Trenholm, 2007).

Many universities and colleges around the country cooperate to offer students the opportunity to take proctored examinations close to their homes. Proctors should be approved by the faculty in advance to observe students taking the examination online (Hart & Morgan, 2009) and should sign an agreement to keep all test materials secure and maintain confidentiality. While the administration of proctored examinations is not as convenient as an asynchronous non-proctored test, it offers a greater level of assurance that students are taking examinations independently.

Course Assignments

Course assignments may require adjustment for online learning to suit the electronic medium. Online course assignments can be crafted to provide opportunities for students to develop and demonstrate cognitive, affective, and psychomotor abilities. Table 11.1 provides specific examples of learning products in the cognitive, affective, and psychomotor domains that can be used for formative and summative evaluation. Assignments such as analyses of cases and critical thinking vignettes, discussion boards, and classroom assessment techniques may be used for formative evaluation, while papers,

☐Table 11.1

EXAMPLES OF METHODS FOR ONLINE ASSESSMENT OF LEARNING

COGNITIVE DOMAIN	AFFECTIVE DOMAIN	PSYCHOMOTOR DOMAIN
Discussion boards	Discussion boards	Creating videos
Online chats	Online chats	Virtual simulations
Case analysis	Case analysis	Developing web pages
Term papers	Debates	Web page presentations
Research or evidence-based practice papers	Role play	Interactive modules
Short written assignments	Discussions of ethical issues	Presentations
Journals	Interviews	
Electronic portfolios	Journals	
	Developing blogs	

debates, electronic presentations, portfolios, and tests are more frequently used to provide information for summative evaluation (O'Neil et al., 2009). Online course assignments may be used for formative or summative evaluation of student learning outcomes. However, the teacher should make it clear to the students how the assignments are being used for evaluation. No matter what type of assignment the faculty member assesses, the student must have clearly defined criteria for the assignment and its evaluation.

Feedback

As in traditional courses, feedback during the learning process and following teacher evaluation of assignments facilitates learning. Students need more feedback in online learning than in the traditional environment because of the lack of face-to-face interaction and subsequent lack of nonverbal communication. Teachers should give timely feedback about each assignment to verify that they are in the process of or have finished assessing it, or to inform the student when to expect more detailed feedback. O'Neil et al. (2009) suggested that feedback should be given within 24 to 48 hours, but it may not be reasonable to expect teachers to give detailed, meaningful feedback to a large group of students or on a lengthy assignment within that timeframe. For this reason, the syllabus for an online or a hybrid course should include information about reasonable expectations regarding the timing of feedback from the teacher. For example, the syllabus might state, "I will acknowledge receipt of submitted assignments via email within 24 hours, and I will e-mail [or post as a private message on the course management system, or other means] more detailed, specific feedback [along with a score or grade if appropriate] within [specify timeframe]."

Feedback to students can occur through a variety of methods. Many faculty members provide electronic feedback on written assignments using the Track Changes feature of Microsoft Word (or similar feature of other word processing software) or by inserting comments into the document. Feedback also may occur through email or orally using vodcasting, Skype, or scheduled phone conferences.

As discussed in Chapter 9, the teacher may also incorporate peer critique within the process of completing an assignment. For example, for a lengthy written formal paper, the teacher may assign each student a peer-review partner, or each student may ask a peer to critique an early draft. The peer reviewer's written feedback and the resulting revision should then be submitted for the faculty member to assess.

When an assignment involves participation in discussion using the course management system's discussion board, the teacher may also assign groups or partners to critique each other's posted responses to questions posed by the teacher or other students. Although peer feedback is important to identify areas in which a student's discussion contribution is unclear or incomplete, the course faculty member should also post summarized feedback to the student group periodically to identify gaps in knowledge, correct misinformation, and help students construct new knowledge.

No matter which types of feedback a teacher chooses to use in an online course, clear guidelines and expectations should be established and clearly communicated to the learners, including due dates for peer feedback. Students should understand the overall purpose of feedback to effectively engage in these processes. Structured feedback forms may be used for individual or group work. O'Neil et al. (2009) recommended multidimensional feedback that:

- addresses the content of the assignment, quality of the presentation, and grammar and other technical writing qualities,
- provides supportive statements highlighting the strengths and areas of improvement, and
- conveys a clear, thorough, consistent, equitable, constructive, and professional message.

Development of a scoring rubric provides an assessment tool that uses clearly defined criteria for the assignment and gauges student achievement (Isaacson & Stacy, 2008). Rubrics enhance assessment reliability among multiple graders (Bonnel, 2009), communicate specific goals to students, describe behaviors that constitute a specific grade, and serve as a feedback tool (Isaacson & Stacy). Table 11.2 provides a sample rubric for an online discussion board assignment and evaluation criteria.

❏Table 11.2

EXAMPLE OF DISCUSSION BOARD FEEDBACK AND ASSIGNMENT RUBRIC

CRITERIA	EXEMPLARY (3 POINTS)	GOOD (2 POINTS)	SATISFACTORY (1 POINTS)	UNSATISFACTORY (0 POINTS)	SCORE
Frequency	Participates 4–5 times during a week	Participates 2–3 times during the week	Participates during the week	No participation on discussion board	
Initial assignment posting	Posts a well-developed discussion that addresses 3 or more concepts related to the topic	Posts a well-developed discussion addressing at least 1 or 2 key concepts related to the topic	Posts a summary with superficial preparation and unsupported discussion	No assignment posted	
Peer feedback postings	Posts an analysis of a peer's post extending the discussion with supporting references	Posts a response that elaborates on a peer's comments with references	Posts superficial responses such as "I agree" or "great idea"	Does not post feedback to peers	
Content	Post provides a reflective contribution with evidence-based references extending the discussion	Post provides evidence-based facts supporting the topic	Post does not add substantive information to the discussion	Post does not apply to the related topic	
References	Provides personal experiences and reflection with 2 or more supporting references	Provides personal experiences and only 1 supporting reference	Provides personal experiences and no references	Provides no personal experience or references	
Grammar, clarity, writing style	Responses organized, no grammatical or spelling errors, correct style	Responses organized, 1–2 grammatical and spelling errors, uses correct style	Responses organized, 3–4 grammatical and spelling errors, 1–2 minor style errors	Responses are not organized, 5–6 grammatical and spelling errors, many style errors	

SUMMARY

This chapter discussed methods of assessing learning in online courses, including testing and course assignments, to determine if course goals have been met. Online assessment principles do not differ substantially from the approaches used in the traditional classroom environment, but courses and programs that are offered only online or in a hybrid format depend heavily or entirely on technological methods to assess learning.

The use of online testing usually raises concerns among teachers about academic dishonesty. Faculty members want to be confident that students who are enrolled in the course are the ones who are taking the tests, and they want to prevent students from using unauthorized sources of information during a test or sharing test information with students who have not yet taken it. A number of low technology and high technology solutions have been proposed to deter cheating on online tests. One low technology solution involves creating a climate conducive to academic integrity based on positive relationships with students and clearly communicating expectations about cheating on online tests, plagiarism, and other forms of academic dishonesty. Other low technology approaches include administering tightly timed examinations, using timed synchronous examinations, randomizing the test items and response options, displaying one item at a time, creating different versions of the examination for the same group of learners, and developing open-book tests. Each of these options has disadvantages that were discussed in the chapter.

High technology solutions for unproctored examinations include webcams to assure students' identities to the instructor; browser security programs to keep students from searching the Internet while taking the examination; course management systems with password-protected access and codes to prevent printing, copying, and pasting test content; and remote proctoring that incorporates a web camera, biometric scanner, and microphone. Disadvantages to these approaches were discussed in the chapter. One solution to these dilemmas may be the use of proctored testing centers.

Course assignments usually require some adaptation for online learning. The teacher should make it clear to the students how the assignments are being used for evaluation and clearly define the criteria for each assignment. Students need more feedback during the learning process in online learning than in traditional courses because of the lack of face-to-face interaction. Teachers should give timely feedback about each assignment, and the syllabus for an online or hybrid course should include information about reasonable expectations regarding the timing of feedback from the faculty member. Feedback to students about assignments can be provided through a variety of methods. Teachers also may incorporate peer critique within the process of completing an assignment; strategies for this were discussed in the chapter. Scoring rubrics that clearly define criteria for the assignment enhance assessment reliability, communicate specific goals to students, describe what behaviors constitute a specific grade, and serve as a feedback tool.

REFERENCES

Allen, I. E., & Seaman, J. (2007). *Online nation: Five years of growth in online learning.* Needham, MA: Babson Survey Research Group and The Sloan Consortium.

Allen, I. E., & Seaman, J. (2010). *Class differences: Online education in the United States.* Needham, MA: The Sloan Consortium.

Bonnel, W. (2009). Clinical performance evaluation. In D. M. Billings & J. A. Halstead (Eds.), *Teaching in nursing* (3rd ed., pp. 449–466). St. Louis, MO: Saunders.

Christe, B. (2003). Designing online courses to discourage dishonesty. *EDUCAUSE Quarterly, 26*(4), 54–58.

Conway-Klaassen, J., & Keil, D. (2010). Discouraging academic dishonesty in online courses. *Clinical Laboratory Science, 23*, 194–200.

Dunn, T. P., Meine, M. F., & McCarley, J. (2010). The remote proctor: An innovative technological solution for online course integrity. *The International Journal of Technology, Knowledge, and Society, 6*(1), 1–7.

Gronlund, N. E. (2006). *Assessment of student achievement* (8th ed.). Boston, MA: Allyn & Bacon.

Hart, L., & Morgan, L. (2009). Strategies for online test security. *Nurse Educator, 34*, 249–253.

Isaacson, J. J., & Stacy, A. S. (2008). Rubrics for clinical evaluation: Objectifying the subjective experience. *Nurse Education in Practice, 9*, 134–140.

Jones, D., & Wolf, D. (2010). Shaping the future of nursing education today using distance education and technology. *ABNF Journal, 21*(2), 44–47.

Kolitsky, M. A. (2008). Analysis of non-proctored anti-cheating and formative assessment strategies. *E-Mentor, 26*(4), 84–88.

Krsak, A. M. (2007). Curbing academic dishonesty in online courses. *TCC 2007 Proceedings,* 159–170.

Miller, M. D., Linn, R. L., & Gronlund, N. E. (2009). *Measurement and assessment in teaching* (10th ed.). Upper Saddle River, NJ: Prentice Hall.

Moore, M., & Kearsley, G. (2005). *Distance education: A systems view* (2nd ed.). Belmont, CA: Thompson Wadsworth.

Nitko, A. J., & Brookhart, S. M. (2011). *Educational assessment of students* (6th ed.). Upper Saddle River, NJ: Pearson Education.

O'Neil, C. A., Fisher, C. A., & Newbold, S. K. (2009). *Developing an online course: Best practices for nurse educators* (2nd ed.). New York, NY: Springer Publishing.

Trenholm, S. (2007). A review of cheating in fully asynchronous online courses: A math or fact-based course perspective. *Journal of Educational Technology Systems, 35*, 281–300.

Wideman, M. (2011). Caring or collusion? Academic dishonesty in a school of nursing. *Canadian Journal of Higher Education, 41*(2), 28–43.

Zerwekh, J. (2011). E-learning defined. In T. J. Bristol & J. Zerwekh (Eds.), *Essentials of e-learning for nurse educators* (pp. 3–13). Philadelphia, PA: F. A. Davis.

TWELVE

Scoring and

Analyzing Tests

After administering a test, the teacher's responsibility is to score it or arrange to have it scored. The teacher then interprets the results and uses these interpretations to make grading, selection, placement, or other decisions. To accurately interpret test scores, however, the teacher needs to analyze the performance of the test as a whole and of the individual test items, and to use these data to draw valid inferences about student performance. This information also helps teachers prepare for posttest discussions with students about the exam. This chapter discusses the processes of obtaining scores and performing test and item analysis. It also suggests ways in which teachers can use posttest discussions to contribute to student learning and seek student feedback that can lead to test item improvement.

SCORING

Many teachers say that they "grade" tests, when in fact it would be more accurate to say that they "score" tests. Scoring is the process of determining the first direct, unconverted, uninterpreted measure of performance on a test, usually called the raw, obtained, or observed score. The raw score represents the number of correct answers or number of points awarded to separate parts of an assessment (Nitko & Brookhart, 2011). On the other hand, grading or marking is the process of assigning a symbol to represent the quality of the student's performance. Symbols can be letters (A, B, C, D, F, which may also include + or –); categories (pass–fail, satisfactory–unsatisfactory); integers (9 through 1); or percentages (100, 99, 98...), among other options.

In most cases, test scores should not be converted to grades for the purpose of later computing a final average grade. Instead the teacher should record actual test scores and then combine all scores into a composite score that can be converted to a final grade. Recording scores contributes to greater measurement accuracy because information is lost each time scores are converted to symbols. For example, if scores from 70 to 79 all are converted to a grade of C, each score in this range receives the same grade, although scores of 71 and 78 may represent important differences in achievement. If the C grades all are converted to the same numerical grade, for example, C = 2.0, then such distinctions are lost when the teacher computes the final grade for the course. Various grading systems and their uses are discussed in Chapter 17.

Weighting Items

As a general rule, each objectively scored test item should have equal weight. Most electronic scoring systems assign 1 point to each correct answer unless the teacher specifies a different item weight; this seems reasonable for hand-scored tests as well. It is difficult for teachers to justify that one item is worth 2 points while another is worth 1 point; such a weighting system also motivates students to argue for partial credit for some answers.

Differential weighting implies that the teacher believes knowledge of one concept to be more important than knowledge of another concept. When this is true, the better approach is to write more items about the important concept; this emphasis would be reflected in the test blueprint, which specifies the number of items for each content area. When a combination of selection-type items and supply-type items is used on a test, a variable number of points can be assigned to short-answer and essay items to reflect the complexity of the required task and the value of the student's response (Miller, Linn, & Gronlund, 2009). It is not necessary to adjust the numerical weight of items to achieve a total of 100 points. Although a test of 100 points allows the teacher to calculate a percentage score quickly, this step is not necessary to make valid interpretations of students' scores.

Correction for Guessing

The raw score sometimes is adjusted or corrected before it is interpreted. One procedure involves applying a formula intended to eliminate any advantage that a student might have gained by guessing correctly. The correction formula reduces the raw score by some fraction of the number of the student's wrong answers (Miller et al., 2009; Nitko & Brookhart, 2011). The formula can be used only with simple true–false, multiple-choice, and some matching items, and is dependent on the number of alternatives per item. The general formula is:

$$\text{Corrected score} = R - \frac{W}{n - 1} \quad \text{[Equation 12.1]}$$

where R is the number of right answers, W is the number of wrong answers, and n is the number of options in each item (Miller et al., 2009). Thus, for two-option items like true–false, the teacher merely subtracts the number of wrong answers from the number of right answers (or raw score); for four-option items, the raw score is reduced by one third of the number of wrong answers. A correction formula is obviously difficult to use for a test that contains several different item formats.

The use of a correction formula usually is appropriate only when students do not have sufficient time to complete all test items and when they have been instructed not to answer any item for which they are uncertain of the answer (Miller et al., 2009). Even under these circumstances, students may differ in their interpretation of "certainty" and therefore may interpret the advice differently. Some students will guess regardless of the instructions given and the threat of a penalty; the risk-taking or testwise student is likely to be rewarded with a higher score than the risk-avoiding or non-testwise student because of guessing some answers correctly. These personality differences cannot be equalized by instructions not to guess and penalties for guessing.

The use of a correction formula also is based on the assumption that the student who does not know the answer will guess blindly. However, Nitko and Brookhart (2011) suggested that the chance of getting a high score by random guessing was slim, though many students choose correct answers through informed guesses based on some knowledge of the content. Based on these limitations and the fact that most tests in nursing education settings are not speeded, the best approach is to advise all students to answer every item, even if they are uncertain about their answers, and apply no correction for guessing.

ITEM ANALYSIS

Computer software for item analysis is widely available for use with electronic answer sheet scanning equipment. Exhibit 12.1 is an example of a computer-generated item-analysis report. For teachers who do not have access to such equipment and software, procedures for analyzing student responses to test items by hand are described in detail later in this section. Regardless of the method used for analysis, teachers should be familiar

☐Exhibit 12.1

Sample Computer-Generated Item-Analysis Report

ITEM STATISTICS
($N = 68$)

Item	Key	A	B	C	D	E	Omit	Multiple Response	Diff. Index	Discrim. Index
1	A	44	0	24	0	0	0	0	.65	.34
2	B	0	62	4	2	0	0	0	.91	.06
3	A	59	1	4	4	0	0	0	.87	.35
4	C	12	4	51	1	0	0	0	.75	.19
5	E	23	8	0	8	29	0	0	.43	.21
6	D	2	3	17	46	0	0	0	.68	.17

Note: Diff. Index = difficulty index; Discrim. Index = discrimination index.

enough with the meaning of each item-analysis statistic to correctly interpret the results. It is important to realize that most item-analysis techniques are designed for items that are scored dichotomously, that is, either right or wrong, from tests that are intended for norm-referenced uses (Nitko & Brookhart, 2011).

Difficulty Index

One useful indication of test-item quality is its difficulty. The most commonly employed index of difficulty is the P-level, the value of which ranges from 0 to 1.00, indicating the percentage of students who answered the item correctly. A P-value of 0 indicates that no one answered the item correctly, and a value of 1.00 indicates that every student answered the item correctly (Nitko & Brookhart, 2011). A simple formula for calculating the P-value is:

$$P = \frac{R}{T} \quad \text{[Equation 12.2]}$$

where R is the number of students who responded correctly and T is the total number of students who took the test (Miller et al., 2009).

The difficulty index commonly is interpreted to mean that items with P-values of .20 and below are difficult, and items with P-values of .80 and above are easy. However, this interpretation may imply that test items are intrinsically easy or difficult and may not take into account the quality of the instruction or the abilities of the students in that group. A group of students who were taught by an expert instructor might tend to answer a test item correctly, whereas a group of students with similar abilities who were taught by an ineffectual instructor might tend to answer it incorrectly. Different P-values might be produced by students with more or less ability. Thus, test items cannot be labeled as easy or difficult without considering how well that content was taught.

The P-value also should be interpreted in relationship to the student's probability of guessing the correct response. For example, if all students guess the answer to a true–false item, on the basis of chance alone, the P-value of that item should be approximately .50. On a four-option multiple-choice item, chance alone should produce a P-value of .25. A four-alternative, multiple-choice item with moderate difficulty therefore would have a P-value approximately halfway between chance (.25) and 1.00, or 0.625. This calculation is explained below:

$1.00 - 0.25 = 0.75$ [range of values between 0.25 and 1.00]

$\dfrac{0.75}{2} = 0.375$ [½ of the range of values between 0.25 and 1.00]

$0.25 + 0.375 = 0.625$ [the chance of guessing correctly plus ½ of the range of values between that value and 1.00]

For most tests whose results will be interpreted in a norm-referenced way, P-values of .30 to .70 for test items are desirable. However, for tests whose results will be interpreted in a criterion-referenced manner, as most tests in nursing education settings are, the difficulty level of test items should be compared between groups (students whose total scores met the criterion and students who didn't). If item difficulty levels indicate a relatively easy (P-value of .70 or above) or relatively difficult (P-value of .30 or below) item, criterion-referenced decisions still will be appropriate if the item correctly classifies students according to the criterion (Miller et al., 2009; Waltz, Strickland, & Lenz, 2005).

Very easy and very difficult items have little power to discriminate between students who know the content and students who do not, and they also decrease the reliability of the test scores. Teachers can use item difficulty information to identify the need for remedial work related to specific content or skills, or to identify test items that are ambiguous (Miller et al., 2009).

Discrimination Index

The discrimination index, D, is a powerful indicator of test-item quality. A positively discriminating item is one that was answered correctly more often by students with high scores on the test than by those whose test scores were low. A negatively discriminating item was answered correctly more often by students with low test scores than by students with high scores. When an equal number of high- and low-scoring students answer the item correctly, the item is nondiscriminating (Miller et al., 2009; Nitko & Brookhart, 2011).

A number of item discrimination indexes are available; a simple method of computing D is:

$$D = P_u - P_1 \quad \text{[Equation 12.3]}$$

where P_u is the fraction of students in the high-scoring group who answered the item correctly and P_1 is the fraction of students in the low-scoring group who answered the item correctly. If the number of test scores is large, it is not necessary to include all scores in this calculation. Instead, the teacher (or computer item analysis software) can use the top 25% and the bottom 25% of scores based on the assumption that the responses of students in the middle group follow essentially the same pattern (Miller et al., 2009; Waltz et al., 2005)

The D-value ranges from –1.00 to +1.00. In general, the higher the positive value, the better the test item. An index of +1.00 means that all students in the upper group answered correctly, and all students in the lower group answered incorrectly; this indication of maximum positive discriminating power is rarely achieved. D-values of +.20 or above are desirable, and the higher the positive value the better. An index of .00 means that equal numbers of students in the upper and lower groups answered the item correctly, and this item has no discriminating power (Miller et al., 2009). Negative D-values signal items that should be reviewed carefully; usually they indicate items that are flawed and need to be revised. One possible interpretation of a negative D-value is that the item was misinterpreted by high scorers or that it provided a clue to low scorers that enabled them to guess the correct answer (Waltz et al., 2005).

When interpreting a D-value, it is important to keep in mind that an item's power to discriminate is highly related to its difficulty index. An item that is answered correctly by all students has a difficulty index of 1.00; the discrimination index for this item is 0.00, because there is no difference in performance on that item between students whose overall test scores were high and those whose scores were low. Similarly, if all students answered the item incorrectly, the difficulty index is 0.00, and the discrimination index is also 0.00 because there is no discrimination power. Thus, very easy and very difficult items have low discriminating power. Items with a difficulty index of .50 make maximum discriminating power possible, but do not guarantee it (Miller et al., 2009).

It is important to keep in mind that item-discriminating power does not indicate item validity. To gather evidence of item validity, the teacher would have to compare each test item to an independent measure of achievement, seldom possible for teacher-constructed tests. Standardized tests in the same content area usually measure the achievement of more general objectives, so they are not appropriate as independent criteria. The best measure of the domain of interest usually is the total score on the test if the test has been constructed to correspond to specific instructional objectives and content. Thus, comparing each item's discriminating power to the performance of the entire test determines how effectively each item measures what the entire test measures. However, retaining very easy or very difficult items despite low discrimination power may be desirable so as to measure a representative sample of learning objectives and content (Miller et al., 2009).

Distractor Analysis

As previously indicated, item-analysis statistics can serve as indicators of test item quality. No teacher, however, should make decisions about retaining a test item in its present form, revising it, or eliminating it from future use on the basis of the item statistics alone. Item difficulty and discrimination indexes are not fixed, unchanging characteristics. Item-analysis data for a given test item will vary from one administration to another because of factors such as students' ability levels, quality of instruction, and the size of the group tested. With very small groups of students, if a few students would have changed their responses to the test item, the difficulty and discrimination indexes could change considerably (Miller et al., 2009). Thus, when using these indexes to identify questionable items, the teacher should carefully examine each test item for evidence of poorly functioning distractors, ambiguous alternatives, and miskeying.

Every distractor should be selected by at least one lower group student, and more lower group students than higher group students should select it. A distractor that is not selected by any student in the lower group may contain a technical flaw or may be so implausible as to be obvious even to students who lack knowledge of the correct answer. A distractor is ambiguous if upper group students tend to choose it with about the same frequency as the keyed, or correct, response. This result usually indicates that there is no single clearly correct or best answer. Poorly functioning and ambiguous distractors may be revised to make them more plausible or to eliminate the ambiguity. If a large number of higher scoring students select a particular incorrect response, the teacher should check to see if the answer key is correct. In each case, the content of the item, not the statistics alone, should guide the teacher's decision making (Nitko & Brookhart, 2011).

Performing an Item Analysis by Hand

The following process for performing item analysis by hand is adapted from Nitko and Brookhart (2011) and Miller et al. (2009):

Step 1. After the test is scored, arrange the test scores in rank order, highest to lowest.

Step 2. Divide the scores into a high-scoring half and a low-scoring half. For large groups of students, the scores may be divided into equal thirds or quarters, with only the top and bottom groups used for analysis.

Step 3. For each item, tally the number of students in each group who chose each alternative. Record these counts on a copy of the test item next to each response option. The keyed response for the following sample item is d; the group of 20 students is divided into 2 groups of 10 students each.

1. What is the most likely explanation for breast asymmetry in an adolescent girl?

	Higher	*Lower*
a. Blocked mammary duct in the larger breast	0	3
b. Endocrine disorder	2	3
c. Mastitis in the larger breast	0	0
d. Normal variation in growth	8	4

Step 4. Calculate the difficulty index for each item. The following formula is a variation of the one presented earlier, to account for the division of scores into two groups:

$$P = \frac{R_h + R_l}{T} \quad \text{[Equation 12.4]}$$

where R_h is the number of students in the high-scoring half who answered correctly, R_l is the number of students in the low-scoring half who answered correctly, and T is the total number of students. For the purpose of calculating the difficulty index, consider omitted responses and multiple responses as incorrect. For the example in Step 4, the P-value is .60, indicating an item of moderate difficulty.

Step 5. Calculate the discrimination index for each item. Using the data from Step 4, divide R_h by the total number of students in that group to obtain P_h. Repeat the process to calculate P_1 from R_1. Subtract P_1 from P_h to obtain D. For the example in Step 4, the discrimination index is .40, indicating that the item discriminates well between high-scoring and low-scoring students.

Step 6. Check each item for implausible distractors, ambiguity, and miskeying. It is obvious that in the sample item, no students chose "Mastitis in the larger breast" as the correct answer. This distractor does not contribute to the discrimination power of the item, and the teacher should consider replacing it with an alternative that might be more plausible.

No test item should be rejected solely on the basis of item-analysis data. The teacher should carefully examine each questionable item and, if there is no obvious structural defect, it may be best to use the item again with a different group. Remember that with small groups of students, item-analysis data can vary widely from one test administration to another.

TEST CHARACTERISTICS

In addition to item-analysis results, information about how the test performed as a whole also helps teachers to interpret test results. Measures of central tendency and variability, reliability estimates, and the shape of the score distribution can assist the teacher in making judgments about the quality of the test; difficulty and discrimination indices are related to these test characteristics. Test statistics are discussed in detail in Chapter 16.

In addition, teachers should examine test items in the aggregate for evidence of bias. For example, although there may be no obvious gender bias in any single test item, such a bias may be apparent when all items are reviewed as a group. Similar cases of ethnic, racial, religious, and cultural bias may be found when items are grouped and examined together. The effect of bias on testing and evaluation is discussed in detail in Chapter 15.

CONDUCTING POSTTEST DISCUSSIONS

Giving students feedback about test results can be an opportunity to reinforce learning, to correct misinformation, and to solicit their input for improvement of test items. But a feedback session also can be an invitation to engage in battle, with students attacking to gain extra points and the teacher defending the honor of the test and, it often seems, the very right to give tests. Discussions with students about the test should be rational rather than opportunities for the teacher to assert power and authority. Posttest discussions can be beneficial to both teachers and students if they are planned in advance and not emotionally charged. The teacher should prepare for a posttest discussion by completing a test analysis and an item analysis and reviewing the items that were most difficult for the majority of students.

Teachers may use this information about item effectiveness as an aid to posttest discussion. The items with the lowest difficulty index (the ones answered incorrectly by the largest number of students) can be discussed at greater length, and the teacher can ask students why they selected the correct or wrong answer for such items. A discussion of the rationale for their choices may reveal common errors and misconceptions that may be corrected at that time, serve as a basis for remedial study, or contribute to a revision of those items (Gronlund, 2006).

Teachers usually assume that students choose correct responses to selection-type items because they know the content at the expected cognitive level, but there could be many other reasons for their selections. For example, a student:

- Has partial knowledge that supports choosing the correct answer
- Uses unintended cues given in the item
- Uses information from other test items
- Makes a lucky blind guess
- Intends to choose a distractor but makes a lucky clerical error in recording the correct answer

Many students who choose incorrect responses lack knowledge of the content, but other reasons for their selections may include:

- Partial knowledge that favors a distractor
- Misinformation that supports a distractor
- Unlucky blind guessing
- Intending to choose the correct answer but making a mistake in recording an incorrect response (Gronlund, 2006)

Discussing why students chose correct or incorrect answers can reveal students' thought processes that can contribute to better teaching, improved test construction skills, and better test-taking skills.

To use time efficiently, the teacher should read the correct answers aloud quickly. If the test is hand-scored, correct answers also may be indicated by the teacher on the students' answer sheets or test booklets. If machine-scoring is used, the answer key may be projected as a scanned document from a computer or via a document camera or overhead projector. Many electronic scoring applications allow an option for marking the correct or incorrect answers directly on each student's answer sheet.

Teachers should continue to protect the security of the test during the posttest discussion by accounting for all test booklets and answer sheets and by eliminating other opportunities for cheating. Some teachers do not allow students to use pens or pencils during the feedback session to prevent answer-changing and subsequent complaints that scoring errors were made. Another approach is to distribute pens with red or green ink and permit only those pens to be used to mark answers. Teachers also should decide in advance whether to permit students to take notes during the session.

During test administration, some teachers allow students to record their answers on the test booklets, where the students also record their names, as well as on a separate answer sheet. At the completion of the exam, students submit the answer sheets and their test booklets to the teacher. When all students have finished the exam, they return to the room to check their answers using only their test booklets. The teacher might project the answers onto a screen as described previously. At the conclusion of this session, the teacher collects the test booklets again. It is important not to review and discuss individual items at this time because the test has not yet been scored and analyzed. However, the teacher may ask students to indicate problematic items and give a rationale for their answers. As discussed above, the teacher can use this item in conjunction with the item-analysis results to evaluate the effectiveness of test items. One disadvantage to this method of giving posttest feedback is that because the test has not yet been scored and analyzed, the teacher would not have an opportunity to thoroughly prepare for the session; feedback consists only of the correct answers, and no discussion takes place. With item effectiveness information, the teacher can identify and point out defective test items and discuss how they will be treated in scoring, rather than feel the need to defend the fairness of the items without data to support it (Gronlund, 2006).

Whatever the structure of the posttest discussion, the teacher should control the session so that it produces maximum benefit for all students. While discussing an item that was answered incorrectly by a majority of students, the teacher should maintain a calm, matter-of-fact, nondefensive attitude. The teacher should avoid arguing with students about individual items and engaging in emotionally charged discussion; instead, the teacher should either invite written comments as described previously or schedule individual appointments to discuss the items in question. Students who need additional help also may be encouraged to make appointments with the teacher for individual review sessions.

Eliminating Items or Adding Points

Teachers often debate the merits of adjusting test scores by eliminating items or adding points to compensate for real or perceived deficiencies in test construction or performance. For example, during a posttest discussion, students may argue that if they all answered an item incorrectly, the item should be omitted or all students should be awarded an extra point to compensate for the "bad item." It is interesting to note that students seldom propose subtracting a point from their scores if they all answer an item correctly. In any case, how should the teacher respond to such requests? In this discussion, a distinction is made between test items that are technically flawed and those that do not function as intended.

If test items are properly constructed, critiqued, and proofread, it is unlikely that serious flaws will appear on the test. However, errors that do appear may have varying effects on students' scores. For example, if the correct answer to a multiple-choice item is inadvertently omitted from the test, no student will be able to answer the item correctly. In this case, the item simply should not be scored. That is, if the error is discovered during or after test administration and before the test is scored, the item is omitted from the answer key; a test that was intended to be worth 73 points then is worth 72 points. If the error is discovered after the tests are scored, they can be re-scored. Students often worry about the effect of this change on their scores and may argue that they should be awarded an extra point in this case. The possible effects of both adjustments on a hypothetical score are shown in Table 12.1.

It is obvious that omitting the flawed item and adding a point to the raw score produce nearly identical results. Although students might view adding a point to their scores as more satisfying, it makes little sense to award a point for an item that was not answered correctly. The "extra" point in fact does not represent knowledge of any content area or achievement of an objective, and therefore it does not contribute to a valid interpretation

▢Table 12.1

EFFECTS OF TEST SCORE ADJUSTMENTS

	TOTAL POSSIBLE POINTS	RAW SCORE	PERCENTAGE CORRECT
Original test	73	62	84.9
Flawed item not scored	72	62	86.1
Point added to raw score	73	63	86.3

of the test scores. Teachers should inform students matter-of-factly that an item was eliminated from the test and reassure them that their relative standing with regard to performance on the test has not changed.

If the technical flaw consists of a misspelled word in a true–false item that does not change the meaning of the statement, no adjustment should be made. The teacher should avoid lengthy debate about item semantics if it is clear that such errors are unlikely to have affected the students' scores. Feedback from students can be used to revise items for later use and sometimes make changes in teaching that concept or skill.

As previously discussed, teachers should resist the temptation to eliminate items from the test solely on the basis of low difficulty and discrimination indices. Omission of items may affect the validity of the scores from the test, particularly if several items related to one content area or objective are eliminated, resulting in inadequate sampling of that content (Miller et al., 2009).

Because identified flaws in test construction do contribute to measurement error, the teacher should consider taking them into account when using the test scores to make grading decisions and set cutoff scores. That is, the teacher should not fix cutoff scores for assigning grades until after all tests have been given and analyzed. The proposed grading scale can then be adjusted if necessary to compensate for deficiencies in test construction. It should be made clear to students that any changes in the grading scale because of flaws in test construction would not adversely affect their grades.

DEVELOPING A TEST-ITEM BANK

Because considerable effort goes into developing, administering, and analyzing test items, teachers should develop a system for maintaining and expanding a pool or bank of items from which to select items for future tests. Teachers can maintain databases of test items on their computers with backups on storage devices. When teachers store test-item databases electronically, the files must be password-protected and test security maintained. When developing test banks, the teacher can record the following data with each test item: (a) the correct response for objective-type items and a brief scoring key for completion or essay items; (b) the course, unit, content area, or objective for which it was designed; and (c) the item-analysis results for a specified period of time. Exhibit 12.2 offers one such example.

Commercially produced software applications can be used in a similar way to develop a database of test items. Each test item is a record in the database. The test items can then be sorted according to the fields in which the data are entered; for example, the teacher could retrieve all items that are classified as Objective 3, with a moderate difficulty index.

▢Exhibit 12.2

Sample Information to Include With Items in Test Bank

Content Area: Physical Assessment
Unit 5
Objective 3

1. What is the most likely explanation for breast asymmetry in an adolescent girl?

    A. Blocked mammary duct in the larger breast
    B. Endocrine disorder
    C. Mastitis in the larger breast
    D. Normal variation in growth*

Test Date	Diff. Index	Discrim. Index
10/22	.72	.25
2/20	.56	.33
10/23	.60	.40

Note: Diff. Index = difficulty index; Discrim. Index = discrimination index.

Many publishers also offer test-item banks that relate to the content contained in their textbooks. However, faculty members need to be cautious about using these items for their own examinations. The purpose of the test, relevant characteristics of the students to be tested, and the balance and emphasis of content as reflected in the teacher's test blueprint are the most important criteria for selecting test items. Although some teachers would consider these item banks to be a shortcut to the development and selection of test items, they should be evaluated carefully before they are used (Miller et al., 2009). There is no guarantee that the quality of test items in a published item bank is superior to that of test items that a skilled teacher can construct. Many of the items may be of questionable quality.

In addition, published test-item banks seldom contain item-analysis information such as difficulty and discrimination indices. However, the teacher can calculate this information for each item used or modified from a published item bank, and can develop and maintain an item file.

SUMMARY

After administering a test, the teacher must score it and interpret the results. To accurately interpret test scores, the teacher needs to analyze the performance of the test as a whole as well as the individual test items.

Information about how the test performed helps teachers to give feedback to students about test results and to improve test items for future use.

Scoring is the process of determining the first direct, uninterpreted measure of performance on a test, usually called the raw score. The raw score usually represents the number of right answers. Test scores should not be converted to grades for the purpose of later computing a final average grade. Instead, the teacher should record actual test scores and then combine them into a composite score that can be converted to a final grade.

As a general rule, each objectively scored test item should have equal weight. If knowledge of one concept is more important than knowledge of another concept, the teacher should sample the more important domain more heavily by writing more items in that area. Most machine-scoring systems assign 1 point to each correct answer; this seems reasonable for hand-scored tests as well.

A raw score sometimes is adjusted or corrected before it is interpreted. One procedure involves applying a formula intended to eliminate any advantage that a student might have gained by guessing correctly. Correcting for guessing is appropriate only when students have been instructed to not answer any item for which they are uncertain of the answer; students may interpret and follow this advice differently. Therefore, the best approach is to advise all students to answer every item, with no correction for guessing applied.

Item analysis can be performed by hand or by the use of a computer program. Teachers should be familiar enough with the meaning of each item-analysis statistic to correctly interpret the results. The difficulty index (P), ranging from 0 to 1.00, indicates the percentage of students who answered the item correctly. Items with P-values of .20 and below are considered to be difficult, and those with P-values of .80 and above are considered to be easy. However, interpretation of the difficulty index should take into account the quality of the instruction and the abilities of the students in the group. The discrimination index (D), ranging from –1.00 to +1.00, is an indication of the extent to which high-scoring students answered the item correctly more often than low-scoring students did. In general, the higher the positive value, the better the test item; desirable discrimination indexes should be at least +.20. An item's power to discriminate is highly related to its difficulty index. An item that is answered correctly by all students has a difficulty index of 1.00; the discrimination index for this item is 0.00, because there is no difference in performance on that item between high scorers and low scorers.

Flaws in test construction may have varying effects on students' scores and therefore should be handled differently. If the correct answer to a multiple-choice item is inadvertently omitted from the test, no student will be able to answer the item correctly. In this case, the item simply should not be scored. If a flaw consists of a misspelled word that does not change the meaning of the item, no adjustment should be made.

Teachers should develop a system for maintaining a pool or bank of items from which to select items for future tests. Item banks can be developed by the faculty and stored electronically. Use of published test-item banks should be based on the teacher's evaluation of the quality of the items as well as on the purpose for testing, relevant characteristics of the students, and the desired emphasis and balance of content as reflected in the teacher's test blueprint. Items selected from a published item bank often must be modified to be technically sound and relevant to how the content area was taught and the characteristics of the students to be tested.

REFERENCES

Gronlund, N. E. (2006). *Assessment of student achievement* (8th ed.). Boston, MA: Pearson Education.

Miller, M. D., Linn, R. L., & Gronlund, N. E. (2009). *Measurement and assessment in teaching* (10th ed.). Upper Saddle River, NJ: Prentice Hall.

Nitko, A. J., & Brookhart, S. M. (2011). *Educational assessment of students* (6th ed.). Upper Saddle River, NJ: Pearson Education.

Waltz, C. F., Strickland, O. L., & Lenz, E. R. (2005). *Measurement in nursing and health research* (3rd ed.). New York NY: Springer Publishing.

PART IV

Clinical Evaluation

THIRTEEN

Clinical Evaluation

Nursing as a practice discipline requires development of higher level cognitive skills, values, and psychomotor and technological skills for care of patients across settings. Acquisition of knowledge alone is not sufficient; professional education includes a practice dimension in which students develop competencies for care of patients and learn to think like professionals. Through clinical evaluation the teacher arrives at judgments about the students' competencies—their performance in practice. This chapter describes the process of clinical evaluation in nursing; in the next chapter specific clinical evaluation methods are presented.

OUTCOMES OF CLINICAL PRACTICE

There are many outcomes that students can achieve through their clinical practice experiences. In clinical courses students acquire knowledge and learn about concepts and theories to guide their patient care. They have an opportunity to transfer learning from readings, face-to-face classes and discussions, online classes, simulations, and other experiences to care of patients.

Clinical experiences provide an opportunity for students to use research findings and other evidence to make decisions about interventions and other aspects of patient care. In the practice setting, students learn the process of evidence-based nursing and how to search for, critique, and use evidence in clinical practice. They also need to acquire knowledge, skills, and attitudes for improving the quality of health care (Cronenwett et al., 2007; Cronenwett, Sherwood, & Gelmon, 2009; McKown, McKeon, & Webb, 2011; Sherwood, 2012). In practice, students deal with ambiguous patient situations and unique cases that do not fit the textbook description; this requires students to think critically about what to do. For this reason, clinical practice, whether in the patient care setting or simulation laboratory, is important for developing higher level cognitive skills and for learning to arrive at clinical judgments based on available information. Schön (1990) emphasized the need for such learning in preparing for professional practice. Clinical experiences present problems and situations that may not lend themselves to resolution through the application of scientific theory learned in class and through one's readings. Schön referred to these problems as ones in the swampy lowlands, problems that may be difficult to identify, may present themselves as unique cases, and may be known by the professional but have no clear solutions. When faced with uncertainties in clinical practice and problems not easily solved, students have an opportunity to develop their thinking and clinical judgment skills—important outcomes of clinical practice (Gaberson & Oermann, 2010).

Through practice experiences with patients and in learning and simulation laboratories, students develop their psychomotor skills, learn how to use technology, and gain necessary skills for implementing nursing and other interventions. This practice is essential for initial learning, to refine competencies, and to maintain them over a period of time. Through practice students also learn the "real world" of nursing, which prepares them for the realities of today's health care environment (Hickey, 2010). As health care systems and patients rely increasingly on information technology, students must acquire informatics competencies. Although many nursing programs have computer and information literacy requirements, fewer provide experiences for students to develop the ability to use informatics in clinical practice (Flood, Gasiewicz, & Delpier, 2010; Skiba & Barton, 2009; Tellez, 2012). The Institute of Medicine reports on health professions education and the future of nursing suggested that one of the core competencies of all health care professionals was the ability to use informatics to manage information, communicate, prevent health care errors, and support decision making (Greiner & Knebel, 2003; Institute of Medicine, 2011). Ability to use informatics is another outcome of clinical practice in nursing programs.

Having technical skills, though, is only one aspect of professional practice. In caring for patients and working with nurses and other health care providers, students gain an understanding of how professionals approach their patients' problems, how they interact with each other, and behaviors important in carrying out their roles and working as a team in the practice setting. Learning to collaborate with other health professionals and function effectively on nursing and interprofessional teams are critical to providing quality and safe care (Cronenwett et al., 2007; Sherwood & Barnsteiner, 2012). Clinical learning activities provide an opportunity for students to develop their individual and team communication skills and learn how to collaborate with others.

Practice as a professional is contingent not only on having knowledge to guide decisions but also on having a value system that recognizes the worth, dignity, and rights of patients and others in the health care system. As part of this value system, students need to develop cultural competence and gain the knowledge and attitudes essential to provide multicultural health care. As society becomes more diverse, it is critical for nursing students to become culturally competent (Giddens, North, Carlson-Sabelli, Rogers, & Fogg, 2012; Hawala-Druy & Hill, 2012). Much of this learning can occur in clinical practice as students care for culturally diverse patients and communities and through simulations in which they can explore cultural differences. Clinical experiences help students develop competencies in patient-centered care: respecting patients' preferences, values, and needs; recognizing patients as partners in care; providing compassionate care; continuously coordinating care; and advocating for patients (Greiner & Knebel, 2003; McKeon, Norris, Cardell, & Britt, 2009; Sherwood & Barnsteiner, 2012). These core competencies, needed by all health professionals, are developed in clinical practice.

Another outcome of clinical practice is developing knowledge, skills, and values to continuously improve the quality and safety of health care. Applying quality improvement in health care is a core competency of all health professionals (Cronenwett, Sherwood, & Gelmon, 2009; Greiner & Knebel, 2003; Institute of Medicine, 2011). Nursing students need to learn quality improvement methods and have experience with them as part of their clinical practice. They also need to understand their role in creating a safe health care system for patients and a safety culture in every clinical setting, learn about health care errors and how to prevent them, and value the importance of error reporting. These are competencies that can be developed in simulation and clinical practice.

Some clinical courses focus on management and leadership outcomes. For those courses, clinical practice provides learning opportunities for students to manage groups of patients, provide leadership in the health care setting, and learn how to delegate, among other competencies.

In clinical practice students learn to accept responsibility for their actions and decisions about patients. They also should be willing to accept errors in judgment and learn from them. These are important outcomes of clinical practice in any nursing and health professions program.

Another outcome of clinical practice is learning to learn. Professionals in any field are learners throughout the duration of their careers. Continually expanding knowledge, developments in health care, and new technology alone create the need for lifelong learners in nursing. In clinical practice, students are faced with situations of which they are unsure; they are challenged to raise questions about patient care and seek further learning. In nursing courses as students are faced with gaps in their learning, they should be guided in the self-assessment process, directed to resources for learning, and supported by the teacher. All too often students are hesitant to express their learning needs to their teachers for fear of the effect it will have on their grade or on the teacher's impression of the student's competence in clinical practice.

These outcomes of clinical practice are listed in Exhibit 13.1. Integrated in this list are the core competencies needed by all health care professionals: patient-centered care, teamwork and collaboration, evidence-based practice, quality improvement, safety, and informatics (Cronenwett et al., 2007; Cronenwett, Sherwood, & Gelmon, 2009; Greiner & Knebel, 2003; Sherwood & Barnsteiner, 2012). The outcomes provide a framework for faculty members to use in planning their clinical courses and deciding how to assess student performance. Not all outcomes are applicable to every nursing course; for instance, some courses may not call for the acquisition of technological or delegation skills, but overall most courses will move students toward achievement of these outcomes as they progress through the nursing program.

❏Exhibit 13.1

Outcomes of Clinical Practice in Nursing Programs

- Acquire concepts, theories, and other knowledge for clinical practice
- Use research and other evidence in clinical practice
- Develop higher level thinking and clinical judgment skills
- Develop psychomotor and technological skills, competence in performing other types of interventions, and informatics competencies
- Communicate effectively with patients, others in the health system, and nursing and interprofessional team members
- Develop values and knowledge essential for providing patient-centered care to a culturally and ethnically diverse patient population
- Develop knowledge, skills, and values essential for continuously improving the quality and safety of health care
- Demonstrate leadership skills and behaviors of a professional
- Accept responsibility for actions and decisions
- Accept the need for continued learning and self-development

CONCEPT OF CLINICAL EVALUATION

Clinical evaluation is a process by which judgments are made about learners' competencies in practice. This practice may involve care of patients, families, and communities; other types of experiences in the clinical setting; simulated experiences; and performance of varied skills. Most frequently, clinical evaluation involves observing performance and arriving at judgments about the student's competence. Judgments influence the data collected, that is, the specific types of observations made to evaluate the student's performance, and the inferences and conclusions drawn from the data about the quality of that performance. Teachers may collect different data to evaluate the same outcomes, and when presented with a series of observations about a student's performance in clinical practice, there may be little consistency in their judgments about how well that student performed.

Clinical evaluation is not an objective process; it is subjective—involving judgments of the teacher and others involved in the process. As discussed in Chapter 1, the teacher's values influence evaluation. This is most apparent in clinical evaluation, where our values influence the observations we make of students and the judgments we make about the quality of their performance. Thus, it is important for teachers to be aware of their own values that might bias their judgments of students.

This is not to suggest that clinical evaluation can be value-free; the teacher's observations of performance and conclusions always will be influenced by her or his values. The key is to develop an awareness of these values so as to avoid their influencing clinical evaluation to a point of unfairness to the student. For example, if the teacher prefers students who initiate discussions and participate actively in conferences, this value should not influence judgments about students' competencies in other areas. The teacher needs to be aware of this preference to avoid an unfair evaluation of other dimensions of the students' clinical performance. Or, if the teacher is used to the fast pace of most acute care settings, when working with beginning students or someone who "moves slowly," the teacher should be cautious not to let this prior experience influence expectations of performance. Faculty members should examine their own values, attitudes, and beliefs so that they are aware of them as they teach and assess students' performance in practice settings.

Clinical Evaluation Versus Grading

Clinical evaluation is not the same as grading. In evaluation the teacher makes observations of performance and collects other types of data, then compares this information to a set of standards to arrive at a judgment. From this assessment, a quantitative symbol or grade may be applied to reflect the evaluation data and judgments made about performance. The clinical grade, such as pass–fail or A through F, is the symbol used to represent the evaluation. Clinical performance may be evaluated and not graded, such as with formative evaluation or feedback to the learner, or it may be graded. Grades, however, should not be assigned without sufficient data about clinical performance.

Norm- and Criterion-Referenced Clinical Evaluation

Clinical evaluation may be either norm-referenced or criterion-referenced, as described in Chapter 1. In norm-referenced evaluation, the student's clinical performance is compared with that of other students, indicating that the performance is better than, worse than, or equivalent to that of others in the comparison group or that the student has more or less knowledge, skill, or ability than the other students. Rating students' clinical competencies in relation to others in the clinical group, for example, indicating that the student was "average," is a norm-referenced interpretation.

In contrast, criterion-referenced clinical evaluation involves comparing the student's clinical performance with predetermined criteria, not to the performance of other students in the group. In this type of clinical evaluation, the criteria are known in advance and used as the basis for evaluation. Indicating that the student has met the clinical outcomes or achieved the clinical competencies, regardless of how other students performed, represents a criterion-referenced interpretation.

Formative and Summative Clinical Evaluation

Clinical evaluation may be formative or summative. Formative evaluation in clinical practice provides feedback to learners about their progress in meeting the outcomes of the clinical course or in developing the clinical competencies. The purposes of formative evaluation are to enable students to develop further their clinical knowledge, skills, and values; indicate areas in which learning and practice are needed; and provide a basis for suggesting additional instruction to improve performance. With this type of evaluation, after identifying the learning needs, instruction is provided to move students forward in their learning. Formative evaluation, therefore, is diagnostic; it should not be graded (Nitko & Brookhart, 2011). For example, the clinical teacher or preceptor might observe a student perform wound care and give feedback on changes to make with the technique. The goal of this assessment is to improve subsequent performance, not to grade how well the student carried out the procedure.

Summative clinical evaluation, however, is designed for determining clinical grades because it summarizes competencies the student has developed in clinical practice. Summative evaluation is done at the end of a period of time, for example, at midterm or at the end of the clinical practicum, to assess the extent to which learners have achieved the clinical outcomes or competencies. Summative evaluation is not diagnostic; it summarizes the performance of students at a particular point in time. For much of clinical practice in a nursing education program, summative evaluation comes too late for students to have an opportunity to improve performance. At the end of a course involving care of mothers and children, for instance, there may be many behaviors the student will not have an opportunity to practice in subsequent courses.

Any protocol for clinical evaluation should include extensive formative evaluation and periodic summative evaluation. Formative evaluation is essential to provide feedback to improve performance while practice experiences are still available. A third type of clinical evaluation, confirmative, determines if learners have maintained their clinical competencies over time.

FAIRNESS IN CLINICAL EVALUATION

Considering that clinical evaluation is not objective, the goal is to establish a *fair* evaluation system. Fairness requires that:

1. the teacher identify her/his own values, attitudes, beliefs, and biases that may influence the evaluation process
2. clinical evaluation be based on predetermined outcomes or competencies
3. the teacher develop a supportive clinical learning environment

Identify One's Own Values

Teachers need to be aware of their personal values, attitudes, beliefs, and biases, which may influence the evaluation process. These can affect both the data collected about students and the judgments made about performance. In addition, students have their own set of values and attitudes that influence their self-evaluations of performance and their responses to the teacher's evaluations and feedback. Students' acceptance of the teacher's guidance in clinical practice and information provided to them for improving performance is affected by their past experiences in clinical courses with other faculty. Students may have had problems in prior clinical courses, receiving only negative feedback and limited support from the teacher, staff members, and others. In situations in which student responses inhibit learning, the teacher may need to intervene to guide students to be more self-aware concerning the student's own values and the effect they are having on learning.

Base Clinical Evaluation on Predetermined Outcomes or Competencies

Clinical evaluation should be based on preset outcomes, clinical objectives, or competencies that are then used to guide the evaluation process. Without these, neither the teacher nor the student has any basis for evaluating clinical performance. What are the outcomes of the clinical course (or in some nursing education programs, the clinical objectives) to be met? What clinical competencies should the student develop? These outcomes or competencies provide a framework for faculty members to use in observing performance and for arriving at judgments about achievement in clinical practice. For example, if the competencies relate to developing communication skills, then the learning activities, whether in the patient care setting, as part of a simulation, or in the learning laboratory, should assist students in learning how to communicate. The teacher's observations and subsequent assessment should focus on communication behaviors, not on other competencies unrelated to the learning activities.

Develop a Supportive Learning Environment

It is up to the teacher to develop a supportive learning environment in which students view the teacher as someone who will facilitate their learning and development of clinical competencies. Students need to be comfortable asking faculty and staff questions and seeking their guidance rather than avoiding them in the clinical setting. A supportive environment is critical to effective assessment because students need to recognize that the teacher's feedback is intended to help them improve performance. Developing a "climate" for learning is also important because clinical practice is stressful for students (Li, Wang, Lin, & Lee, 2011; Manning, Cronin, Monaghan, & Rawlings-Anderson, 2009; Moscaritolo, 2009). Many factors influence the development of this learning climate. The clinical setting needs to provide experiences that foster student learning and development. Staff members need to be supportive of students; work collaboratively with each other, students, and the faculty member; and communicate effectively, both individually and as a team (Gaberson & Oermann, 2010). Most of all, trust and respect must exist between the teacher and the students.

STUDENT STRESS IN CLINICAL PRACTICE

There have been a number of studies in nursing education on student stress in the clinical setting. Some of the stresses students have identified are:

- the fear of making a mistake that would harm the patient
- having insufficient knowledge and skills for patient care
- changing patient conditions and uncertainty about how to respond
- being unfamiliar with the staff, policies, and other aspects of the clinical setting
- caring for difficult patients
- having the teacher observe and evaluate clinical performance
- interacting with the patient, the family, nursing staff, and other health care providers

The stresses that students experience in clinical practice, however, may not be the same in each course. For example, in an early study Oermann and Lukomski (2001) found that students were more stressed in their pediatric nursing course than in other courses in the curriculum. More recently, Fisher, Taylor, and High (2012) examined the outcomes of students participating in parent-led post conferences. One of the findings was that students were apprehensive about talking with parents. The parent-led conferences provided an opportunity for students to better understand their important role in communicating with parents and working with families. Further study is needed about differences in student stress across courses in a nursing program, particularly as this may influence their clinical performance.

Learning in the clinical setting is a *public experience*. Students cannot hide their lack of understanding or skills as they might in class or in an online discussion. In clinical practice the possibility exists for many people to observe the student's performance—the teacher, patient, peers, nursing staff, and other health care providers. Being observed and evaluated by others is stressful for students in any health care field.

The potential stress that students might experience in clinical practice reinforces the need for faculty members to be aware of the learning environment they set when working with students in a clinical course. In a qualitative study by Melincavage (2011), students described behaviors of physicians, staff nurses, and faculty members that contributed to their anxiety. The author recommended that nurse educators realize the power structure in the clinical setting, teach students conflict resolution techniques and coping mechanisms, support them in sharing their perceptions, and work with staff to change their behaviors. The student is a learner, not a nurse, although some educators and staff expect students to perform at an expert level without giving them sufficient time to practice and refine their performance (Gaberson & Oermann, 2010). Simulated experiences may be effective in reducing some of the anxieties students experience by allowing them to practice their skills, both cognitive and psychomotor, prior to care of patients.

FEEDBACK IN CLINICAL EVALUATION

For clinical evaluation to be effective, the teacher should provide continuous feedback to students about their performance and how they can improve it. Feedback is the communication of information to students, based on the teacher's assessment, that enables students to reflect on their performance, identify continued learning needs, and decide how to meet them (Bonnel, 2008). Feedback may be verbal, by describing observations of performance and explaining what to do differently, or visual, by demonstrating correct performance. Feedback should be specific and accompanied by further instruction from the teacher or by working with students to identify appropriate learning activities. The ultimate goal is for students to progress to a point at which they can judge their own performance, identify resources for their learning, and use those resources to further develop competencies. Bonnel emphasized that for feedback to be useful, students need to reflect on the information communicated to them and take an active role in incorporating that feedback in their own learning (p. 290).

Students must have an underlying knowledge base and beginning skills to judge their own performance. Nitko and Brookhart (2011) suggested that feedback on performance also identifies the possible causes or reasons why the student has not mastered the learning outcomes. Sometimes the reason is that the student does not have the prerequisite knowledge and skills for developing the new competencies. As such it is critical for faculty members and preceptors to begin their interactions with students by assessing whether students have learned the necessary concepts and skills and, if not, to start there.

Principles of Providing Feedback as Part of Clinical Evaluation

There are five principles for providing feedback to students as part of the clinical evaluation process. First, the feedback should be precise and specific. General information about performance, such as "You need to work on your assessment" or "You need more practice in the simulation center," does not indicate which behaviors need improvement or how to develop them. Instead of using general statements, the teacher should indicate what specific areas of knowledge are lacking, where there are problems in thinking and clinical judgments, and what particular competencies need more development (Gaberson & Oermann, 2010). Rather than saying to a student, "You need to work on your assessment," the feedback would be more effective if the teacher identified the specific areas of data collection omitted and the physical examination techniques that need improvement. Specific feedback is more valuable to learners than a general description of their behavior.

Second, for procedures, use of technologies, and any psychomotor skill, the teacher should provide both verbal and visual feedback to students. This means that the teacher should explain first, either orally or in writing, where the errors were made in performance and then demonstrate the correct procedure or skill. This should be followed by student practice of the skill with the teacher guiding performance. By allowing immediate practice, with the teacher available to correct problems, students can more easily *use* the feedback to further develop their skills.

Third, feedback about performance should be given to students at the time of learning or immediately following it. Giving prompt feedback is one of the seven core principles for effective teaching in undergraduate programs (Chickering & Gamson, 1987, 1991). Providing prompt and rich feedback is equally important when teaching graduate students, nurses, and other learners regardless of their educational level. The longer the period of time between performance and feedback from the teacher, the less effective the feedback (Gaberson & Oermann, 2010). As time passes, neither student nor teacher may remember specific areas of clinical practice to be improved. This principle holds true whether the performance relates to critical thinking and clinical judgment, a procedure or technical skill, or an attitude or value expressed by the student, among other areas. Whether working with a group of students in a clinical setting, communicating with preceptors about students, or teaching an online course, the teacher needs to develop a strategy for giving focused and immediate feedback to students and following up with further discussion as needed. Recording short notes on paper or with some technology for later discussion with individual students helps the teacher remember important points about performance.

Fourth, students need different amounts of feedback and positive reinforcement. In beginning practice and with clinical situations that are new to learners, most students will need frequent and extensive feedback. As students progress through the program and become more competent, they should be able to assess their own performance and identify personal learning needs. Some students will require more feedback and direction from the teacher than others. As with many aspects of education, one approach does not fit all students. Regardless of the extent of feedback a student may need, feedback should always be given in private, allowing time for discussion about performance and with consideration for the student's feelings (Clynes & Raftery, 2008).

One final principle is that feedback should be diagnostic. This means that after identifying areas in which further learning is needed, the teacher's responsibility is to guide students so that they can improve their performance. The process is cyclical—the teacher observes and assesses performance, gives students feedback about that performance, and then guides their learning and practice so they can become more competent.

Gigante, Dell, and Sharkey (2011) proposed a 5-step process for giving feedback to students:

1. Identify the expectations for the student. Students need to know what is expected of them in the clinical practicum.
2. Set the stage for the student to receive feedback from the teacher and others involved in the learning situation. The authors recommend beginning with this phrase, "I am giving you feedback" because then students realize that the information is to help them improve performance. Feedback must be given promptly and privately.
3. Begin the interaction by asking students to assess their own performance, encouraging reflection and lifelong learning.
4. Describe how the student is performing based on specific observations of behaviors, which should be shared. It is important to provide concrete examples of performance and describe specifically how the learner can improve.
5. Suggest ways the student can improve performance with input from the learner. In some cases, such as when there are concerns about not achieving at a satisfactory level in the course, a written plan for improvement should be developed with consequences outlined. (p. 206)

CLINICAL OUTCOMES AND COMPETENCIES

There are different ways of specifying the outcomes to be achieved in clinical practice, which in turn provide the basis for clinical evaluation. These may be stated in the form of outcomes to be met or as competencies to be demonstrated in clinical practice. The faculties of some nursing education programs specify the outcomes in the form of clinical objectives. Regardless of how these are stated, they represent *what* is evaluated in clinical practice.

The outcomes of clinical practice offered in Exhibit 13.1 can be used for developing specific outcomes or competencies for a clinical course. Not all clinical courses will have outcomes in each of these areas, and in some courses there may be other types of competencies unique to practice in that clinical specialty. Some faculty members identify common outcomes or competencies that are used for each clinical course in the program and then level those to demonstrate their progressive development through the nursing program (Billings & Halstead, 2009; Oermann, Yarbrough, Ard, Saewert, & Charasika, 2009). For example, with this model, each course would have an outcome on communication. In a beginning clinical course, the outcome might be, "Identifies verbal and nonverbal techniques for communicating with patients." In a later course in the curriculum, the communication outcome might focus on the family and working with caregivers, for example, "Develops interpersonal relationships with families and caregivers." Then in the community health course the outcome might be, "Collaborates with other health care providers in care of patients in the community and the community as client."

As another approach, some faculty members state the outcomes broadly and then indicate specific behaviors students should demonstrate to meet those outcomes in a particular course. For example, the outcome on communication might be stated as "Communicates effectively with patients and within nursing and interprofessional teams." Examples of behaviors that indicate achievement of this outcome in a course on care of children include, "Uses appropriate verbal and nonverbal communication based on the child's age, developmental status, and health condition" and "Interacts effectively with parents, caregivers, and the interprofessional team." Generally, the outcomes or competencies are then used for developing the clinical evaluation tool or rating form, which is discussed in the next chapter.

Regardless of how the outcomes are stated for a clinical course, they need to be specific enough to guide the evaluation of students in clinical practice. An outcome such as "Use the nursing process in care of children" is too broad to guide evaluation. More specific outcomes such as "Carries out a systematic assessment of children reflecting their developmental stage," "Evaluates the impact of health problems on the child and family," and "Identifies resources for managing the child's care at home" make clear to students what is expected of them in clinical practice.

Competencies are the abilities to be demonstrated by the learner in clinical practice. Boland (2009) viewed competencies as the knowledge, skills, and attitudes that students need to develop. For nurses in practice, these competencies reflect the expected level of performance for caring for patients in the health care setting. Competencies for nurses are assessed as part of the orientation to the health care setting and on an ongoing basis, ensuring that employees are qualified to practice based on the organization's mission, patient population, and types of services delivered (Bashford, Shaffer, & Young, 2012).

Caution should be exercised in developing clinical outcomes and competencies to avoid having too many for evaluation, considering the number of learners for whom the teacher is responsible, types of clinical learning opportunities available, and time allotted for clinical learning activities. In preparing outcomes or competencies for a clinical course, teachers should keep in mind that they need to collect sufficient data about students' performance of each outcome or competency specified for that course. Too many outcomes make it nearly impossible to collect enough data on the performance of all of the students in the clinical setting whether they are in a small group with a faculty member on-site or are working one-to-one with a clinician. Regardless of how the evaluation system is developed, the clinical outcomes or competencies need to be realistic and useful for guiding the evaluation.

SUMMARY

Through clinical evaluation the teacher arrives at judgments about students' performance in clinical practice. The teacher's observations of performance should focus on the outcomes to be met or competencies to be developed in the clinical course. These provide the framework for learning in clinical practice and the basis for evaluating performance.

Although a framework such as this is essential in clinical evaluation, teachers also need to examine their own beliefs about the evaluation process and the purposes it serves in nursing. Clarifying one's own values, beliefs, attitudes, and biases that may affect evaluation is an important first step. Recognizing the inherent stress of clinical practice for many students and developing a supportive learning environment are also important. Other concepts of evaluation, presented in Chapter 1, apply to clinical evaluation. Specific methods for clinical evaluation are described in the next chapter.

REFERENCES

Bashford, C. W., Shaffer, B. J., & Young, C. M. (2012). Assessment of clinical judgment in nursing orientation: Time well invested. *Journal for Nurses in Staff Development, 28*, 62–65.

Billings, D. M., & Halstead, J. A. (2009). *Teaching in nursing: A guide for faculty*. St. Louis, MO: Saunders.

Boland, D. L. (2009). Developing curriculum frameworks, outcomes, and competencies. In D. M. Billings & J. A. Halstead (Eds.), *Teaching in nursing: A guide for faculty* (3rd ed., pp. 137–153). St. Louis, MO: Saunders.

Bonnel, W. (2008). Improving feedback to students in online courses. *Nursing Education Perspectives, 29*, 290–294.

Chickering, A. W., & Gamson, Z. F. (1987). Seven principles for good practice in undergraduate education. *AAHE Bulletin, 39*(7), 3–7.

Chickering, A. W., & Gamson, Z. F. (1991). Applying the seven principles for good practice in undergraduate education. In *New directions in teaching and learning* (No. 47). San Francisco, CA: Jossey-Bass.

Clynes, M. P., & Raftery, S. E. C. (2008). Feedback: An essential element of student learning in clinical practice. *Nurse Education in Practice, 8*, 405–411.

Cronenwett, L., Sherwood, G., Barnsteiner, J., Disch, J., Johnson, J., Mitchell, P., ... Warren, J. (2007). Quality and safety education for nurses. *Nursing Outlook, 55*, 122–131.

Cronenwett, L., Sherwood, G., & Gelmon, S. B. (2009). Improving quality and safety education: The QSEN Learning Collaborative. *Nursing Outlook, 57*, 304–312.

Fisher, M. J., Taylor, E. A., & High, P. L. (2012). Parent-nursing student communication practice: Role-play and learning outcomes. *Journal of Nursing Education, 51*, 115–119.

Flood, L. S., Gasiewicz, N., & Delpier, T. (2010). Integrating information literacy across a BSN curriculum. *Journal of Nursing Education, 49*, 101–104.

Gaberson, K. B., & Oermann, M. H. (2010). *Clinical teaching strategies in nursing* (3rd ed.). New York, NY: Springer.

Giddens, J. F., North, S., Carlson-Sabelli, L., Rogers, E., & Fogg, L. (2012). Using a virtual community to enhance cultural awareness. *Journal of Transcultural Nursing, 23*, 198–204.

Gigante, J., Dell, M., & Sharkey, A. (2011). Getting beyond "good job": How to give effective feedback. *Pediatrics, 127*, 205–207.

Greiner, A. C., & Knebel, E. (Eds.). (2003). *Health professions education: A bridge to quality.* Washington, DC: National Academies Press.

Hawala-Druy, S., & Hill, M. H. (2012). Interdisciplinary: Cultural competency and culturally congruent education for millennials in health professions. *Nurse Education Today, 32*, 772–778.

Hickey, M. T. (2010). Baccalaureate nursing graduates' perceptions of their clinical instructional experiences and preparation for practice. *Journal of Professional Nursing, 26*, 35–41.

Institute of Medicine. (2011). *The future of nursing: Leading change, advancing health.* Washington, DC: The National Academies Press.

Li, H. C., Wang, L. S., Lin, Y. H., & Lee, I. (2011). The effect of a peer-mentoring strategy on student nurse stress reduction in clinical practice. *International Nursing Review, 58*, 203–210.

Manning, A., Cronin, P., Monaghan, A., & Rawlings-Anderson, K. (2009). Supporting students in practice: An exploration of reflective groups as a means of support. *Nurse Education in Practice, 9*, 176–183.

McKeon, L. M., Norris, T., Cardell, B., & Britt, T. (2009). Developing patient-centered care competencies among prelicensure nursing students using simulation. *Journal of Nursing Education, 48*, 711–715.

McKown, T., McKeon, L., & Webb, S. (2011). Using quality and safety education for nurses to guide clinical teaching on a new dedicated education unit. *Journal of Nursing Education, 50*, 706–710.

Melincavage, S. M. (2011). Student nurses' experiences of anxiety in the clinical setting. *Nurse Education Today, 31*, 785–789.

Moscaritolo, L. M. (2009). Interventional strategies to decrease nursing student anxiety in the clinical learning environment. *Journal of Nursing Education, 48*, 17–23.

Nitko, A. J., & Brookhart, S. M. (2011). *Educational assessment of students* (6th ed.). Upper Saddle River, NJ: Pearson Education.

Oermann, M. H., & Lukomski, A. P. (2001). Experiences of students in pediatric nursing clinical courses. *Journal of the Society of Pediatric Nurses, 9*(2), 65–72.

Oermann, M. H., Yarbrough, S. S., Ard, N., Saewert, K. J., & Charasika, M. (2009). Clinical evaluation and grading practices in schools of nursing: National survey findings Part II. *Nursing Education Perspectives, 30*, 352–357.

Schön, D. A. (1990). *Educating the reflective practitioner*. San Francisco, CA: Jossey-Bass.

Sherwood, G. (2012). Driving forces for quality and safety: Changing mindsets to improve health care. In G. Sherwood & J. Barnsteiner (Eds.), *Quality and safety in nursing: A competency approach to improving outcomes* (pp. 3–22). Oxford, England: John Wiley & Sons.

Sherwood, G., & Barnsteiner, J. (Eds.). (2012). *Quality and safety in nursing: A competency approach to improving outcomes*. Oxford, UK: John Wiley & Sons.

Skiba, D. J., & Barton, A. J. (2009). Using social software to transform informatics education. *Studies in Health Technology and Informatics, 146,* 608–612.

Tellez, M. (2012). Nursing informatics education past, present, and future. *CIN: Computers, Informatics, Nursing, 30,* 229–233.

FOURTEEN

Clinical Evaluation Methods

After establishing a framework for evaluating students in clinical practice and exploring one's own values, attitudes, and biases that may influence evaluation, the teacher identifies a variety of methods for collecting data on student performance. Clinical evaluation methods are strategies for assessing learning outcomes and performance in clinical practice. That practice may be with patients in hospitals and other health care facilities, with families and communities, in simulation and learning laboratories, or involving other activities using multimedia. Some evaluation methods are most appropriate for use by faculty or preceptors who are on-site with students and can observe their performance; other evaluation methods assess students' knowledge, cognitive skills, and other competencies but do not involve direct observation of their performance.

There are many evaluation methods for use in nursing education. Some methods, such as reflective writing assignments, are most appropriate for formative evaluation, whereas others are useful for either formative or summative evaluation. In this chapter varied strategies are presented for evaluating clinical performance.

SELECTING CLINICAL EVALUATION METHODS

There are several factors to consider when selecting clinical evaluation methods to use in a course. First, the evaluation methods should provide information on student performance of the clinical competencies associated with the course. With the evaluation methods, the teacher collects data on performance to judge if students are developing the clinical competencies or have achieved them by the end of the course. For many outcomes of a course, there are different strategies that can be used, thereby providing flexibility in choosing methods for evaluation. Most evaluation methods provide data on multiple clinical outcomes. For example, a written assignment in which students compare two different data sets might relate to outcomes on assessment, analysis, and writing. In planning the evaluation for a clinical course, the teacher reviews the outcomes or competencies to be developed and decides which evaluation methods will be used for assessing them, recognizing that most methods provide information on more than one outcome or competency.

In clinical courses in nursing programs, students are evaluated typically on the outcomes of clinical practice, as identified in Exhibit 13.1 in Chapter 13. These relate to students' knowledge; use of evidence in practice; higher level thinking skills; psychomotor, technological, and informatics competencies; communication and teamwork skills; values and professional behaviors; quality and safety competencies; leadership skills; responsibility; and self-assessment and development. Some of these competencies are easier to assess than others, but all aspects should be addressed in the evaluation process. Because of the breadth of competencies students need to develop, multiple strategies should be used for assessment in clinical courses.

Second, there are many different clinical evaluation strategies that might be used to assess performance. Varying the methods maintains student interest and takes into account individual needs, abilities, and characteristics of learners. Some students may be more proficient in methods that depend on writing, whereas others prefer strategies such as conferences and other discussion forms. Planning for multiple evaluation methods in clinical courses, as long as they are congruent with the outcomes to be evaluated, reflects these differences among students. It also avoids relying on one method, such as a rating scale, for determining the entire clinical grade. Although there is limited research on the effectiveness of many evaluation methods used in nursing education, teachers should examine studies that have been done and other literature. A review of the literature may provide faculty members with ideas about how to assess particular competencies in their courses and methods already developed by other nurse educators. In one study, fewer than half of the nurse faculty respondents considered research on the effectiveness of various assessment strategies as very important in their decisions on assessment in a course (Oermann, Saewert, Charasika, & Yarbrough, 2009).

Third, the teacher should always select evaluation methods that are realistic considering the number of students to be evaluated, available practice or simulation activities, and constraints such as the teacher's or preceptor's time. Planning for an evaluation method that depends on patients with specific health problems or particular clinical situations is not realistic considering the types of experiences with actual patients available to students. For that goal, a simulation or use of standardized patients would be more appropriate. Some methods are not feasible because of the number of students who would need to use them within the time frame of the course. Others may be too costly or require resources not available in the nursing education program or health care setting.

Fourth, evaluation methods can be used for either formative or summative evaluation. In the process of deciding how to evaluate students' clinical performance, the teacher should identify whether the methods will be used to provide feedback to learners (formative) or for grading (summative). With formative clinical evaluation, the focus is on the progression of students in meeting the learning goals (Clynes & Raftery, 2008; Gigante, Dell, & Sharkey, 2011). At the end of the rotation, course, or semester, summative evaluation establishes whether the student met those goals and is competent (Bourke & Ihrke, 2009; Gaberson & Oermann, 2010). In clinical practice, students should know ahead of time whether the assessment by the teacher is for formative or summative purposes. Some of the methods designed for clinical evaluation provide feedback to students on areas for improvement and should not be graded. Other methods such as rating scales and written assignments can be used for summative purposes and therefore can be computed as part of the course or clinical grade.

Fifth, before finalizing the protocol for evaluating clinical performance in a course, the teacher should review the purpose of each assignment completed by students in clinical practice and should decide on how many assignments will be in the course. What are the purposes of these assignments, and how many are needed to demonstrate competency? In some clinical courses, students complete an excessive number of written assignments. How many assignments, regardless of whether they are for formative or summative purposes, are needed to meet the outcomes of the course? Students benefit from continuous feedback from the teacher, not from repetitive assignments that contribute little to their development of clinical knowledge and skills. Rather than daily or weekly care plans or other assignments, which may not even be consistent with current practice, once students develop the competencies, they can progress to other, more relevant learning activities.

Sixth, in deciding how to evaluate clinical performance, the teacher should consider the time needed to complete the evaluation, provide feedback, and grade the assignment. Instead of requiring a series of written assignments in a clinical course, the same outcomes might be met through discussions with students, case analysis by students in clinical conferences, group-writing activities, and other methods requiring less teacher time that accomplish the same purposes. Considering the demands on nursing faculty members, it is important to consider one's own time when planning how to evaluate students' performance in clinical practice (Oermann, 2004).

The rest of the chapter presents clinical evaluation methods for use in nursing education programs. Some of these methods such as written assignments were examined in earlier chapters.

OBSERVATION

The predominant strategy for evaluating clinical performance is observing students in clinical practice, simulation and learning laboratories, and other settings. In a survey of 1,573 faculty members representing all types of prelicensure nursing programs (diploma, 128; associate degree, 866; baccalaureate, 563; and other entry-level, 16), observation of student performance was the predominant strategy used across programs (93%) (Oermann, Yarbrough, Ard, Saewert, & Charasika, 2009). Although observation is widely used, there are threats to its validity and reliability. First, observations of students may be influenced by the teacher's values, attitudes, and biases, as discussed in the last chapter. There also may be over-reliance on first impressions, which might change as the teacher or preceptor observes the student over a period of time and in different situations. In any performance assessment there needs to be a series of observations made before drawing conclusions about performance.

Second, in observing performance, there are many aspects of that performance on which the teacher may focus attention. For example, while observing a student administer an IV medication, the teacher may focus mainly on the technique used for its administration, ask limited questions about the purpose of the medication, and make no observations of how the student interacts with the patient. Another teacher observing this same student may focus on those other aspects. The same practice situation, therefore, may yield different observations.

Third, the teacher may arrive at incorrect judgments about the observation, such as inferring that a student is inattentive during conference when in fact the student is thinking about the comments made by others in the group. It is important to discuss observations with students, obtain their perceptions of their behavior, and be willing to modify one's own inferences when new data are presented. In discussing observations and impressions with students, the teacher can learn about their perceptions of performance; this, in turn, may provide additional information that influences the teacher's judgment about competencies (Oermann, 2008).

Fourth, every observation in the clinical setting reflects only a sampling of the learner's performance during a clinical activity. An observation of the same student at another time may reveal a different level of performance. The same holds true for observations of the teacher; on some clinical days and for some classes the teacher's behaviors do not represent a typical level of performance. An observation of the same teacher during another clinical activity and class may reveal a different quality of teaching.

Finally, similar to other clinical evaluation methods, the outcomes or competencies guide the teacher on *what* to observe. They help the teacher focus the observations of performance. However, all observations should be shared with the students.

Notes About Performance

It is difficult if not impossible to remember the observations made of each student for each clinical activity. For this reason teachers need a strategy to help them remember their observations and the context in which the performance occurred. There are several ways of recording observations of students in clinical settings, simulation and learning laboratories, and other settings such as notes about performance, checklists, and rating scales. These are summarized in Table 14.1.

The teacher can make notes that describe the observations made of students in the clinical setting; these are sometimes called anecdotal notes. Some teachers include only a description of the observed performance and then, after a series of observations, review the pattern of the performance and draw conclusions about it. Other teachers record their observations and include a judgment about how well the student performed (Di Leonardi & Oermann, 2010). Notes about observations of performance should be recorded as close to the time of the observation as possible; otherwise it is difficult to remember what was observed and the context, for example, the patient and clinical situation, of that observation. In a study of clinical nurse educators from six schools of nursing, 97% reported they use anecdotal notes as part of the evaluation process (Hall, Daly, & Madigan, 2010).

⊔Table 14.1

METHODS FOR RECORDING OBSERVATIONS	
Notes About Performance	Used for recording descriptions of observations made of students in the clinical setting, simulation laboratory, and other learning activities in which teachers, preceptors, and others observe performance. May also include interpretations or conclusions about the performance. Often referred to as anecdotal notes.
Checklists	Used primarily for recording observations of specific competencies, procedures, and skills performed by students; includes list of behaviors to demonstrate competency and steps for carrying out the procedure or skill. May also include errors in performance to check.
Rating Scales	Used for recording judgments about students' performance in clinical practice. Includes a set of defined clinical outcomes and competencies and scale for rating the degree of competence (with multiple levels or pass–fail).

Areas of performance identified as essential for use of anecdotal notes were medication accuracy, patient safety, and professional behaviors. In the clinical setting, notes can be handwritten or recorded in Personal Digital Assistants (PDAs) or by using other portable devices such as a tablet computer or an iPad (Apple Inc., Cupertino, CA). These technologies can lead to more accurate student evaluation because the observations can be recorded in real time (Zurmehly, 2010). With these types of devices teachers can keep a running record for each student and share it easily with students. The notes can then be exported to the computer for formatting and printing.

The goal of the anecdotal note is to provide a description of the student's performance as observed by the teacher or preceptor. Liberto, Roncher, and Shellenbarger (1999) identified five key areas to include in an anecdotal note:

- Date of the observation
- Student name
- Faculty signature
- Setting of the observation
- Record of student actions, with an objective and a detailed description of the observed performance (p. 16)

Notes should be shared with students as frequently as possible; otherwise they are not effective for feedback. Considering the issues associated with observations of clinical performance, the teacher should discuss observations with the students and be willing to incorporate their own judgments about the performance. Notes about performance also are useful in conferences with students, for example, at midterm and end-of-term, as a way of reviewing a pattern of performance over time. When there are sufficient observations about performance, the notes can serve as documentation for ratings on the clinical evaluation tool.

Checklists

A checklist is a list of specific behaviors or actions to be observed with a place for marking whether or not they were present during the performance (Nitko & Brookhart, 2011). A checklist often lists the steps to be followed in performing a procedure or demonstrating a skill. Some checklists also include errors in performance that are commonly made. Checklists not only facilitate the teacher's observations, but they also provide a way for learners to assess their own performance. With checklists, learners can review and evaluate their performance prior to assessment by the teacher.

Checklists are used frequently in health care settings to assess skills of nurses and document their continuing competence in performing them. They also are used to assess performance in simulations. Many checklists and tools have been developed for evaluating the performance of students, nurses, and other health professionals in simulations. For example, Liaw, Scherpbier, Klainin-Yobas, and Rethans (2011) developed and tested a tool that can be used for evaluating students' performance in a simulation in managing and reporting clinical deterioration of a patient. When skills are assessed in an Objective Structured Clinical Examination (OSCE) or by using standardized patients, checklists are often included to guide observations of performance of those skills.

For common procedures and skills, teachers often can find checklists already prepared that can be used for evaluation, and some nursing textbooks have accompanying skills checklists. When these resources are not available, teachers can develop their own checklists. Initially, it is important to review the procedure or competency to understand the steps in the procedure and critical elements in its performance. The steps that follow indicate how to develop a checklist for rating performance:

1. List each step or action to be demonstrated in the correct order
2. Add to the list specific errors students often make (to alert the assessor to observe for these)
3. Develop the list into a form to check off the steps or actions as they are performed in the proper sequence (Nitko & Brookhart, 2011)

In designing checklists, it is important not to include every possible step, which makes the checklist too cumbersome to use, but to focus instead on critical actions and where they fit into the sequence. The goal is for students to learn how to perform a procedure and use technology safely. When there are different ways of performing a procedure, the students should be allowed that flexibility when evaluated. Exhibit 14.1 provides an example of a checklist.

Rating Scales

Rating scales, also referred to as clinical evaluation tools or instruments, provide a means of recording judgments about the observed performance of students in clinical practice. A rating scale has two parts: (a) a list of outcomes or competencies the student is to demonstrate in clinical practice and (b) a scale for rating the student's performance of them.

Rating scales are most useful for summative evaluation of performance; after observing students over a period of time, the teacher arrives at conclusions about performance, rating it according to the scale provided with the tool. They also may be used to evaluate specific activities that the students complete in clinical practice, for example, rating a student's presentation of a case in clinical conference. Other uses of rating scales are to: (a) help students focus their attention on important competencies to be

☐Exhibit 14.1

Sample Checklist

Student Name _____

_____

Instructions to teacher/examiner: Observe the student performing the following procedure and check the steps completed properly by the student. Check only those steps that the student performed properly. After completing the checklist, discuss performance with the student, reviewing aspects of the procedure to be improved.

IV Medication Administration

Checklist:

- ☐ Checks provider's order
- ☐ Checks medication administration record
- ☐ Adheres to rights of medication administration
- ☐ Assembles appropriate equipment
- ☐ Checks compatibility with existing IV if present
- ☐ Explains procedure to patient
- ☐ Positions patient appropriately
- ☐ Checks patency of administration port or line
- ☐ Administers medication at proper rate and concentration
- ☐ Monitors patient response
- ☐ Flushes tubing as necessary
- ☐ Documents IV medication correctly

---

developed, (b) give specific feedback to students about their performance, and (c) demonstrate growth in clinical competencies over a designated time period if the same rating scale is used. Rating scales also are used to assess performance in simulations. Generally in simulations the goal of the assessment is formative, providing feedback to students on their judgments and actions taken in the simulation. However, some educators are using simulations for high-stakes evaluation, determining students' achievement of end-of-program competencies (Bensfield, Olech, & Horsley, 2012).

The same rating scale can be used for multiple purposes. Exhibit 14.2 shows sample competencies from a rating scale that is used midway through a course; in Exhibit 14.3 those same competencies are used for the final evaluation, but the performance is rated as "satisfactory" or "unsatisfactory" as a summative rating. Alternately, one form, designed to rate performance at both midterm and the end of the course, can be used. An example of this format can be seen in exhibits later in this chapter.

Types of Rating Scales

Many types of rating scales are used for evaluating clinical performance. The scales may have multiple levels for rating performance, such as 1 to 5 or exceptional to below average, or have two levels, such as pass–fail or

☐Exhibit 14.2

Sample Competencies from Rating Scale for Formative Evaluation

Maternal–Newborn Nursing
Mid-Term Progress Report

Name _____

Date _____

OBJECTIVE	Yes	No	Not Obs.
1. Provides patient-centered care to mothers and newborns			
A. Assesses the individual needs of mothers and newborns			
B. Plans care to meet the patient's needs			
C. Implements nursing interventions based on evidence			
D. Evaluates the outcomes of care			
E. Includes the family in planning and implementing care for the mother and newborn			
2. Participates in health teaching for maternal–newborn patients and families			
A. Identifies learning needs of mothers and families			
B. Identifies processes for improving the quality of health teaching in the setting			

Note: Not obs. = not observed.

❏Exhibit 14.3

Sample Competencies From Same Rating Scale for Final Evaluation

Maternal–Newborn Nursing
Clinical Performance Evaluation

Name _____

Date _____

COMPETENCIES	S	U
1. Provides patient-centered care to mothers and newborns		
A. Assesses the individual needs of mothers and newborns		
B. Plans care to meet the patient's needs		
C. Implements nursing interventions based on evidence		
D. Evaluates the outcomes of care		
E. Includes the family in planning and implementing care for the mother and newborn		
2. Participates in health teaching for maternal–newborn patients and families		
A. Identifies learning needs of mothers and families		
B. Identifies processes for improving the quality of health teaching in the setting		

Note: S = Satisfactory, U = Unsatisfactory.

satisfactory-unsatisfactory. Types of scales with multiple levels for rating performance include:

- Letters: A, B, C, D, E or A, B, C, D, F
- Numbers: 1, 2, 3, 4, 5
- Qualitative labels: Excellent, very good, good, fair, and poor; Exceptional, above average, average, and below average
- Frequency labels: Always, often, sometimes, and never

Exhibit 14.4 provides an example of a rating scale for clinical evaluation that has multiple levels for rating performance.

❑Exhibit 14.4

Clinical Evaluation Tool with Multiple Levels for Rating Performance

Community Health Nursing (RN section)
CLINICAL EVALUATION FORM

Total Raw Score: _____   Student Name: _____

Mean Score: _____   Faculty Name: _____

Letter Grade: _____   Agency: _____

Uses a theoretical framework in care of individuals, families, and groups in the community	4	3	2	1	NO
A. Applies concepts and theories in the practice of community health nursing					
B. Examines multicultural concepts of care as they apply to the community					
C. Analyzes family theory as a basis for care of clients in a community setting					
D. Examines relationships of family members within a community setting					
E. Examines the community as a client through ongoing assessment					
F. Evaluates health care delivery systems within a community setting					
Uses the nursing process for care of individuals, families, and groups in the community and the community as client					
A. Adapts assessment skills in the collection of data from individuals, families, and groups in a community setting					
B. Uses relevant resources in the collection of data in the community					
C. Analyzes client and community data*					
D. Develops nursing diagnoses for individuals, families, and groups within the community and the community as client					
E. Develops measurable outcome criteria and plan of action					

(continued)

Exhibit 14.4 *(continued)*

	4	3	2	1	NO
F. Uses outcome criteria for evaluating plans and effectiveness of interventions					
G. Assumes accountability for own practice in the community*					
H. Uses research findings and standards for community-based care					
I. Accepts differences among clients and communities*					
Is responsible for identifying and meeting own learning needs					
A. Evaluates own development as a professional*					
B. Meets own learning needs in community practice*					
Collaborates with others in providing community care					
A. Interacts effectively with clients and others in the community					
B. Uses community resources effectively					

FACULTY–STUDENT NARRATIVE

Faculty Comments:

Signature: _____

Date: _____

Student Comments:

Signature: _____

Date: _____

*Critical behaviors must be passed at 2.0 to pass clinical practicum.
Note: NO = Not Observed
4 = Consistently excels in performance of behavior
3 = Is competent in performance
2 = Performs behavior safely
1 = Unable to perform behavior

Tool developed by Judith M. Fouladbakhsh, PhD, RN, APRN, BC, AHN-BC, CHTP. Adapted by permission of J. Fouladbakhsh, 2012.

Some instruments for rating clinical performance combine different types of scales. For example, Holaday and Buckley (2008) developed a tool for rating performance at five levels of competence: from dependent (0) to self-directed (4). A score is generated from the ratings and can be used to convert to a grade.

A short description included with the letters, numbers, and labels for each of the outcomes or competencies rated improves objectivity and consistency (Nitko & Brookhart, 2011). For example, if teachers were using a scale of exceptional, above average, average, and below average, or based on the numbers 4, 3, 2, and 1, short descriptions of each level in the scale could be written to clarify the performance expected at each level. For the clinical outcome "Collects relevant data from patient," the descriptors might be:

Exceptional (or 4): Differentiates relevant from irrelevant data, analyzes multiple sources of data, establishes comprehensive database, identifies data needed for evaluating all possible patient problems.

Above Average (or 3): Collects significant data from patients, uses multiple sources of data as part of assessment, identifies possible patient problems based on the data.

Average (or 2): Collects significant data from patients, uses data to develop main patient problems.

Below Average (or 1): Does not collect significant data and misses important cues in data; unable to explain relevance of data for patient problems.

Rating scales for clinical evaluation also may have two levels such as pass–fail and satisfactory–unsatisfactory. A survey of nursing faculty from all types of programs indicated that most faculty members ($n = 1,116$; 83%) used pass–fail or satisfactory-unsatisfactory in their clinical courses (Oermann, Yarbrough, et al., 2009). Exhibits 14.5 and 14.6 are examples of clinical evaluation tools that have two levels for rating performance: satisfactory–unsatisfactory. For midterm evaluation, which is formative, a column can be added that indicates for students the competencies that need improvement, as shown in these exhibits. With the aim of preparing students with the knowledge, skills, and values for improving the quality and safety of health care, clinical courses should reflect these competencies. Exhibits 14.5 and 14.6 illustrate tools that were developed based on the Quality and Safety Education for Nurses (QSEN) competencies (QSEN, 2012). They also demonstrate how the competencies are developed progressively in a nursing program: the core competencies in Exhibit 14.6, a course in the second level of the nursing program, are a higher level than the performance expected of students in the level I course in Exhibit 14.5.

❑Exhibit 14.5

Clinical Evaluation Tool With Two Levels for Rating Performance (Based on QSEN Competencies)

NICHOLLS STATE UNIVERSITY
DEPARTMENT OF NURSING
BSN PROGRAM

Clinical Performance Evaluation Tool
NURS 225 Level I

Self Evaluation _____
Faculty Evaluation _____

Student Name_____

Faculty_____   Course: NURS 225   Semester_____

Fill in appropriate fields to the right & below:

Student must obtain a Satisfactory "S" grade in all competencies at the Final Evaluation to pass the Course.

Core Competencies	Midterm			Final	
	S	NI	U	S	U
Focusing on wellness, health promotion, illness and disease management across the lifespan in a variety of settings while recognizing the diverse uniqueness of individuals, providing directed care to individuals with well-defined health alterations, the student at the end of N225, should be able to:					
I. Patient-Centered Care					
a. Develop an individualized plan of care with a focus on assessment and planning utilizing the nursing process					
b. Demonstrate caring behaviors					
c. Conduct a comprehensive assessment while eliciting patient values, preferences and needs					
d. Respect diversity of individuals					
e. Assess the presence and extent of pain and suffering					
f. Demonstrate beginning competency in skills					

Exhibit 14.5 *(continued)*

II. Teamwork and Collaboration

Core Competencies	Midterm			Final	
	S	NI	U	S	U
a. Develop effective communication skills (orally and through charting) with patients, team members, and family					
b. Identify relevant data for communication in pre and post conferences					
c. Identify intra- and inter-professional team member roles and scopes of practice					
d. Establish appropriate relationships with team members					
e. Identify need for help when appropriate to situation					

III. Evidence-Based Practice

a. Locate evidence-based literature related to clinical practice and guideline activities					
b Reference clinical related activities with evidence-based literature					
c Value the concept of evidence-based practice in determining best clinical practice					

IV. Quality Improvement

a. Deliver care in timely and cost effective manner					
b. Seek information about processes/projects to improve care (QI)					
c. Value the significance of variance reporting					

V. Safety

a. Demonstrate effective use of technology and standardized practices that support safety and quality					
b. Implement strategies to reduce risk of harm to self or others					
c. Demonstrate appropriate clinical decision making					

(continued)

Exhibit 14.5 *(continued)*

Core Competencies	Midterm			Final	
	S	NI	U	S	U
d. Identify national patient safety goals and quality measures					
e. Use appropriate strategies to reduce reliance on memory					
f. Communicate observations or concerns related to hazards and errors to patient, families, and the health care team					
g. Organize multiple responsibilities and provide care in a timely manner					
VI. Informatics					
a. Navigate the electronic health record for patient information where appropriate for clinical setting					
b. Document clear and concise responses to care in the electronic health record, where appropriate for clinical setting					
c. Identify information and clinical technology using critical thinking to collect, process, and communicate data					
d. Manage data, information, and knowledge of technology in an ethical manner					
e. Protect confidentiality of electronic health records					
VII. Professionalism					
a. Demonstrate core professional values (caring, altruism, autonomy, integrity, human dignity, and social justice)					
b. Maintain professional behavior and appearance					
c. Comply with the Code of Ethics, Standards of Practice, and policies and procedures of Nicholls State University, Department of Nursing, and clinical agencies					
d. Accept constructive criticism and develop plan of action for improvement					

Exhibit 14.5 *(continued)*

Core Competencies	Midterm			Final	
	S	NI	U	S	U
e. Maintain a positive attitude and interact with inter-professional team members, faculty, and fellow students in a positive, professional manner					
f. Provide evidence of preparation for clinical learning experiences					
g. Arrive to clinical experiences at assigned times					
h. Demonstrate expected behaviors and complete tasks in a timely manner					
i. Accept individual responsibility and accountability for nursing interventions, outcomes, and other actions					
j. Engage in self evaluation					
k. Assume responsibility for learning					

Midterm Comments (Address strengths and weaknesses)

Faculty

Student

Student Signature _____   **Date** _____

Faculty Signature _____   **Date** _____

Final Comments (Address strengths and weaknesses)

Faculty

Student

Student Signature _____   **Date** _____

Faculty Signature _____   **Date** _____

(continued)

Exhibit 14.5 *(continued)*

Mid-clinical Evaluation: faculty and student *must* complete documentation for remediation of unsatisfactory areas. CPR Tool[a] must be initiated for any unsatisfactory areas.

Unsatisfactory Area	Remediation Strategy

Student Signature _____   Date _____

Faculty Signature _____   Date _____

Developed collaboratively by Nicholls State University Nursing Faculty. Reprinted by permission, 2012.

Two copies on file – 1 for student self evaluation; 1 for clinical faculty
*Content based upon QSEN Competencies and KSA's.
[a] Clinical Performance Remediation tool.   S = Satisfactory
NI = Needs Improvement
U = Unsatisfactory

©2012 Nicholls State University Department of Nursing, Thibodaux, LA.

As the goal is to guide students in improving performance, other tools can be developed to accompany the rating forms. For example, if a student is not performing at a satisfactory level in any of the core competencies in those exhibits, the teacher initiates a Clinical Performance Remediation tool that has the same competencies as the clinical evaluation tool but provides a means for faculty to document student progress in developing them.

Any rating form used in a school of nursing or health system must be clear to all stakeholders. Students, educators, preceptors, and others need to understand the meaning of the competencies and scale levels. They also need to be able to determine examples of clinical performance that reflect each level in the scale. For example, what is satisfactory and unsatisfactory performance in establishing relationships with team members? If a scale with 5 levels is used, what are the differences in establishing relationships with team members at each of those levels? All too often the meaning of the competencies in the tool and levels to rate observed performance are not fully understood by the clinical educators using it. Teachers should be prepared for use of the form through faculty development. The meaning of the competencies and examples of performance that reflect each level can be discussed, and teachers might

❏Exhibit 14.6

Clinical Evaluation Tool for Higher Level Course in Same Nursing Program

NICHOLLS STATE UNIVERSITY
DEPARTMENT OF NURSING
BSN PROGRAM

Clinical Performance Evaluation Tool
NURS 355 Level II

Self Evaluation _____

Faculty Evaluation _____

Student Name _____

Faculty _____   Course: NURS 355   Semester_____

Fill in appropriate fields to the right and below:

Student must obtain a Satisfactory "S" grade in all competencies at the Final Evaluation to pass the Course.

Core Competencies	Midterm			Final	
	S	NI	U	S	U
Focusing on wellness, health promotion, illness, and disease management across the lifespan in a variety of settings while recognizing the diverse uniqueness of individuals, providing collaborative care to individuals and families with multiple health alterations, the student at the end of N355, should be able to:					
I. Patient-Centered Care					
a. Institute an individualized plan of care including assessment, planning, intervention, and evaluation of multiple patients with multiple health alterations					
b. Assess health status, health potential, and learning needs of adult individuals and their families using appropriate data collection tools					
c. Deliver care based on knowledge of pathophysiology and pharmacotherapy with respect for individual values, preferences, needs, and diversity					
d. Modify the established goals and/or time frame based on interpretation of individual's achievement of objectives/outcomes					
e. Recommend interventions to address physical and emotional comfort, pain, and/or suffering					

(continued)

Exhibit 14.6 *(continued)*

Core Competencies	Midterm			Final	
	S	NI	U	S	U
II. Teamwork and Collaboration					
a. Communicate effectively with the patient and inter-professional team to acquire and convey information about the patient					
b. Participate in conferences/discussions using SBAR to communicate relevant data to inter-professional team					
c. Collaborate with members of intra- and inter-professional team to identify patient needs and deliver care					
d. Collaborate with fellow students to establish team approach that delivers timely administration of care					
e. Function competently within own scope of practice as a member of the intra- and inter-professional team					
f. Distinguish between professional nursing roles appropriate to meet the needs of individuals and family with multiple health alterations					
g. Initiate requests for help when appropriate to situation					
III. Evidence-Based Practice					
a. Integrate evidence-based practice in the formulation of an individualized plan of care for the adult patient with multiple health alterations					
b. Differentiate clinical opinion from research and evidence					
c. Implement evidence-based care					
d. Inform intra-professional team members of current evidence-based practice					

Exhibit 14.6 *(continued)*

IV. Quality Improvement

Core Competencies	Midterm			Final	
	S	NI	U	S	U
a. Promote cost containment through an understanding of the development and use of managed care systems while providing quality care					
b. Participate in quality improvement processes in the health care setting					

V. Safety

a. Integrate effective use of technology and standardized practices that support safety and quality					
b. Perform nursing tasks/skills safely and timely					
c. Demonstrate safe, timely administration of medications, stating pharmacologic implications as they relate to the adult patient with multiple health alterations					
d. Recommend interventions to improve safety hazards and concerns to patient, families, and inter-professional team					
e. Incorporate national patient safety goals in the delivery of care					

VI. Informatics

a. Navigate and document within the electronic health record where applicable to clinical setting					
b. Simulate accurate, thorough documentation of adult health assessment with computer documentation program					
c. Document medication administration in medication delivery system where applicable					
d. Utilize technology and information management tools using critical thinking for clinical reasoning and quality improvement to support safe processes of care					

(continued)

Exhibit 14.6 *(continued)*

Core Competencies	Midterm			Final	
	S	NI	U	S	U
e. Manage data, information, and knowledge of technology in an ethical manner					
f. Protect confidentiality of electronic health records					
VII. Professionalism					
a. Demonstrate core professional values (caring, altruism, autonomy, integrity, human dignity, and social justice)					
b. Maintain professional behavior and appearance					
c. Comply with the Code of Ethics, Standards of Practice, and policies and procedures of Nicholls State University, Department of Nursing, and clinical agencies					
d. Accept constructive criticism and develop plan of action for improvement					
e. Maintain a positive attitude and interact with inter-professional team members, faculty, and fellow students in a positive, professional manner					
f. Provide evidence of preparation for clinical learning experiences					
g. Arrive to clinical experiences at assigned times					
h. Demonstrate expected behaviors and complete tasks in a timely manner					
i. Accept individual responsibility and accountability for nursing interventions, outcomes, and other actions					
j. Engage in self evaluation					
k. Assume responsibility for learning					

Midterm Comments (Address Strengths and weaknesses)

Faculty

Student

Student Signature _____   **Date** _____

Faculty Signature _____   **Date** _____

Exhibit 14.6 *(continued)*

Final Comments (Address strengths and weaknesses)

Faculty

Student

Student Signature _____   Date _____

Faculty Signature _____   Date _____

Mid-Clinical Evaluation: Faculty and student *must* complete documentation for remediation of unsatisfactory areas. CPR Tool[a] must be initiated for any unsatisfactory areas.

Unsatisfactory Area	Remediation Strategy

Student Signature _____   Date _____

Faculty Signature _____   Date _____

Developed collaboratively by Nicholls State University Nursing Faculty. Reprinted by permission, 2012.

Two copies on file – 1 for student self evaluation; 1 for clinical faculty
*Content based upon QSEN Competencies and KSA's.
[a] Clinical Performance Remediation tool.

S = Satisfactory
NI = Needs Improvement
U = Unsatisfactory

©2012 Nicholls State University Department of Nursing, Thibodaux, LA.

practice using the form to evaluate performance of students in digitally recorded simulations. In addition to teacher preparation, there should be guidelines that accompany the tool to improve consistency in its use across educators. Exhibit 14.7 presents the guidelines that accompany the tools shown in Exhibits 14.5 and 14.6.

❏Exhibit 14.7

Guidelines for Using Clinical Evaluation Tools in Exhibits 14.5 and 14.6

NICHOLLS STATE UNIVERSITY
DEPARTMENT OF NURSING
BSN PROGRAM

Clinical Performance Evaluation Tool Guidelines

Tool Guidelines

- The clinical evaluation tool is used for all clinical nursing courses. Each nursing course builds on prior knowledge, skills, and attitudes.
- All clinical learning experiences will be evaluated upon completion and/or as deemed necessary by the faculty. Students who are not meeting clinical outcomes will be counseled individually as needed.
- Each student will fill out a self-evaluation at (1) midterm (2) final.
- Each faculty member will fill out an evaluation at (1) midterm (2) final.
- Each row item (boxes) must be checked by placing a"√" in appropriate box at (1) midterm (2) final.
- The score for Clinical Evaluation will be either "S" "NI" or "U" at mid-term.
- The score for Clinical Evaluation will be either "S" or "U" at final.
- A score of "NI" cannot be awarded as a grade post mid-clinical or as a final grade.
- Clinical faculty will initiate the Clinical Performance Remediation (CPR) Tool for a student who receives a score of "U" on the mid-clinical evaluation. The CPR Tool may also be initiated for a score of "NI," at the discretion of the clinical faculty.
- Final grades for any nursing clinical related component must be "S" or "U."
- A passing grade will only be assigned if **all** the items are checked "S" at the time of the final evaluation.
- An unsatisfactory "U" for **any** clinical learning experience at final evaluation constitutes **failure** of the course.

Core Competency Statements

- Each core competency (as outlined in **BOLD**) has associated statements, which specifies individual guidelines.
- The core competency statements are based upon level of matriculation in each clinical course.
- Each clinical course has a unique clinical evaluation tool specific to the course and level.

Grading Guidelines

- Clinical Performance will be evaluated with a Clinical Performance Tool, and will be scored either "S" "NI" or "U".
- Every student must receive a score of "S" on the Clinical Performance Tool during the final clinical evaluation to pass the course.

Exhibit 14.7 *(continued)*

■ If a student receives a "U" on the Clinical Performance Tool during the final clinical evaluation, the student will <u>FAIL</u> the course and receive a grade of no higher than "D" for the course.

Grade Descriptions

A grade of "S" means the student:

■ Functions satisfactorily with minimum guidance in the clinical situation
■ Demonstrates accurate and appropriate knowledge and integrates knowledge with skills and attitudes
■ Engages consistently in self direction in approach to learning
■ Provides evidence of preparation for all clinical learning experiences
■ Follows directions and performs safely
■ Identifies own learning needs and seeks appropriate assistance
■ Demonstrates continued improvement during the semester
■ Uses nursing process and applies scientific rationale

A grade of "NI" means the student:

■ Functions safely with moderate amount of guidance in the clinical situation
■ Demonstrates adequate knowledge and requires moderate assistance in integrating knowledge with skills
■ Requires some direction in recognizing and utilizing learning opportunities

A grade of "U" means the student:

■ Requires intense guidance for the performance of activities at a safe level
■ Clinical performance reflects difficulty in the provision of nursing care
■ Demonstrates gaps in necessary knowledge and requires frequent or almost constant assistance in integrating knowledge and skills
■ Requires frequent and detailed instructions regarding learning opportunities and is often unable to utilize them
■ Is often unprepared and has limited insight into own behavior
■ Is unable to identify own learning needs and neglects to seek appropriate assistance
■ Not dependable
■ Breaches in professional or ethical conduct such as falsification of records and failure to maintain confidentiality

Developed collaboratively by Nicholls State University Nursing Faculty. Reprinted by permission, 2012.

©2012 Nicholls State University Department of Nursing, Thibodaux, LA

Walsh, Jairath, Paterson, and Grandjean (2010) reported on the development of their Clinical Performance Evaluation Tool (CPET), based on the QSEN competencies. The CPET has three parts: (1) a 1-page checklist for teachers to evaluate student performance related to the QSEN competencies, (2) a key that explains the application of the competencies to the specific clinical course, and (3) guidelines for grading performance.

Issues With Rating Scales

One problem in using rating scales with multiple levels is apparent by a review of the sample scale descriptors. What are the differences between above average and average? Between a "2" and "1"? Is there consensus among faculty members using the rating scale as to what constitutes different levels of performance for each outcome or competency evaluated? This problem exists even when descriptions are provided for each level of the rating scale. Teachers may differ in their judgments of whether the student collected *relevant* data, whether *multiple* sources of data were used, whether the database was *comprehensive* or not, whether *all possible* patient problems were considered, and so forth. Scales based on frequency labels are often difficult to implement because of limited opportunities for students to practice and demonstrate a level of skill rated as "always, often, sometimes, and never." How should teachers rate students' performance in situations in which they practiced the skill perhaps once or twice? Even with two-dimensional scales such as pass–fail, there is room for variability among educators.

Nitko and Brookhart (2011) identified eight common errors that can occur with rating scales applicable to rating clinical performance. Three of these can occur with tools that have multiple points on the scale for rating performance, such as 1 to 5 or below average to exceptional:

1. *Leniency error* results when the teacher tends to rate all students toward the high end of the scale.

2. *Severity error* is the opposite of leniency, tending to rate all students toward the low end of the scale.

3. *Central tendency error* is hesitancy to mark either end of the rating scale and instead use only the midpoint of the scale. Rating students only at the extremes or only at the midpoint of the scale limits the validity of the ratings for all students and introduces the teacher's own biases into the evaluation (Nitko & Brookhart, 2011).

Three other errors that can occur with any type of clinical performance rating scale are a halo effect, personal bias, and a logical error:

4. *Halo effect* is a judgment based on a general impression of the student. With this error the teacher lets an overall impression of the student influence the ratings of specific aspects of the student's performance. This impression is considered a "halo" around the student that affects the teacher's ability to objectively evaluate and rate specific competencies on the tool. This halo may be positive, giving the student a higher rating than is deserved, or negative, letting a general negative impression of the student result in lower ratings of specific aspects of the performance. In a study with medical residents, positive impressions of the student were associated with a significant increase in ratings of observed performance (Stroud, Herold, Tomlinson, & Cavalcanti, 2011).

5. *Personal bias* occurs when the teacher's biases influence ratings such as favoring nursing students who do not work while attending school over those who are employed while attending school.

6. *Logical error* results when similar ratings are given for items on the scale that are logically related to one another. This is a problem with rating scales in nursing that are too long and often too detailed. For example, there may be multiple competencies related to communication skills to be rated. The teacher observes some of these competencies but not all of them. In completing the clinical evaluation form, the teacher gives the same rating to all competencies related to communication on the tool. When this occurs, often some of the items on the rating scale can be combined.

Two other errors that can occur with performance ratings are rater drift and reliability decay (Nitko & Brookhart, 2011):

7. *Rater drift* can occur when teachers redefine the performance behaviors to be observed and assessed. Initially in developing a clinical evaluation form, teachers agree on the competencies to be rated and the scale to be used. However, over a period of time, educators may interpret them differently, drifting away from the original intent. For this reason faculty members in a course should discuss as a group each competency on their clinical evaluation tool at the beginning of the course and at the mid-point. This discussion should include the meaning of the competency and what a student's performance would "look like" at each rating level in the tool. Simulated experiences in observing a performance, rating it with the tool, and discussing the rationale for the rating are valuable to prevent rater drift as the course progresses.

8. *Reliability decay* is a similar issue that can occur. Nitko and Brookhart (2011) indicated that immediately following training on using a performance rating tool, educators tend to use the tool consistently across students and with each other. As the course continues, though, faculty members may become less consistent in their ratings. Discussion of the clinical evaluation tool among course faculty, as indicated earlier, may improve consistency in use of the tool.

Although there are issues with rating scales, they remain an important clinical evaluation method because they allow teachers, preceptors, and others to rate performance over time and to note patterns of performance. Exhibit 14.8 provides guidelines for using rating scales for clinical evaluation in nursing.

❑Exhibit 14.8

Guidelines for Using Rating Scales for Clinical Evaluation

1. Be alert to the possible influence of your own values, attitudes, beliefs, and biases in observing performance and drawing conclusions about it.
2. Use the clinical outcomes or competencies to focus your observations. Give students feedback on other observations made about their performance.
3. Collect sufficient data on students' performance before drawing conclusions about it.
4. Observe the student more than one time before rating performance. Rating scales when used for clinical evaluation should represent a *pattern* of the student's performance over a period of time.
5. If possible, observe students' performance in different clinical situations, either in the patient care setting or simulation. When not possible, develop additional strategies for evaluation so that performance is evaluated with different methods and at different times.
6. Do not rely on first impressions; they may not be accurate.
7. Always discuss observations with students, obtain their perceptions of performance, and be willing to modify own judgments and ratings when new data are presented.
8. Review the available clinical learning activities and opportunities in the simulation and learning laboratories. Are they providing sufficient data for completing the rating scale? If not, new learning activities may need to be developed, or the competencies on the tool may need to be modified to be more realistic considering the clinical teaching circumstances.
9. Avoid using rating scales as the only source of data about a student's performance—use multiple evaluation methods for clinical practice.
10. Rate each competency individually based on the observations made of performance and conclusions drawn. If you have insufficient information about achievement of a particular competency, do not rate it—leave it blank.
11. Do not rate all students high, low, or in the middle; similarly, do not let your general impression of the student or personal biases influence the ratings.
12. If the rating form is ineffective for judging student performance, then revise and re-evaluate it. Consider these questions: Does use of the form yield data that can be used to make valid decisions about students' competence? Does it yield reliable, stable data? Is it easy to use? Is it realistic for the types of learning activities students complete and that are available in clinical and simulation settings?
13. Discuss as a group (with other educators and preceptors involved in the evaluation) each competency on the rating scale. Come to agreement as to the meaning of the competencies and what a student's performance would look like at each rating level in the tool. Share examples of performance, how you would rate them, and your rationale. As a group exercise observe a video clip or other simulation of a student's performance, rate it with the tool, and come to agreement as to the rating. Exercises and discussions such as these should be held before the course begins and periodically throughout to ensure reliability across teachers and settings.

Most nursing faculty use some type of clinical evaluation tool to evaluate students' performance in their courses (n = 1,534; 98%) (Oermann, Yarbrough, et al., 2009). Seventy percent of nursing faculty (n = 1,095) reported in a survey that they used one basic tool for their nursing courses that was adapted for the competencies of each particular course. Only 242 (16%) faculty members reported having a unique evaluation tool for each clinical course (Oermann, Yarbrough, et al.).

SIMULATIONS

Simulation allows learners to experience a clinical situation without the risks. With simulations students can develop their psychomotor and technological skills and practice those skills to maintain their competence. Simulations, particularly those involving high-fidelity simulators, enable students to think through clinical situations and make independent decision. With human patient simulators and complex scenarios, students can assess a patient and clinical situation, analyze data, make decisions about priority problems and actions to take, implement those interventions, practice complex technologies, and evaluate outcomes. Lasater (2007, 2011) suggested that high-fidelity simulation can be used to guide students' development of clinical judgment skills, especially when combined with high quality debriefing following the simulation (Dreifuerst, 2012).

Research suggests that simulations promote learning of both knowledge and skills (Nickless, 2011; Norman, 2012; Pascual et al., 2011; Yuan, Williams, Fang, & Ye, 2012). Another outcome of instruction with simulations is the opportunity to have deliberate practice of skills. Simulations allow students to practice skills, both cognitive and motor, until competent and receive immediate feedback on performance (Oermann, 2011; Oermann, Kardong-Edgren, & Odom-Maryon, 2011; Oermann et al., 2011). Through simulations students can develop their communication and teamwork skills and apply quality and safety guidelines to practice (Aebersold, Tschannen, & Bathish, 2012; Ironside, Jeffries, & Martin, 2009; Kameg, Howard, Clochesy, Mitchell, & Suresky, 2010; Kaplan, Holmes, Mott, & Atallah, 2011; Norman, 2012; Sears, Goldsworthy, & Goodman, 2010).

Simulations are increasingly important as a clinical teaching strategy, given the limited time for clinical practice in many programs and the complexity of skills to be developed by students. Brown (2008) suggested that simulated scenarios ease the shortage of clinical experiences for students because of clinical agency restrictions and fewer practice hours in a curriculum. In a simulation laboratory, students can practice skills without the constraints of a real-life situation.

Using Simulations for Clinical Evaluation

Simulations not only are effective for instruction in nursing, but they also are useful for clinical evaluation. Students can demonstrate procedures and technologies, conduct assessments, analyze scenarios, make decisions about problems and actions to take, carry out interventions, and evaluate the effects of their decisions. Each of these outcomes can be evaluated for feedback to students or for summative grading.

There are different types of simulations that can be used for clinical evaluation. Case scenarios that students analyze can be presented in paper-and-pencil format or through multimedia. Many computer simulations are available for use in evaluation. Simulations can be developed with models and manikins for evaluating skills and procedures, and for evaluation with standardized patients. With human patient simulators, teachers can identify outcomes and clinical competencies to be assessed, present various clinical events and scenarios for students to analyze and then take action, and evaluate student decision making and performance in these scenarios. In the debriefing session that follows, the students as a group can analyze the scenario and critique their actions and decisions, with faculty members providing feedback. The debriefing guides students in reflecting on their learning and promotes development of their clinical judgment skills (Dreifuerst, 2012; Lasater, 2011).

Many nursing education programs have simulation laboratories with high-fidelity and other types of simulators, clinically equipped examination rooms, manikins and models for skill practice and assessment, areas for standardized patients, and a wide range of multimedia that facilitate performance evaluations. The rooms can be equipped with two-way mirrors, video cameras, microphones, and other media for observing and performance rating by faculty and others. Videoconferencing technology can be used to conduct clinical evaluations of students in settings at a distance from the nursing education program, replacing onsite performance evaluations by faculty.

For simulations to be used effectively for clinical evaluation, though, teachers need to be adequately prepared for their role. In a project to prepare nurse educators for simulation, 12 nursing programs and practice partners collaborated to provide faculty development. By preparing educators, the use of simulation increased in their nursing programs, and 30% reported expanded student enrollment with the use of more simulated experiences in the curriculum (Bentley & Seaback, 2011).

Incorporating Simulations Into Clinical Evaluation Protocol

The same principles used for evaluating student performance in the clinical setting apply to using simulations. The first task is to identify which clinical outcomes will be assessed with a simulation. This decision should be made during the course planning phase as part of the protocol developed for clinical evaluation in the course. When deciding on evaluation methods, it is important to remember that assessment can be done for feedback to students and thus remain ungraded, or be used for grading purposes.

Once the outcomes or clinical competencies to be evaluated with simulations are identified, the teacher can plan the specifics of the evaluation. Some questions to guide teachers in using simulations for clinical evaluation are:

■ What are the specific clinical outcomes or competencies to be evaluated using simulations? These should be designated in the plan or protocol for clinical evaluation in a course.
■ What types of simulations are needed to assess the designated outcomes, for example, simulations to demonstrate psychomotor and technological skills; ability to identify problems, treatments, and interventions; and critical thinking skills?
■ Do the scenarios need to be developed by the faculty, or are they available?
■ If the scenarios need to be developed, who will be responsible for their development? Who will manage their implementation?
■ Are the simulations for formative evaluation only? If so, how many practice sessions should be planned? What is the extent of faculty and expert guidance needed? Who will provide that supervision and guidance?
■ Are the simulations for summative evaluation (i.e., for grading purposes and high-stakes evaluation such as verifying that students have met the end-of-program outcomes)? If used for summative evaluation, then faculty need to determine the process for rating performance and use an evaluation tool that produces valid and reliable results.
■ When will the simulations be implemented in the course?
■ How will the outcomes of the simulations be evaluated, and who will be responsible?

A key point in evaluating student performance in simulation for high-stakes assessment and other summative decisions is the need for a tool that produces valid and reliable results. An example of a rating scale for evaluating students in the simulated clinical environment, with demonstrated measurement validity and reliability, is the Creighton Simulation Evaluation Instrument© (C-SEI) (Todd, Manz, Hawkins, Parsons, & Hercinger, 2008). The C-SEI is shown in Exhibit 14.9. Even with a validated tool, however, evaluators using it may not interpret the competencies nor

☐Exhibit 14.9

Creighton U N I V E R S I T Y	**Creighton Simulation Evaluation Instrument™ (C-SEI)**	

Scenario:	0 = Does not demonstrate
	       competency
	1 = Demonstrates
	       competency
		Date: M M D D Y Y Y Y

ASSESSMENT	(Circle Appropriate Score for All Applicable Criteria)		**GROUP COMMENTS***
Obtains Pertinent Subjective Data	0	1	
Obtains Pertinent Objective Data	0	1	
Performs Follow-Up Assessments as Needed	0	1	
Assesses in a Systematic & Orderly Manner Using the Correct Technique	0	1	
COMMUNICATION			
Communicates Effectively With Providers (delegation, medical terms, SBAR, WRBO)	0	1	
Communicates Effectively With Patient and S. O. (verbal, nonverbal, teaching)	0	1	
Writes Documentation Clearly, Concisely, & Accurately	0	1	
Responds to Abnormal Findings Appropriately	0	1	
Promotes Realism/ Professionalism	0	1	
CRITICAL THINKING			
Interprets Vital Signs (T, P, R, BP, Pain)	0	1	
Interprets Lab Results	0	1	

Exhibit 14.9 *(continued)*

CRITICAL THINKING *(continued)*

Interprets Subjective/ Objective Data (recognizes relevant from irrelevant data)	0	1
Formulates Measurable Priority Outcomes	0	1
Performs Outcome-Driven Interventions	0	1
Provides Specific Rationale for Interventions	0	1
Evaluates Interventions and Outcomes	0	1
Reflects on Simulation Experience		

TECHNICAL SKILLS

Uses Patient Identifiers	0	1
Utilizes Standard Precautions Including Hand Washing	0	1
Administers Medications Safely	0	1
Manages Equipment, Tubes, & Drains Therapeutically	0	1
Performs Procedures Correctly	0	1

Student Participants	**Total Score**		If not applicable, no score is given.	* Individual comments on clinical evaluation
_____ _____ _____ _____	**Passing Score**		Passing score = 0.75 × number of items used.	
Faculty Evaluator:				

Developed by Martha Todd, MS, APRN; Julie Manz, MS, RN; Kimberly Hawkins, MS, APRN; Mary Parsons, PhD, RN; Maribeth Hercinger, PhD, RN, BC. Copyright by Authors. Reprinted with permission, 2012.

score them as intended. For this reason Parsons, Hawkins, Hercinger, Todd, Manz, and Fang (2012) developed a formal educational program for all faculty members who were going to use the C-SEI. As part of this program, they reviewed the individual components of the tool and achieved consensus on the minimum expectations of student performance to indicate achievement of each competency. Findings suggested that education of faculty members and dialogue about the tool and its use in a particular scenario improve consistency of ratings.

Standardized Patients

One type of simulation for clinical evaluation uses standardized patients. Standardized patients are individuals who have been trained to accurately portray the role of a patient with a specific diagnosis or condition. With simulations using standardized patients, students can be evaluated on a history and physical examination, related skills and procedures, and communication abilities, among other outcomes. Standardized patients are effective for evaluation because the actors are trained to recreate the same patient condition and clinical situation each time they are with a student, providing for consistency in the performance evaluation.

When standardized patients are used for formative evaluation, they provide feedback to the students on their performance, an important aid to their learning. Standardized patients are trained to provide both written and oral feedback to students and evaluate their performance (McWilliam & Botwinski, 2012). Because they are trained for their role, standardized patients are well suited for summative evaluation of students' assessment, clinical, interpersonal, and communication skills as long as there is evidence that the evaluation tools produce valid and reliable results.

Objective Structured Clinical Examination

An Objective Structured Clinical Examination (OSCE) provides a means of evaluating performance in a simulation laboratory rather than in the clinical setting. In an OSCE students rotate through a series of stations; at each station they complete an activity or perform a task, which is then evaluated. Some stations assess the student's ability to take a patient's history, perform a physical examination, and implement other interventions while being observed by the teacher or an examiner. The student's performance then can be rated using a rating scale or checklist. At other stations, students might be tested on their knowledge and cognitive skills—they might be asked to analyze data, select interventions and treatments, and manage the patient's condition. Most often OSCEs are used for summative clinical evaluation; however, they also can be used formatively to assess performance and provide feedback to students. Based on a review of the research in nursing, Walsh, Bailey, and Koren (2009) suggested that the complexities of evaluating clinical competence can be addressed with OSCEs as long as the goals of the evaluation are clear and the OSCEs are carefully designed. They also recommended a multi-method approach to clinical evaluation to assess the wide range of competencies students need to develop.

Different types of stations can be used in an OSCE. At one type of station the student may interact with a standardized patient as if interviewing or examining the patient (Hawkins & Boulet, 2008). At these stations the teacher or examiner can evaluate students' understanding of varied patient conditions and management of them and can rate the students' performance. At other stations students may demonstrate skills, perform procedures, use technologies, and demonstrate other technical competencies. Performance at these stations may be evaluated by the teacher or examiner, usually with checklists.

There also may be post-encounter stations to facilitate the evaluation of cognitive skills such as interpreting lab results and other data, developing management plans, and making other types of decisions about patient care. Students may be asked to document their findings with the standardized patient, answer questions about the clinical situation, and provide evidence for their decisions, among other competencies (Hawkins & Boulet, 2008). At these stations the teacher or examiner is not present to observe students.

GAMES

Games are teaching methods that involve competition, rules (structure), and collaboration among team members. There are individual games such as crossword puzzles or games played against other students either individually or in teams; many games require props or other equipment and are available online. In a survey of 218 nursing students, findings indicated that students supported use of video gaming and multi-player online health care simulations in nursing education (Lynch-Sauer et al., 2011). Games actively involve learners, promote teamwork, may require problem-solving skills, motivate, stimulate interest in a topic, and support learning (Blakely, Skirton, Cooper, Allum, & Nelmes, 2010; Royse & Newton, 2007; Skiba, 2008; Thompson, Ford, & Webster, 2011). Games, however, are not intended for grading; they should be used only for instructional purposes and formative evaluation.

MEDIA CLIPS

Media clips, short segments of a digital recording, a DVD, a video from YouTube, and other forms of multimedia, may be viewed by students as a basis for discussions in postclinical conferences, on discussion boards, and for other online activities; used for small-group activities; and critiqued by students as an assignment. Media clips often are more effective than written descriptions of a scenario because they allow the student to visualize the patient and clinical situation. The segment viewed by the students should be short so they can focus on critical aspects related to the outcomes to be evaluated. Media clips are appropriate for assessing whether students can apply concepts and theories to the patient or clinical situation depicted in the media clip, observe and collect data, identify possible problems, identify priority actions and interventions, and explore own feelings and responses.

Students can answer questions about the media clips as part of a graded learning activity. Otherwise, media clips are valuable for formative evaluation, particularly in a group format in which students discuss their ideas and receive feedback from the teacher and their peers.

WRITTEN ASSIGNMENTS

Written assignments accompanying the clinical experience are effective methods for assessing students' problem solving, critical thinking, and higher level learning; their understanding of content relevant to clinical practice; and their ability to express ideas in writing. Evaluation of written assignments was described in Chapter 9. There are many types of written assignments appropriate for clinical evaluation. The teacher should first specify the outcomes to be evaluated with written assignments and then decide which assignments would best assess whether those outcomes were met. The final decision is how many assignments will be required in a clinical course.

Written assignments are valuable for evaluating outcomes in face-to-face, clinical practice, and distance education courses in nursing. However, they are misused when students complete the same assignments repetitively throughout a course once the outcomes have been met. At that point students should progress to other, more challenging learning activities. Some of the written assignments might be done in postclinical conferences, in class, or online as small-group activities—teachers still can assess student progress toward meeting the outcomes but with fewer demands on their time for reviewing the assignments and providing prompt feedback on them.

Journal Writing

Journals provide an opportunity for students to describe events and experiences in their clinical practice and to reflect on them. With journals students can "think aloud" and share their feelings with teachers. Journals are not intended to develop students' writing skills; instead they provide a means of expressing feelings and reflections on clinical practice and engaging in a dialogue with the teacher about them. When journals are used for reflection, students develop an awareness of their environment and develop skills in self assessment (Schuessler, Wilder, & Byrd, 2012). Other outcomes of using journals are connecting theory and practice, assessing own strengths and weaknesses, and integrating new ideas. Issues, however, are the amount of time needed for reflection and for faculty comments, and the need to have trust between students and the teacher (Langley & Brown, 2010). Journals can be submitted in electronic formats, but should be password protected. Electronic submission of journals makes it easier for teachers to provide prompt feedback and engage in dialogue with learners, and it simplifies storing the journals.

Journals are not the same as diaries and logs. In a diary, students document their experiences in clinical practice with personal reflections; these reflections are meant to remain "personal" and thus are not shared with the teacher or others. A log is typically a structured record of activities completed in the clinical course without reflections about the experience. Students may complete any or all of these activities in a nursing program.

When journals are used in a clinical course, students need to be clear about the objectives—what are the purposes of the journal? For example, a journal intended for reflection in practice would require different entries than one for documenting events and activities in the clinical setting as a means of communicating them to faculty. Students also need written guidelines for journal entries, including how many and what types of entries to make. Depending on the outcomes, journals may be done throughout a clinical course or at periodic intervals. Regardless of the frequency, students need immediate and meaningful feedback about their reflections and entries.

One of the issues in using journals is whether they should be graded or used solely for reflection and growth. For those educators who support grading journals, a number of strategies have been used, such as:

- indicating a grade based on the number of journals submitted rather than on the comments and reflections in them
- grading papers written from the journals
- incorporating journals as part of portfolios, which then are graded

- having students evaluate their own journals based on preset criteria developed by the students themselves
- requiring a journal as one component among others for passing a clinical course

There are some teachers who grade the entries of a journal similar to other written assignments. However, when the purpose of the journal is to reflect on experiences in clinical practice and on the students' own behaviors, beliefs, and values, journals should not be graded. By grading journals the teacher inhibits the student's reflection and dialogue about feelings and perceptions of clinical experiences.

Nursing Care Plans

Nursing care plans enable the student to learn the components of the nursing process and how to use the literature and other resources for writing the plan. However, a linear kind of care planning does not help students learn how problems interrelate nor does it encourage the complex thinking that nurses must do in clinical practice (Kern, Bush, & McCleish, 2006). If care plans are used for clinical evaluation, teachers should be cautious about the number of plans required in a course and the outcomes of such an assignment. Short assignments in which students analyze data, examine competing diagnoses, evaluate different interventions and their evidence for practice, suggest alternative approaches, and evaluate outcomes of care are more effective than a care plan that students often paraphrase from their textbooks.

Concept Maps

Concept maps are tools used to visually display relationships among concepts. An example is provided in Figure 14.1. With a concept map students can develop their understanding of how concepts relate to one another and can organize information into a framework for improved learning and retention (Noonan, 2011). It has been suggested that concept maps develop learners' critical thinking and decision-making skills (Pilcher, 2011; Vacek, 2009). Concept maps are an effective way of helping students organize data as they plan for their clinical experience; the map can be developed in a preclinical conference based on the patient's admitting diagnosis, revised during the clinical day as the student collects data and cares for the patient, and then assessed and discussed in postclinical conference (Hill, 2006). With a concept map students can "see" graphically how assessment data, patient problems, interventions, and other aspects of care are related to one another.

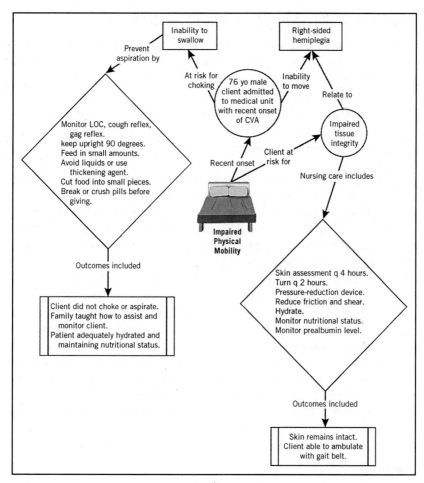

Figure 14.1 An example of a concept map.
Developed by Deanne Blach, MSN, RN. Reprinted by permission of Deanne Blach, 2012.

In most cases, concept maps are best used for formative evaluation. However, with criteria established for evaluation, they also can be graded. For example students could be asked to explain in a paper how the concepts in the map relate to one another. They could write short papers that accompany the concept map, which are then graded by the teacher similar to other written assignments. Other areas to assess in a concept map for patient care, depending on the goal of the assignment, are: whether the assessment data are comprehensive, whether the data are linked with the correct diagnoses and problems, whether nursing interventions and treatments are specific and relevant, and whether the relationships among the concepts are indicated and accurate.

Case Method, Unfolding Cases, and Case Study

Case method, unfolding cases, and case study were described in Chapter 7 because they are strategies for assessing problem solving, clinical judgment, and higher level learning. Cases that require application of knowledge from readings and the classroom or an online component of the course can be developed for analysis by students. The scenarios can focus on patients, families, communities, the health care system, and other clinical situations that students might encounter in their clinical practice.

Although these assignments may be completed as individual activities, they are also appropriate for group work. Cases may be presented for group discussion and peer review in clinical conferences and for online discussions. In online courses, the case scenario can be presented with open-ended questions and, based on student responses, other questions can be introduced for discussion. Using this approach, cases are effective for encouraging critical thinking. By discussing cases as a clinical group, students are exposed to other possible approaches and perspectives that they may not have identified themselves. With this method, the teacher can provide feedback on the content and thought process used by students to arrive at their answers.

One advantage of short cases, unfolding cases, and case studies is that they can be graded. By using the principles described for scoring essay tests, the teacher can establish criteria for grading, develop a rubric, and score responses to the questions with the case. Otherwise cases are useful for formative evaluation and student self-assessment.

Papers

Short papers for assessing critical thinking and other cognitive skills were described in Chapter 9. In short papers about clinical practice, students can:

- Given a data set, identify patient problems and what additional data need to be collected
- Compare data and problems of patients for whom they have provided nursing care, identifying similarities and differences
- Given a hypothetical patient or community problem, identify possible interventions with supporting evidence
- Select a patient, family, or community problem, and describe relevant interventions with evidence for their use
- Identify one intervention they used with a patient, family, or community; identify alternative approaches that could be used; and provide a rationale

- Identify a decision made in clinical practice involving patients or staff, describe why they made that decision, and propose one other approach that could be used
- Identify a problem or an issue they had in clinical practice, critique the approaches they used for resolving it, and identify alternate approaches

Short written assignments in clinical courses may be more beneficial than longer assignments because with long papers students often summarize from the textbook and other literature without engaging in any of their own thinking about the content (Oermann, 2006). Short papers can be used for formative evaluation or graded.

Term papers also may be written about clinical practice. With term papers, students can critique and synthesize relevant literature and write a paper about how that literature relates to patient care. Or they might prepare a paper on the use of selected concepts and theories in clinical practice. If the term paper includes the submission of drafts combined with prompt feedback on writing from the teacher, it can be used as a strategy for improving writing skills. Although drafts of papers are assessed but not graded, the final product is graded by the teacher.

There are many other written assignments that can be used for clinical evaluation in a nursing course. Similar to any assignment in a course, requirements for papers should be carefully thought out: What outcomes will be met with the assignment, how will they contribute to clinical evaluation in the course, and how many of those assignments does a student need to complete for competency? In planning the clinical evaluation protocol, the teacher should exercise caution in the type and number of written assignments so that they promote learning without unnecessary repetition. Guidelines for evaluating written assignments were presented in Chapter 9 and therefore are not repeated here.

PORTFOLIO

A portfolio is a collection of projects and materials developed by the student that document achievement of the objectives of the clinical course. With a portfolio, students can demonstrate what they have learned in clinical practice and the competencies they have developed. Portfolios are valuable for clinical evaluation because students provide evidence in their portfolios to confirm their clinical competencies and document new learning and skills acquired in a course. The portfolio can include evidence of student learning for a series of clinical experiences or over the duration of a clinical course. Portfolios also can be developed for program evaluation purposes to document achievement of curriculum or program outcomes and provide data for revising the curriculum (Rossetti et al., 2012).

Portfolios can be evaluated and graded by faculty members based on predetermined criteria. They also can be used for students' self-assessment of their progress in meeting personal and professional goals. Students can continue using their portfolios after graduation—for career development, for job applications, as part of their annual performance appraisals, for applications for educational programs, and as documentation of continuing competence (Oermann, 2002).

Nitko and Brookhart (2011) identified two types of portfolios: best work and growth. Best-work portfolios contain the student's best final products. These provide evidence that the student has demonstrated certain competencies and achievements in clinical practice, and thus are appropriate for summative clinical evaluation. Growth portfolios are designed for monitoring students' progress and for self-reflection on learning outcomes at several points in time. These contain products and work of the students in process and at the intermediate stages, for the teacher to review and provide feedback (Nitko & Brookhart, 2011).

For clinical evaluation, these purposes can be combined. The portfolio can be developed initially for growth and learning, with products and entries reviewed periodically by the teacher for formative evaluation, and then as a best-work portfolio with completed products providing evidence of clinical competencies. The best-work portfolio then can be graded.

The contents of the portfolio depend on the outcomes of the clinical course and competencies to be developed. Many types of materials and documentation can be included in a portfolio. For example, students can include short papers they completed in the course, a term paper, reports of group work, reports and analyses of observations made in the clinical setting, self-reflections on clinical experiences, concept maps, and other products they developed in their clinical practice. The key is for students to choose materials that demonstrate their learning and development of clinical competencies. By assessing the portfolio, the teacher should be able to determine whether the students met the outcomes of the course.

There are several steps to follow in using portfolios for clinical evaluation in nursing. Nitko and Brookhart (2011) emphasized that the first step guides faculty members in deciding whether a portfolio is an appropriate evaluation method for the course.

Step 1: Identify the purpose of the portfolio.

- Why is a portfolio useful in the course? What goals will it serve?
- Will the portfolio serve as a means of assessing students' development of clinical competencies, focusing predominantly on the

growth of the students? Will the portfolio provide evidence of the students' best work in clinical practice, including products that reflect their learning over a period of time? Or, will the portfolio meet both demands, enabling the teacher to give continual feedback to students on the process of learning and projects on which they are working, as well as providing evidence of their accomplishments and achievements in clinical practice?

- Will the portfolio be used for formative or for summative evaluation? Or both?
- Will the portfolio provide assessment data for use in a clinical course? Or will it be used for curriculum and program evaluation?
- Will the portfolio serve as a means of assessing prior learning and therefore have an impact on the types of learning activities or courses that students complete, for instance, for assessing the prior learning of registered nurses entering a higher degree program or for licensed practical nurses entering an associate degree program?
- What is the role of the students, if any, in defining the focus and content of the portfolio?

Step 2: Identify the type of entries and content to be included in the portfolio.

- What types of entries are required in the portfolio, for example, products developed by students, descriptions of projects with which the students are involved, descriptions of clinical learning activities and reflections, observations made in clinical practice and analysis of them, and papers completed by the students, among others?
- In addition to required entries, what other types of content and entries might be included in the portfolio?
- Who determines the content of the portfolio and the types of entries? Teacher only? Student only? Or both?
- Will the entries be the same for all students or individualized by the student?
- What is the minimum number of entries to be considered satisfactory?
- How should the entries in the portfolio be organized, or will the students choose how to organize them?
- Are there required times for entries to be made in the portfolio, and when should the portfolio be submitted to the teacher for review and feedback?
- Will teacher and student meet in a conference to discuss the portfolio?

Step 3: Decide on the evaluation of the portfolio entries including criteria for evaluation of individual entries and the portfolio overall.

- How will the portfolio be integrated within the clinical evaluation grade and course grade, if at all?
- What criteria will be used to evaluate, and perhaps score, each type of entry and the portfolio as a whole?
- Will only the teacher evaluate the portfolio and its entries? Will only the students evaluate their own progress and work? Or will the evaluation be a collaborative effort?
- Should a rubric be developed for scoring the portfolio and individual entries? Is there one available in the nursing education program that could be used? If not who will develop the rubric?

These steps and questions to be answered provide guidelines for teachers in developing a portfolio system for clinical evaluation in a course or for other purposes in the nursing education program.

Electronic Portfolios

Portfolios can be developed and stored electronically, which facilitates updating and revising entries, as compared with portfolios that include hard copies of materials. In addition to easy updating, prior versions of the portfolio can be archived. Students can develop an electronic portfolio (e-portfolio) in a nursing course and then reformat it for a job application. The electronic portfolio can be saved on a local computer, course website, or other type of website, and can be easily sent to others for feedback or scoring. In a study by Garrett, Macphee, and Jackson (2012), clinical teachers valued the convenience and improved ability to monitor student progress and assess clinical competencies, among other outcomes, of e-portfolios. Students also valued their convenience but were concerned about the openness of information in the portfolio. When using an e-portfolio for assessment, teachers need to provide security for the documents.

Some other reasons for using electronic portfolios in a course:

- They can be shared with others at limited or no cost (e.g., on the Web) and updated easily.
- They can document learning and development over a period of time.
- They can be modified for class and program assessment, graduation requirements, or a job search.
- They can include a variety of multimedia.

- They are interactive, and through use of hypertext, students can connect ideas, projects, and links.
- They can be designed for review by the student for self-assessment, by the teacher and student, by other students in the clinical course or nursing program, or by prospective employers, depending on the purpose of the portfolio (Ring, Weaver, & Jones, 2008).

CONFERENCES

The ability to present ideas orally is an important outcome of clinical practice. Sharing information about a patient, leading others in discussions about clinical practice, presenting ideas in a group format, and giving various types of presentations are skills that students need to develop in a nursing program. Working with nursing staff members and the health care team requires the ability to communicate effectively. Conferences provide a method for developing oral communication skills and for evaluating competency in this area. Discussions also lead to problem solving and higher-level thinking if questions are open-ended and geared to these outcomes, as discussed in Chapter 7.

Many types of conferences are appropriate for clinical evaluation, depending on the outcomes to be met. Preclinical conferences take place prior to beginning a clinical learning activity and allow students to clarify their understanding of patient problems, interventions, and other aspects of clinical practice. Similar types of conferences can be held prior to a simulation. In these conferences, the teacher can assess students' knowledge and provide feedback to them. Postclinical conferences, held at the end of a clinical learning activity or at a predetermined time during the clinical practicum, provide an opportunity for the teacher to assess students' ability to use concepts and theories in patient care, plan care, assess the outcomes of interventions, problem solve and think critically, collaborate with peers and team members, and achieve other outcomes, depending on the focus of the discussion. In clinical conferences students also can examine ethical dilemmas; cultural aspects of care; and issues facing patients, families, communities, providers, and the health care system. In discussions such as these, students can examine different perspectives and approaches that could be taken. One other conference in which students might participate is an interprofessional conference, providing an opportunity to work with other health providers in planning and evaluating care of patients and families.

Debriefing is the discussion that follows a simulation, allowing students to reflect on their experiences. It must be carried out in a safe environment.

Through this discussion, students gain new meanings from the simulation (Campbell, 2010; Dreifuerst, 2012). Other outcomes of learning can also be met. In a debriefing of a leadership scenario of a routine day in a hospital, students were able to identify their errors in performance and decisions, cues that they missed about the status of a patient, and errors they made in delegation (Schultz, Shinnick, & Judson, 2012). Although many clinical conferences will be face-to-face with the teacher or preceptor onsite with the students, conferences also can be conducted online. In a study by Cooper, Taft, and Thelen (2004), students identified "flexibility" and "an opportunity for equal participation" as two benefits of holding clinical conferences online versus face-to-face.

Criteria for evaluating conferences include the ability of students to:

- Present ideas clearly and in a logical sequence to the group
- Participate actively in the group discussion
- Offer ideas relevant to the topic
- Demonstrate knowledge of the content discussed in the conference
- Offer different perspectives to the topic or share their reflections to encourage new learning among the group
- Assume a leadership role, if relevant, in promoting group discussion and arriving at group decisions

Most conferences are evaluated for formative purposes, with the teacher giving feedback to students as a group or to the individual who led the group discussion. When conferences are evaluated as a portion of the clinical or course grade, the teacher should have specific criteria to guide the evaluation and should use a scoring rubric. Exhibit 14.10 provides a sample form that can be used to evaluate how well a student leads a clinical conference or to assess student participation in a conference.

GROUP PROJECTS

Most of the clinical evaluation methods presented in this chapter focus on individual student performance, but group projects also can be assessed as part of the clinical evaluation in a course. Some group work is short term—only for the time it takes to develop a product such as a poster or group presentation. Other groups may be formed for the purpose of cooperative learning with students working in small groups or teams in clinical practice over a longer period of time. With any of these group formats, both the products developed by the group and the ability of the students to work cooperatively can be assessed.

☐Exhibit 14.10

Evaluation of Participation in Clinical Conference

Student's name _____

Conference topic _____

Date _____

Rate the behaviors listed below by circling the appropriate number. Some behaviors will not be applicable depending on student role in conference; mark those as not applicable (na).

BEHAVIORS	RATING					
	POOR				EXCELLENT	
States goals of conference	1	2	3	4	5	na
Leads group in discussion	1	2	3	4	5	na
Asks thought-provoking questions	1	2	3	4	5	na
Uses strategies that encourage all students to participate	1	2	3	4	5	na
Participates actively in discussion	1	2	3	4	5	na
Includes important content	1	2	3	4	5	na
Bases interventions on evidence for practice	1	2	3	4	5	na
Offers new perspectives to group	1	2	3	4	5	na
Considers different points of view	1	2	3	4	5	na
Assists group members in recognizing biases and values that may influence decision making	1	2	3	4	5	na
Is enthusiastic about conference topic	1	2	3	4	5	na
Is well prepared for conference discussion	1	2	3	4	5	na
If leading group, monitors time	1	2	3	4	5	na
Develops quality materials to support discussion	1	2	3	4	5	na
Summarizes major points discussed at end of conference	1	2	3	4	5	na

There are different approaches for grading group projects. The same grade can be given to every student in the group, that is, a group grade, although this does not take into consideration individual student effort and contribution to the group product. Another approach is for the students to indicate in the finished product the parts they contributed, providing a way of assigning individual student grades, with or without a group grade. Students also can provide a self-assessment of how much they contributed to the group project, which can then be integrated into their grade.

Alternatively, students can prepare both a group and an individual product. Rubrics should be used for assessing group projects and should be geared specifically to the project. An example of a scoring rubric for assessing a paper was provided in Table 9.1. This rubric could be used for grading a paper prepared by either a group or an individual student.

To assess students' participation and collaboration in the group, the rubric also needs to reflect the goals of group work. With small groups, the teacher can observe and rate individual student cooperation and contributions to the group. However, this is often difficult because the teacher is not a member of the group, and the group dynamics change when the teacher is present. As another approach, students can assess the participation and cooperation of their peers. These peer evaluations can be used for the students' own development, and shared among peers but not with the teacher, or can be incorporated by the teacher in the grade for the group project. In one study nursing students supported the opportunity to grade individual student contributions to a group project because it reduced the chance of some students not contributing (Shiu, Chan, Lam, Lee, & Kwong, 2012). Students also can be asked to assess their own participation in the group. An easy-to-use form for peer evaluation of group participation is found in Exhibit 14.11.

⊒Exhibit 14.11

Rubric for Peer Evaluation of Participation in Group Project

Participation Rubric

Directions: Complete for each group member. NAME _____

Score	Area Assessed	Excellent = 4	Good = 3	Poor = 2	Unacceptable = 1
_____	Amount of group work	Did a full share of the work and often more than required; willingly helped others	Did an equal share of the work; did additional work when asked	Did less than an equal share of the work; rarely helped others	Did not complete all of assigned group work; never helped others
_____	Quality of group work	Contributions to the group and products met outcomes and were of high quality	Contributions to the group and products met most outcomes and were satisfactory	Some of the contributions and products did not meet outcomes and were of poor quality	Contributions to the group were limited and were consistently of poor quality

Exhibit 14.11 (continued)

_____	Organization	Led group in getting organized; arranged meeting times and places	Helped others with organizing group; was flexible with meeting times and places	Did not contribute to organizing group; was not flexible with meeting times and places	Never participated in organizing group or arranging meeting times and places
_____	Attendance at Group Meetings	Attended all meetings; was on time	Attended most meetings; was on time	Missed some meetings or was consistently late	Missed many meetings; did not provide group with reasons
_____	Group Participation	Provided many valuable ideas with rationale; considered views of others and was willing to modify own perspective	Provided good suggestions; considered views of others but did not readily change own perspective	Listened to group and occasionally shared own ideas	Participated minimally in discussions; ideas were often not relevant to topic
_____	Deadlines	Completed group work prior to deadline or on time	Completed most group work on time	Was late with group work; required constant reminders from group	Did not complete all of assigned group work or was always late
_____	Providing and Receiving Feedback	Always provided specific, clear feedback to the group in a respectful manner; accepted feedback and used for revision	Provided general feedback to the group in a respectful manner; listened to feedback from others	Provided some feedback to the group; occasionally was offensive in how feedback was given; did not accept feedback from group	Did not provide any specific feedback to group; was occasionally rude when providing feedback; never listened to feedback form group

Total Score: _____

SELF-ASSESSMENT

Self-assessment is the ability of students to evaluate their own clinical competencies and identify where further learning is needed. Self-assessment begins with the first clinical course and develops throughout the nursing education program, continuing into professional practice. Through self-assessment, students examine their clinical performance and identify both strengths and areas for improvement. Using students' self-assessments, teachers can develop plans to assist students in gaining the knowledge and skills they need to meet the outcomes of the course. It is important for teachers to establish a positive climate for learning in the course, or students will not be likely to share their self-assessments with them.

In addition to developing a supportive learning environment, the teacher should hold planned conferences with each student to review performance. In these conferences, the teacher can

- give specific and instructional feedback on performance
- obtain the student's own perceptions of competencies and progress
- identify strengths and areas for learning from the teacher's and student's perspectives
- plan with the student learning activities for improving performance, which is critical if the student is not passing the clinical course
- enhance communication between teacher and student

Some students have difficulty assessing their own performance. This is a developmental process, and in the beginning of a nursing education program, students need more guidance in assessing their performance than at the end. Self-evaluation is appropriate only for formative evaluation and should never be graded.

CLINICAL EVALUATION IN DISTANCE EDUCATION

Nursing education programs use different strategies for offering the clinical component of distance education courses. Often preceptors in the local area guide student learning in the clinical setting and evaluate performance. If cohorts of students are available in an area, adjunct or part-time faculty members might be hired to teach a small group of students in the clinical setting. In other programs, students independently complete clinical learning activities to gain the clinical knowledge and competencies of a course. Regardless of how the clinical component is structured, the course syllabus, competencies to be developed, rating forms, guidelines for clinical practice, and other materials associated with the clinical course should be available electronically. This provides easy access for students, their preceptors, other individuals with whom they are working, and agency personnel. Course management systems facilitate communication among students, preceptors, course faculty, and others involved in the students' clinical activities.

The clinical evaluation methods presented in this chapter can be used for distance education. The critical decision for the teacher is to identify which clinical competencies and skills, if any, need to be observed and the performance rated because that decision suggests different evaluation methods than if the focus of the evaluation is on the cognitive outcomes of the clinical course. In programs in which preceptors or adjunct faculty are available on-site, any of the clinical evaluation methods presented in this chapter can be used as long as they are congruent with the course outcomes and competencies. There should be consistency, though, in how the evaluation is done across preceptors and clinical settings.

Strategies should be implemented in the course for preceptors and other educators involved in the performance evaluation to discuss as a group the competencies to be rated, what each competency means, and the performance of those competencies at different levels on the rating scale. This is a critical activity to ensure reliability across preceptors and other evaluators. Activities can be provided in which preceptors observe media clips of performances of students and rate their quality using the clinical evaluation tool. Preceptors and course faculty members then can discuss the performance and rating. Alternately, discussions about levels of performance and their characteristics and how those levels would be reflected in ratings of the performance can be held with preceptors and course faculty members. Preceptor development activities of this type should be done before the course begins and at least once during the course to ensure that evaluators are using the tool as intended and are consistent across student populations and clinical settings. Even in clinical courses involving preceptors, faculty members may decide to evaluate clinical skills themselves by reviewing digital recordings of performance or observing students by using other technology with faculty at the receiving end. Digitally recording performance is valuable not only as a strategy for summative evaluation, to assess competencies at the end of a clinical course or another designated point in time, but also for review by students for self-assessment and by faculty to give feedback.

Simulations and standardized patients are other strategies useful in assessing clinical performance in distance education. Performance with standardized patients can be digitally recorded, and students can submit their patient assessments and other written documentation that would commonly be done in practice in that situation. Students also can complete case analyses related to the standardized patient encounter for assessing their knowledge base and rationale for their decisions.

Some nursing education programs incorporate intensive skill acquisitions workshops in centralized settings for formative evaluation followed by end-of-course ratings by preceptors and others guiding the clinical practicum. In areas where there are regional simulation centers, students can travel to those settings for assessment of clinical competencies.

Students can demonstrate clinical skills and perform procedures on manikins and models, with their performance digitally recorded and transmitted to faculty for evaluation. In distance education courses a portfolio would be a useful evaluation method because it would allow the students to provide materials that indicate their achievement of the course outcomes and clinical competencies.

Simulations, analyses of cases, case presentations, written assignments, and other strategies presented in this chapter can be used to evaluate students' cognitive skills in distance education courses. Similar to clinical evaluation in general, a combination of approaches is more effective than one method alone. Exhibit 14.12 summarizes clinical evaluation methods useful for distance education courses.

SUMMARY

This chapter built on concepts of clinical evaluation examined in Chapter 13. Many clinical evaluation methods are available for assessing student competencies in clinical practice. The teacher should choose evaluation methods that provide information on how well students are performing the clinical competencies. The teacher also decides if the evaluation method is intended for formative or for summative evaluation. Some of the methods designed for clinical evaluation are strictly to provide feedback to students on areas for improvement and are not graded. Other methods, such as rating forms and certain written assignments, may be used for summative purposes.

The predominant method for clinical evaluation is in observing the performance of students in clinical practice. Although observation is widely used, there are threats to its validity and reliability. Observations of students may be influenced by the values, attitudes, and biases of the teacher or preceptor, as discussed in the previous chapter. In observing clinical performance, there are many aspects of that performance on which the teacher may focus attention. Every observation reflects only a sampling of the learner's performance during a clinical learning activity. Issues such as these point to the need for a series of observations before arriving at conclusions about performance. There are several ways of recording

⊔Exhibit 14.12

Clinical Evaluation Methods for Distance Education Courses

Evaluation of Psychomotor, Technological, and Other Clinical Skills

Observation of performance (by faculty members on-site or at distance, preceptors, examiners, others):

- With patients, patient simulators and other virtual-reality devices, models, manikins, standardized patients
- Objective Structured Clinical Examinations and simulations (in laboratories on-site, regional centers, other settings)

Rating of performance:

- Using rating scales, checklists, performance algorithms
- By faculty members, preceptors, examiners, others on-site

Notes about clinical performance by preceptor, examiner, others in local area

---

Evaluation of Cognitive Outcomes and Skills

Test items on clinical knowledge and higher level cognitive skills

Analyses of clinical situations in own practice, of cases and of media clips:

- Reported in a paper, in discussion board, as part of other online activities

Written assignments:

- Write-ups of cases, analyses of patient care, and other clinical experiences
- Electronic journals
- Analyses of interactions in clinical setting and simulated experiences
- Short written assignments
- Nursing care and management plans
- Sample documentation
- Term papers
- Development of teaching materials, and others

Case presentations (can be recorded for faculty members at a distance)

Online conferences, discussions

Portfolio (with materials documenting clinical competencies developed in practicum)

Evaluation of Affective Outcomes

Online conferences and discussions about values, attitudes, and biases that might influence patient care and decisions; about cultural dimensions of care

Analyses and discussions of cases presented online, of clinical scenarios shown in media clips and other multimedia

Written assignments (e.g., reflective papers, journals, others)

Debates about ethical decisions

Value clarification strategies

Reflective journals

observations of students—notes about performance, checklists, and rating scales. These were described in the chapter.

A simulation creates a situation that represents reality. A major advantage of simulation is that it provides a clinical learning activity for students without the constraints of a real-life situation. With high fidelity simulations, students can respond to changing situations and conduct assessments, analyze physiological and other types of data, give medications, and observe the outcomes of interventions and treatments they select. With simulation students can develop their clinical judgment. One type of simulation for clinical evaluation uses standardized patients, that is, individuals who have been trained to accurately portray the role of a patient with a specific diagnosis or condition. Another form of simulation for clinical evaluation is an Objective Structured Clinical Examination, in which students can rotate through a series of stations completing activities or performing skills that are then evaluated.

There are many types of written assignments useful for clinical evaluation depending on the outcomes to be assessed: journal writing, nursing care plan, concept map, case analysis, and a paper on some aspect of clinical practice. Written assignments can be developed as a learning activity and reviewed by the teacher and/or peers for formative evaluation, or they can be graded.

A portfolio is a collection of materials that students develop in clinical practice over a period of time. With a portfolio, students provide evidence to confirm their clinical competencies and document the learning that occurred in clinical practice. Other clinical evaluation methods are the conference, group project, and self-assessment. The evaluation methods presented in this chapter provide the teacher with a wealth of methods from which to choose in evaluating students' clinical performance.

REFERENCES

Aebersold, M., Tschannen, D., & Bathish, M. (2012). Innovative simulation strategies in education. *Nursing Research and Practice, 2012,* Article ID 765212.

Bensfield, L. A., Olech, M. J., & Horsley, T. L. (2012). Simulation for high-stakes evaluation in nursing. *Nurse Educator, 37,* 71–74.

Bentley, R., & Seaback, C. (2011). A faculty development collaborative in interprofessional simulation. *Journal of Professional Nursing, 27*(6), e1–e7.

Blakely, G., Skirton, H., Cooper, S., Allum, P., & Nelmes, P. (2010). Use of educational games in the health professions: A mixed-methods study of educators' perspectives in the UK. *Nursing & Health Sciences, 12*(1), 27–32.

Bourke, M. P., & Ihrke, B. A. (2009). The evaluation process: An overview. In D. M. Billings & J. Halstead (Eds.), *Teaching in nursing* (3rd ed., pp. 391–408). St. Louis, MO: Saunders Elsevier.

Brown, J. (2008). Applications of simulation technology in psychiatric mental health nursing education. *Journal of Psychiatric & Mental Health Nursing, 15,* 638–644.

Campbell, S. H. (2010). Clinical simulation. In K. B. Gaberson & M. H. Oermann (Eds.), *Clinical teaching strategies in nursing* (3rd ed., pp. 151–181). New York, NY: Springer.

Clynes, M. P., & Raftery, S. E. (2008). Feedback: An essential element of student learning in clinical practice. *Nurse Education in Practice, 8,* 405–411.

Cooper, C., Taft, L. B., & Thelen, M. (2004). Examining the role of technology in learning: An evaluation of online clinical conferencing. *Journal of Professional Nursing, 20,* 160–166.

Di Leonardi Case, B., & Oermann, M. H. (2010). Clinical teaching and evaluation. In L. Caputi (Ed.), *Teaching nursing: The art and science* (2nd ed., pp. 82–141). Glen Ellyn, IL: College of DuPage.

Dreifuerst, K. T. (2012). Using debriefing for meaningful learning to foster development of clinical reasoning in simulation. *Journal of Nursing Education, 51,* 326–333.

Gaberson, K. B., & Oermann, M. H. (2010). *Clinical teaching strategies in nursing* (3rd ed.). New York, NY: Springer Publishing.

Garrett, B. M., Macphee, M., & Jackson, C. (2012). Evaluation of an eportfolio for the assessment of clinical competence in a baccalaureate nursing program. *Nurse Education Today.* July 10 [Epub ahead of print].

Gigante, J., Dell, M., & Sharkey, A. (2011). Getting beyond "Good job": How to give effective feedback. *Pediatrics, 127,* 205–207.

Hall, M., Daly, B., & Madigan, E. (2010). Use of anecdotal notes by clinical nursing faculty: A descriptive study. *Journal of Nursing Education, 49,* 156–159.

Hawkins, R. E., & Boulet, J. R. (2008). Direct observation: Standardized patients. In E. S. Holmboe & R. E. Hawkins (Eds.), *Practical guide to the evaluation of clinical competencies* (pp. 102–118). Philadelphia, PA: Mosby.

Hill, C. (2006). Integrating clinical experiences into the concept mapping process. *Nurse Educator, 31,* 36–39.

Holaday, S. D., & Buckley, K. M. (2008). A standardized clinical evaluation tool-kit: Improving nursing education and practice. In M. H. Oermann (Ed.), *Annual review of nursing education* (Vol. 6, pp. 123–149). New York, NY: Springer Publishing.

Ironside, P. M., Jeffries, P. R., & Martin, A. (2009). Fostering patient safety competencies using multiple-patient simulation experiences. *Nursing Outlook, 57,* 332–337.

Kameg, K., Howard, V. M., Clochesy, J., Mitchell, A. M., & Suresky, J. M. (2010). The impact of high fidelity human simulation on self-efficacy of communication skills. *Issues in Mental Health Nursing, 31,* 315–323.

Kaplan, B. G., Holmes, L., Mott, M., & Atallah, H. (2011). Design and implementation of an interdisciplinary pediatric mock code for undergraduate and graduate nursing students. *CIN: Computers, Informatics, Nursing, 29,* 531–538.

Kern, C., Bush, K., & McCleish, J. (2006). Mind-mapped care plans: Integrating an innovative educational tool as an alternative to traditional care plans. *Journal of Nursing Education, 45,* 112–119.

Langley, M. E., & Brown, S. T. (2010). Perceptions of the use of reflective learning journals in online graduate nursing education. *Nursing Education Perspectives, 31,* 12–17.

Lasater, K. (2007). High-fidelity simulation and the development of clinical judgment: Students' experiences. *Journal of Nursing Education, 46,* 269–276.

Lasater, K. (2011). Clinical judgment: The last frontier for evaluation. *Nurse Education in Practice, 11,* 86–92

Liaw, S. Y., Scherpbier, A., Klainin-Yobas, P., & Rethans, J. J. (2011). Rescuing A Patient In Deteriorating Situations (RAPIDS): An evaluation tool for assessing simulation performance on clinical deterioration. *Resuscitation, 82,* 1434–1439.

Liberto, T., Roncher, M., & Shellenbarger, T. (1999). Anecdotal notes: Effective clinical evaluation and record keeping. *Nurse Educator, 24*, 15–18.

Lynch-Sauer, J., Vandenbosch, T. M., Kron, F., Gjerde, C. L., Arato, N., Sen, A., & Fetters, M. D. (2011). Nursing students' attitudes toward video games and related new media technologies. *Journal of Nursing Education, 50*, 513–523.

McWilliam, P. L., & Botwinski, C. A. (2012). Identifying strengths and weaknesses in the utilization of Objective Structured Clinical Examination (OSCE) in a nursing program. *Nursing Education Perspectives, 33*, 35–39.

Nickless, L. (2011). The use of simulation to address the acute care skills deficit in pre-registration nursing students: A clinical skill perspective. *Nurse Education in Practice, 11*, 199–205.

Nitko, A. J., & Brookhart, S. M. (2011). *Educational assessment of students* (6th ed.). Upper Saddle River, NJ: Pearson Education.

Noonan, P. (2011). Using concept maps in perioperative education. *AORN Journal, 94*, 469–478.

Norman, J. (2012). Systematic review of the literature on simulation in nursing education. *ABNF Journal, 23*(2), 24–28.

Oermann, M. H. (2002). Developing a professional portfolio. *Orthopaedic Nursing, 21*, 73–78.

Oermann, M. H. (2004). Reflections on undergraduate nursing education: A look to the future. *International Journal of Nursing Education Scholarship, 1*(article 5).

Oermann, M. H. (2006). Short written assignments for clinical nursing courses. *Nurse Educator, 31*, 228–231.

Oermann, M. H. (2008). Clinical evaluation. In B. Penn (Ed.), *Mastering the teaching role: A guide for nurse educators* (pp. 299–313). Philadelphia, PA: F.A. Davis.

Oermann, M. H. (2011). Toward evidence-based nursing education: Deliberate practice and motor skill learning. *Journal of Nursing Education, 50*, 63–64.

Oermann, M. H., Kardong-Edgren, S., Odom-Maryon, T., Hallmark, B., Hurd, D., Rogers N., … Smart, D. (2011). Deliberate practice of motor skills in nursing education: CPR as exemplar. *Nursing Education Perspectives, 32*, 311–315.

Oermann, M. H., Kardong-Edgren, S., & Odom-Maryon, T. (2011). Effects of monthly practice on nursing students' CPR psychomotor skill performance. *Resuscitation, 82*, 447–453.

Oermann, M. H., Saewert, K. J., Charasika, M., & Yarbrough, S. S. (2009). Assessment and grading practices in schools of nursing: National survey findings Part I. *Nursing Education Perspectives, 30*, 274–278.

Oermann, M. H., Yarbrough, S. S., Ard, N., Saewert, K. J., & Charasika, M. (2009). Clinical evaluation and grading practices in schools of nursing: Findings of the Evaluation of Learning Advisory Council Survey. *Nursing Education Perspectives, 30*, 252–257.

Parsons, M. E., Hawkins, K. S., Hercinger, M., Todd, M., Manz, J. A., & Fang, X. (2012). Improvement in scoring consistency for the Creighton Simulation Evaluation Instrument. *Clinical Simulation in Nursing, 8*(6), e233–e238.

Pascual, J., Holena, D., Vella, M., Palmieri, J., Sicoutris, C., Selvan, B., … Schwab, C. (2011). Short simulation training improves objective skills in established advanced practitioners managing emergencies on the ward and surgical intensive care unit. *Journal of Trauma, 71*, 330–338.

Pilcher, J. (2011). Teaching and learning with concept maps. *Neonatal Network, 30*, 336–339.

Quality and Safety Education for Nurses. (2012). Quality and Safety Competencies. Retrieved from http://www.qsen.org/competencies.php

Ring, G., Weaver, B. M., & Jones, J. H., Jr. (2008). Electronic portfolios: Engaged students create multimedia-rich artifacts. *Journal for the Research Center for Educational Technology, 4*(2), 103–114.

Rossetti, J., Oldenburg, N., Fisher Robertson, J., Coyer, S. M., Koren, M. E., Peters, B., ... Musker, K. (2012). Creating a culture of evidence in nursing education using student portfolios. *International Journal of Nursing Education Scholarship, 9*(1).

Royse, M., & Newton, S. (2007). How gaming is used as an innovative strategy for nursing education. *Nursing Education Perspectives, 28*, 263–267.

Schuessler, J. B., Wilder, S., & Byrd, L. W. (2012). Reflective journaling and development of cultural humility in students. *Nursing Education Perspectives, 33*, 96–99.

Schultz, M. A., Shinnick, M. A., & Judson, L. H. (2012). Learning from mistakes in a simulated nursing leadership laboratory. *CIN: Computers, Informatics, Nursing, 30*, 456–462.

Sears, K., Goldsworthy, S., & Goodman, W. M. (2010). The relationship between simulation in nursing education and medication safety. *Journal of Nursing Education, 49*, 52–55.

Shiu, A. T. Y., Chan, C. W. H., Lam, P., Lee, J., & Kwong, A. N. L. (2012). Baccalaureate nursing students' perceptions of peer assessment of individual contributions to a group project: A case study. *Nurse Education Today, 32*, 214–218.

Skiba, D. (2008). Emerging technologies center. Nursing education 2.0: Games as pedagogical platforms. *Nursing Education Perspectives, 29*, 174–175.

Stroud, L., Herold, J., Tomlinson, G., & Cavalcanti, R. B. (2011). Who you know or what you know? Effect of examiner familiarity with residents on OSCE scores. *Academic Medicine, 86*(10), S8–S11.

Thompson, M. E., Ford, R., & Webster, A. (2011). Effectiveness of interactive, online games in learning neuroscience and students' perception of the games as learning tools. A pre-experimental study. *Journal of Allied Health, 40*, 150–155.

Todd, M., Manz, J., Hawkins, K., Parsons, M., & Hercinger, M. (2008). The development of a quantitative evaluation tool for simulations in nursing education. *International Journal of Nursing Education Scholarship, 5*, Article 41.

Vacek, J. E. (2009). Using a conceptual approach with concept mapping to promote critical thinking. *Journal of Nursing Education, 48*, 45–48.

Walsh, M., Bailey, P. H., & Koren, I. (2009). Objective structured clinical evaluation of clinical competence: An integrative review. *Journal of Advanced Nursing, 65*, 1584–1595.

Walsh, T., Jairath, N., Paterson, M., & Grandjean, C. (2010). Quality and safety education for nurses clinical evaluation tool. *Journal of Nursing Education, 49*, 517–522.

Yuan, H., Williams, B. A., Fang, J., & Ye, Q. (2012). A systematic review of selected evidence on improving knowledge and skills through high-fidelity simulation. *Nurse Education Today, 32*, 294–298.

Zurmehly, J. (2010). Personal Digital Assistants (PDAs): Review and evaluation. *Nursing Education Perspectives, 31*, 179–182.

PART V

Issues Related to Testing, Grading,

and Other Evaluation Concepts

FIFTEEN

Social, Ethical, and

Legal Issues

Educational testing and assessment have grown in use and importance for students in general, and nursing students in particular, over the last decade. One only has to read the newspapers and watch television to appreciate the prevalence of testing and assessment in contemporary American society. With policies and laws such as the No Child Left Behind Act, mandatory high school graduation tests in some states, and the emphasis on standardized achievement tests in many schools, testing and assessment have taken a prominent role in the educational system. From the moment of birth, when we are weighed, measured, and rated according to the Apgar scale, throughout all of our educational and work experiences, and even in our personal and social lives, we are used to being tested and evaluated. In addition, nursing and other professional disciplines have come under increasing public pressure to be accountable for the quality of educational programs and the competency of their practitioners; thus testing and assessment often are used to provide evidence of quality and competence.

With the increasing use of assessment and testing come intensified interest and concern about fairness, appropriateness, and impact. This chapter discusses selected social, ethical, and legal issues related to testing and assessment practices in nursing education.

SOCIAL ISSUES

Testing has tremendous social impact because test scores can have positive and negative consequences for individuals. Tests can provide information to assist in decision making; some of these decisions have more importance to society and to individuals than other decisions. The licensure of drivers is a good example. Written and performance tests provide information for deciding who may drive a vehicle. Society has a vested interest in the outcome because a bad decision can affect the safety of a great many people. Licensure to drive a vehicle also may be an important issue to an individual; some jobs require the employee to drive a car or truck, so a person who lacks a valid operator's license will not have access to these employment opportunities.

Tests also are used to help place individuals into professional and occupational roles. These placement decisions have important implications because a person's profession or occupation to some extent determines status and economic and political power. Because modern society depends heavily on scientific knowledge and technical competence, occupational and professional role selection is based to a significant degree on what individuals know and can do. Therefore, by controlling who enters certain educational programs, institutions have a role in determining the possible career path of an individual.

The way in which schools should select candidates for occupational and professional roles is a matter of controversy, however. Some individuals and groups hold the view that schools should provide equal opportunity and access to educational programs. Others believe that equal opportunity is not sufficient to allow some groups of people to overcome discrimination and oppression that has handicapped their ability and opportunity.

Decisions about which individuals should be admitted to a nursing education program are important because of the nursing profession's commitment to the good of society and to the health and welfare of current and future patients (American Nurses Association, 2010). Nursing faculties must select individuals for admission to nursing programs who are likely to practice nursing competently and safely; tests frequently are used to assist educators in selecting candidates for admission. Improper use of testing or the misinterpretation of test scores can result in two types of poor admission decisions. If an individual is selected who is later found to be incompetent to practice nursing safely, the public might be at risk; if an individual who would be competent to practice nursing is not admitted, that individual is denied access to a professional role.

The use of testing in employment situations and for the purpose of professional certification can produce similar results. Employers have a stake in making these decisions because they are responsible for ensuring the competence of their employees. Tests for employment, to ensure competencies at the end of orientation, and to certify continuing knowledge and skills are important not only to the employee but also to the employer. Through assessments such as these, the employer verifies that the individual is competent for the role. Selection decisions therefore have social implications for individuals, institutions, and society as a whole.

Although educational and occupational uses of testing are growing in frequency and importance, the public often expresses concerns about testing. Some of these concerns are rational and relevant; others are unjustified.

Assessment Bias

One common concern is that assessments are biased or unfair to certain groups of test-takers. A major purpose of assessment is to discriminate among people, that is, to identify important differences among them with regard to their knowledge, skills, or attitudes. To the extent that differences in scores represent real differences in achievement of objectives, this discrimination is not necessarily unfair. Bias can occur, however, when scores from an assessment are misinterpreted, or conclusions are drawn about performance that go well beyond the assessment. For example, if a test is found to discriminate between men and women on variables that are not relevant to educational or occupational success, it would be unfair to use that test to select applicants for admission to a program or for a job. Thus, the question of test bias really is one of measurement validity, the degree to which inferences about test results are justifiable in relation to the purpose and intended use of the test (Miller, Linn, & Gronlund, 2009; Nitko & Brookhart, 2011).

Assessment bias also has been defined as the differential validity of an assessment result for a group of student or other people being assessed. With assessment bias, a given score does not have the same meaning for all students who were assessed. The teacher may interpret a low test score to mean inadequate knowledge of the content, but there may be a relevant subgroup of individuals, for example, students with learning disabilities, for whom that score interpretation is not accurate. The test score may be low for a student with a learning disability because he or she did not have enough time to complete the exam or because there was too much environmental noise, not because of a lack of knowledge about the content.

Individual test items also can discriminate against subgroups of test-takers, such as students from ethnic minority groups; this is termed differential item functioning (Nitko & Brookhart, 2011). Test items are considered to function differentially when students of different subgroups but of equal ability, as evidenced by equal total test scores, perform differently on the item. However, differences in item functioning do not necessarily confirm item bias (Nitko & Brookhart, 2011).

Item bias (and collectively, test bias) also can be construed as content and experience differential. Bias is produced by test or item content that differs substantially from one subgroup's life experiences *and* when these differences are not taken into account when the assessment results are interpreted (Nitko & Brookhart, 2011). S. D. Boscher (2009) proposed that this type of item bias exists in two forms, cultural bias and linguistic/structural bias.

A culturally biased item contains references to a particular culture and is more likely to be answered incorrectly by students from a minority group. An example of a culturally biased test item follows:

1. While discussing her health patterns with the nurse, a patient says that she enjoys all of the following leisure activities. Which one is an aerobic activity?
   a. Attending ballet performances
   b. Cultivating house plants
   c. Line dancing
   d. Singing in the church choir

The correct answer is "line dancing," but students who are non-native English speakers or English-language learners, students from cultural minority groups, and even domestic students from certain regions of the country may be unfamiliar with this term and therefore may not select this response. In this case, an incorrect response may mean that the student is unfamiliar with this type of dancing, not that the student is unable to differentiate between aerobic and nonaerobic activities. As discussed in Chapter 2, cultural bias of this type contributes to construct-irrelevant variance that can reduce measurement validity (S. Boscher & Bowles, 2008; Miller et al., 2009). The *Standards for Educational and Psychological Testing* (American Educational Research Association, American Psychological Association, & National Council on Measurement in Education [NCME], 1999) specify that test developers should "reduce threats to the reliability and validity of test score inferences that may arise from language differences" (p. 97).

Careful peer review of test items for discernible bias allows the teacher to reword items to remove references to American or English literature, music, art, history, customs, or regional terminology that are not essential to the nursing content being tested. The inclusion of jokes, puns, and other forms of humor also may contribute to cultural bias because these forms of expression may not be interpreted correctly by international students, non-native English speakers, and English-language learners. It is appropriate, however, to include content related to cultural differences that are essential to safe nursing practice. Students and graduate nurses must be culturally competent if they are to meet the needs of patients from a variety of cultures.

A test item with linguistic/structural bias is poorly written. It may be lengthy, unclear, or awkwardly worded, interfering with the student's understanding of the teacher's intent (S. D. Boscher, 2009). Structurally biased items create problems for all students, but they are more likely to discriminate against English as a second language (ESL) students or those with learning disabilities. Additionally, students from minority cultures may be less likely than dominant-culture students to ask the test proctor to clarify a poorly written item, usually because it is inappropriate to question a teacher in certain cultures. Following the general rules for writing test items in this book will help the teacher to avoid structural bias.

An assessment practice that helps to protect students from potential bias is anonymous or blinded scoring and grading. The importance of scoring essay items and written assignments anonymously was discussed earlier in the book. Anonymous grading also can be used for an entire course. The process is similar to that of peer review of manuscripts and grant proposals: the teacher is unaware of the student's identity until the end of the course. Students choose a number or are randomly assigned an anonymous grading system number at the beginning of a course. That number is recorded on every test, quiz, written assignment, and other assessments during the semester, and scores are recorded according to these code numbers. The teacher does not know the identity of the students until the end of the course. This method of grading prevents the influence of a teacher's previous impressions of a student on the scoring of a test or written assignment.

Grade and Test Score Inflation

Another common criticism of testing concerns the general trend toward inflation of test scores and grades at all educational levels. Scanlan and Care (2008) found that grade inflation occurred throughout their university but more so in their nursing program, and that inflated clinical practice grades give students an unrealistic perspective of their ability to practice nursing safely. Grade inflation distorts the meaning of test scores, making it difficult for teachers to use them wisely in decision making. If an A is intended to represent exceptional or superior performance, then all students cannot earn A grades because if everyone is exceptional, then no one is. With grade inflation all grades are compressed near the top, which makes it difficult to discriminate among students (Scanlan & Care, 2008; Walsh & Seldomridge, 2005). When there is no distribution of scores or grades, there is little value in testing. Most faculty members believe that grade inflation exists, but that their own assessment methods do not contribute to it (Scanlan & Care, 2008). Issues common to the problem of grade inflation include:

- Students' expectations related to the belief that they are consumers of the educational program
- Institutional policies related to late course withdrawal dates and mandatory faculty evaluation

- Increase in number of older students who bring more life experiences to the nursing education program and approach learning activities with more focus
- Faculty beliefs about the effect of grading on student self-esteem, what constitutes satisfactory performance, and the subjective nature of grading
- Clinical grading issues
- Increasing use of part-time faculty members in nursing education programs (Scanlan & Care, 2008)

The relationship between the last two factors is especially relevant in nursing education. Most part-time faculty members teach in the clinical area, and many are skilled clinicians with little or no formal academic preparation for the role of educator. Many nursing faculty members are reluctant to assign failing grades in clinical courses, giving students the benefit of the doubt especially in beginning courses. This belief is easily communicated to part-time faculty members, who may have additional concerns about their job security because most of them are hired on limited-term contracts. Where student evaluation of faculty members is mandatory, part-time teachers may be unwilling to assign lower clinical grades because of possible repercussions related to continued employment in that role (Scanlan & Care, 2008).

Additionally, grading discrepancies between theory and related clinical courses frequently occur. Scanlan and Care (2008) found a wide discrepancy between grades awarded in theory courses and grades in clinical courses. Especially in nursing education programs where clinical practice is assigned a letter grade (instead of a pass–fail or similar grading system), higher clinical grades tend to inflate the overall grade point average. This discrepancy is difficult to explain or defend on the basis of the assumption that theory informs clinical practice; why would a student with a grade of C in a theory course be likely to earn an A grade in the corresponding clinical course? Clinical grade inflation of this sort may result in more students with marginal ability "slipping through the cracks" and failing the final clinical course of the nursing education program, or graduating only to fail the NCLEX-RN® (Scanlan & Care, 2008).

Clinical grading also may be governed by the "rule of C," where the D grade is virtually eliminated as a grading option because of program policies that require a minimum grade of C to pass a clinical course. As previously mentioned, faculty members who are reluctant to assign failing grades to students then may award C grades to students with marginal performance, and the B grade becomes the symbol for average or acceptable performance. This grade compression (only three grade levels instead of five) contributes to grade inflation (Walsh & Seldomridge, 2005).

Another factor contributing to grade inflation is the increasing pressure of accountability for educational outcomes. When the effectiveness of a teacher's instruction is judged on the basis of students' test performance, the teacher may "teach to the test." Teaching to the test may involve using actual test items as practice exercises, distributing copies of a previously used test for review and then using the same test, or focusing exclusively on test content in teaching.

Because regulatory and accreditation standards for nursing education programs commonly include expectations of an acceptable first-time NCLEX pass rate for graduates each year, and the quality of graduate nursing programs is judged by graduates' pass rates on certification exams, these test results have significant implications for the educational institutions as well as the individual test-takers. When faculty members and educational programs are judged by how well their graduates perform on these high-stakes assessments, "direct preparation for the tests and assessments is likely to enter into classroom activities and thereby distort the curriculum" (Miller et al., 2009, p. 14).

It is important, however, to distinguish between teaching to the test and purposeful teaching of content to be sampled by the test and the practice of relevant test-taking skills. However, nursing faculty members who understand the NCLEX test plan and ensure that their nursing curricula include content and learning activities that will enable students to be successful on the NCLEX are not teaching to the test.

Effect of Tests and Grades on Self-Esteem

Some critics of tests claim that testing results in emotional or psychological harm to students. The concern is that tests threaten students and make them anxious, fearful, and discouraged, resulting in harm to their self-esteem. There is no empirical evidence to support these claims. Feelings of anxiety about an upcoming test are both normal and helpful to the extent that they motivate students to prepare thoroughly so as to demonstrate their best performance. Because testing is a common life event, learning how to cope with these challenges is a necessary part of student development. Giving effuse praise for every performance whether or not it is praiseworthy (i.e., "ovation inflation"), while temporarily raising self-esteem, does little to produce students who can realistically assess their own efforts and persist despite challenges.

Nitko and Brookhart (2011) identified three types of test-anxious students: (a) students who have poor study skills and become anxious prior to a test because they do not understand the content that will be tested, (b) students who have good study skills and understand the content but fear they will do poorly no matter how much they prepare for the exam, and (c) students who believe that they have good study skills but in essence do not. If teachers can identify why students are anxious about testing, they can direct them to specific resources such as those on study skills, test-taking strategies, and techniques to reduce their stress.

Most nursing students will benefit from developing good test-taking skills, particularly learners who are anxious. For example, students should be told to follow the directions carefully, read the item stems and questions without rushing to avoid misreading critical information, read each option for multiple-choice items before choosing one, manage time during the test, answer easy items first, and check their answers. Arranging the test with the easy items first often helps relieve anxiety as students begin the test. Because highly anxious students are easily distracted (Nitko & Brookhart, 2011), the teacher should ensure quiet during the testing session.

General guidelines for the teacher to intervene with students who have test anxiety include:

1. Identify the problem to be certain it is test anxiety and not a learning disability or a problem such as depression
2. Give specific detailed feedback about the student's performance on each test
3. Help the student to develop testwiseness skills (e.g., using time well, avoiding technical and clerical errors, how to make informed guesses, using unintended cues in item content or structure)
4. Refer the student to outside resources as needed
5. Advise students to concentrate on the assessment tasks and not allow themselves to be distracted (Nitko & Brookhart, 2011)

Although it is probably true that a certain level of self-esteem is necessary before a student will attempt the challenges associated with nursing education, high self-esteem is not essential to perform well on a test. In fact, if students are able to perform at their best, their self-esteem is enhanced. An important part of a teacher's role is to prepare students to do well on tests by helping them improve their study and test-taking skills and to learn to manage their anxiety.

Testing as a Means of Social Control

All societies sanction some form of social control of behavior; some teachers use the threat of tests and the implied threat of low test grades to control student behavior. In an attempt to motivate students to prepare for and attend class, a teacher may decide to give unannounced tests; the student who is absent that day will earn a score of zero, and the student who does not do the assigned readings will likely earn a low score. This practice is unfair to students because they need sufficient time to prepare for a test to demonstrate their maximum performance, as discussed in Chapter 3. Using tests in a punitive, threatening, or vindictive way is unethical (Nitko & Brookhart, 2011).

ETHICAL ISSUES

Ethical standards make it possible for nurses and patients to achieve understanding of and respect for each other (Husted & Husted, 2007). These standards also should govern the relationships of teachers and students. Contemporary bioethical standards include those of autonomy, freedom, veracity, privacy, beneficence, nonmaleficence, and fidelity. Several of these standards are discussed here as they apply to common issues in testing and evaluation.

The standards of privacy, autonomy, and veracity relate to the ownership and security of tests and test results. Some of the questions that have been raised are: Who owns the test? Who owns the test results? Who has or should have access to the test results? Should test-takers have access to standardized test items and their own responses?

Because educational institutions and employers started using standardized tests to make decisions about admission and employment, the public has been concerned about the potential discriminatory use of test results. The result of this public concern was the passage of federal and state "Truth in Testing" laws, requiring greater access to tests and test results. Some of these laws require publishers of standardized tests to supply copies of the test, the answer key, and the test-taker's own responses on request, allowing the student to verify the accuracy of the test score (Nitko & Brookhart, 2011).

Test-takers have the right to expect that certain information about them will be held in confidence. Teachers, therefore, have an obligation to maintain a privacy standard regarding students' test scores. Such practices as public posting of test scores and grades should be examined in light of this privacy standard. Teachers should not post assessment results if individual students' identities can be linked with their results; for this reason, many educational programs do not allow scores to be posted with student names or identification numbers. During posttest discussions, teachers should not ask students to raise their hands to indicate if they answered an item correctly or incorrectly; this practice can be considered an invasion of students' privacy (Nitko & Brookhart, 2011).

An additional privacy concern relates to the practice of keeping student records that include test scores and other assessment results. Questions often arise about who should have access to these files and the information they contain. Access to a student's test scores and other assessment results is limited by laws such as the Family Educational Rights and Privacy Act of 1974 (FERPA). This federal law gives students certain rights with respect to their education records. For example, they can review their education records maintained by the school and request that the school correct records they believe to be inaccurate or misleading. Schools must have written permission from the student to release information from the student's record except in selected situations such as accreditation or for program assessment purposes (U.S. Department of Education, n.d.). The FERPA limits access to a student's records to those who have legitimate rights to the information to meet the educational needs of the student. This law also specifies that a student's assessment results may not be transferred to another institution without written authorization from the student. In addition to these limits on access to student records, teachers should assure that the information in the records is accurate and should correct errors when they are discovered. Files should be purged of anecdotal material when this information is no longer needed (Nitko & Brookhart, 2011).

Another way to violate students' privacy is to share confidential information about their assessment results with other teachers. To a certain extent, a teacher should communicate information about a student's strengths and weaknesses to other teachers to help them meet that student's learning needs. In most cases, however, this information can be communicated through student records to which other teachers have legitimate access. Informal conversations about students, especially if those conversations center on the teacher's impressions and judgments rather than on verifiable data such as test scores, can be construed as gossip.

Test results sometimes are used for research and program evaluation purposes. As long as students' identities are not revealed, their scores usually can be used for these purposes (Nitko & Brookhart, 2011). One way to assure that this use of test results is ethical is to announce to the students when they enter an educational program that test results occasionally will be used to assess program effectiveness. Students may be asked for their informed consent for their scores to be used, or their consent may be implied by their voluntary participation in optional program evaluation activities. For example, if a questionnaire about student satisfaction with the program is distributed or mailed to students, those who wish to participate simply complete the questionnaire and return it; no written consent form is required. In many institutions of higher education, however, this use of test results may require review by the Institutional Review Board.

The ethical principle of fidelity requires faithfulness in relationships and matters of trust (Bosek & Savage, 2007; Husted & Husted, 2007). In nursing education programs, adherence to this principle requires that faculty members act in the best interest of students. By virtue of their education, experience, and academic position, faculty members hold power over their students. They have the ability to influence students' progress through the nursing education program and their ability to gain employment after graduation. Violations of professional boundaries may occur and affect students' ability to trust faculty members. Teachers who have personal relationships with students may be accused of awarding grades based on favoritism, or conversely, may be accused of using failing grades to retaliate against students who rebuff a sexual or emotional advance (Bosek & Savage, 2007).

Standards for Ethical Testing Practice

Several codes of ethical conduct in using tests and other assessments have been published by professional associations. These include the *Code of Fair Testing Practices in Education* (Joint Committee on Testing Practices, 2004) and the *Code of Professional Responsibilities in Educational Measurement* (NCME, 1995). These are reproduced in Appendices A and C, respectively. The *Standards for Educational and Psychological Testing* (American Educational Research Association et al., 1999) describe standards for test construction, administration, scoring, and reporting; supporting documentation for tests; fairness in testing; and a range of testing applications. The *Standards* also address testing individuals with disabilities and different linguistic backgrounds. Common elements of these codes and standards are:

- Teachers are responsible for the quality of the tests they develop and for selecting tests that are appropriate for the intended use
- Test administration procedures must be fair to all students and protect their safety, health, and welfare
- Teachers are responsible for the accurate scoring of tests and reporting test results to students in a timely manner
- Students should receive prompt and meaningful feedback
- Test results should be interpreted and used in valid ways
- Teachers also must communicate test results accurately and anticipate the consequences of using results to minimize negative results to students (Nitko & Brookhart, 2011)

High-Stakes Assessments

High-stakes assessments are used for decision making that results in serious consequences for the test-takers, teachers, and administrators of educational programs (Nitko & Brookhart, 2011). As mentioned in the introduction to this chapter, public demands for accountability have influenced a growing use of assessments intended to demonstrate that students and graduates meet knowledge and performance standards. In nursing as in many other health professions, an ongoing concern is the need to protect the public through the use of standardized licensure examinations to assure competence to practice. State boards of nursing, which have regulatory authority to license nurses, share accountability with nursing education programs to assure the competence of program graduates. A state board of nursing's oversight of nursing education programs gives it the authority to curtail programs that have low licensure examination first-time pass rates. Therefore, licensure examinations are high-stakes assessments not only for nursing students and new graduates, but also for faculty members and administrators of nursing education programs (National Council of State Boards of Nursing [NCSBN], 2007, 2011; National League for Nursing [NLN], 2010, 2012b).

Adding to the pressure on nursing education programs to meet state board of nursing minimum first-time pass rate requirements is a board of nursing's responsibility and authority also to sanction programs that have high attrition rates (NCSBN, 2007). The need to meet both standards (high NCLEX-RN pass rate and low attrition rate) is a double-edged sword that has motivated increasing numbers of nursing education programs to use standardized end-of-program tests to identify students at risk of NCLEX-RN failure, and to deny program progression or graduation to students who are predicted to fail the licensure examination. According to Giddens and Morton (2010), this type of high-stakes assessment "borders on unethical educational practice" (p. 374) based on the need for multiple approaches to assessment of knowledge and skill when high-stakes decisions are based on the assessment (NLN, 2012b). Additionally, use of a single standardized test as a basis for progression and graduation decisions raises concerns about whether any such test reliably predicts success among various subgroups of an increasingly diverse group of learners (Nitko & Brookhart, 2011).

Requiring students to achieve a predetermined score on a standardized test to graduate from the nursing education program or to be authorized to take the NCLEX-RN so that program's first-time pass rates meet or exceed a state board-mandated level is a complex problem for those who have successfully met all other program requirements. If this "exit exam" is a required component of a nursing course, students who cannot achieve the required score may fail the course, endangering their academic status. Students may need to take the exit examination repeatedly until they meet the standard, delaying graduation or licensure and thus adversely affecting them economically (NLN, 2012b). Additionally, most of the standardized tests being used as exit examinations are intended to predict whether an individual student is likely to *pass* the NCLEX-RN. Such tests are much less accurate in predicting the likelihood of failure (Spurlock, 2006).

Progression or graduation policies requiring high-stakes testing also can distort the intended purpose of NCLEX-RN pass-rate requirements as a measure of program quality. A nursing program that achieves a high first-time pass rate by allowing only the highest performing students to progress in the program, graduate, and take the NCLEX-RN illustrates the effect of selection bias. Thus, the use of high-stakes assessments in progression and graduation policies raises concern about the extent to which the nursing education program provides equal opportunity and access to diverse groups of students. As Giddens (2009) observed, "Is there really anything to celebrate when a nursing program with only a 50% persistence to graduation rate boasts of a 100% first-time NCLEX-RN pass rate?" (p. 124).

The National League for Nursing's concern about the "prevalent use of standardized tests to block graduation or in some other way deny eligibility to take the licensing exam" (NLN, 2012b) prompted creation of fair testing guidelines to assist nursing faculty members and administrators in developing and implementing ethical academic progression and graduation policies. These guidelines, reprinted in Appendix B, emphasize the obligation of faculty members and administrators to:

- Use multiple approaches for assessment of knowledge and clinical abilities when making high-stakes decisions
- Select tests with evidence of measurement validity, and fairness and equity demonstrated by test performance across cultural, racial, or gender subgroups
- Inform students about how the test results will be used
- Undertake a comprehensive review of factors leading to development and implementation of high-stakes testing
- Review other factors that affect NCLEX-RN pass rates and other measures of program quality, such as admissions policies, instructional effectiveness, remediation requirements, and course-level assessments to identify opportunities for improvement (NLN, 2012a)

LEGAL ASPECTS OF ASSESSMENT

It is beyond the scope of this book to interpret laws that affect the use of tests and other assessments, and the authors are not qualified to give legal advice to teachers concerning their assessment practices. However, it is appropriate to discuss a few legal issues to provide guidance to teachers in using tests.

A number of issues have been raised in the courts by students claiming violations of their rights by testing programs. These issues include race or gender discrimination, violation of due process, unfairness of particular tests, various psychometric aspects such as measurement validity and reliability, and accommodations for students with disabilities (Nitko & Brookhart, 2011).

Assessment of Students With Disabilities

The Americans with Disabilities Act (ADA) of 1990 has influenced testing and assessment practices in nursing education and employment settings. This law prohibits discrimination against qualified individuals with disabilities. A qualified individual with a disability is defined as a person with a physical or mental impairment that substantially limits major life activities. Qualified individuals with disabilities meet the requirements for admission to and participation in a nursing program. Nursing education programs have a legal and an ethical obligation to accept and educate qualified individuals with disabilities (Carroll, 2004). It is up to the nursing education program to provide reasonable accommodations, additional services and aids as needed, and removal of barriers. This does not mean that institutions lower their standards to comply with the ADA.

The ADA requires teachers to make reasonable accommodations for disabled students to assess them properly. Such accommodations may include oral testing, computer testing, modified answer format, extended time for exams, test readers or sign language interpreters, a private testing area, or the use of large type for printed tests (Nitko & Brookhart, 2011). However, nursing faculty members should provide accommodations only if a student submits verification of qualification for such accommodations. This verification should be provided by the institutional officer responsible for disability services, after receipt of evidence of the student's disability and individual needs from an appropriate professional. NCLEX policies permit test-takers with documented learning disabilities to have extended testing time as well as other reasonable accommodations, if approved by the board of nursing in the states in which they apply for initial licensure (NCSBN, 2012). This approval usually is granted only when the educational institution has verified the documentation of a disability and students' use of accommodations during the nursing education program. Because English language proficiency is required for competent nursing practice in the United States of America, non-native English speakers or English language learners are not considered to be qualified persons with disabilities.

A number of concerns have been raised regarding the provision of reasonable testing accommodations for students with disabilities. One issue is the validity of the test result interpretations if the test was administered under standard conditions for one group of students and under accommodating conditions for other students. The privacy rights of students with disabilities is another issue: Should the use of accommodating conditions be noted along with the student's test score? Such a notation would identify the student as disabled to anyone who had access to the record. There are no easy answers to such questions. In general, faculty members should be guided by accommodation policies developed by their institution and have any additional policies reviewed by legal counsel to ensure compliance with the ADA.

SUMMARY

Educational testing and assessment are growing in use and importance for society in general and for nursing in particular. Nursing has come under increasing public pressure to be accountable for the quality of educational programs and the competency of its practitioners, and testing and assessment often are used to provide evidence of quality and competence. With the increasing use of assessment and testing come intensified interest in and concern about fairness, appropriateness, and impact.

The social impact of testing can have positive and negative consequences for individuals. Tests can provide information to assist in decision making, such as selecting individuals for admission to education programs or for employment. The way in which selection decisions are made can be a matter of controversy, however, regarding equality of opportunity and access to educational programs and jobs.

The public often expresses concerns about testing. Common criticisms of tests include: tests are biased or unfair to some groups of test-takers; test scores have little meaning because of grade inflation; testing causes emotional or psychological harm to students; and tests are sometimes used in a punitive, threatening, or vindictive way. By understanding and applying codes for the responsible and ethical use of tests, teachers can assure the proper use of assessment procedures and the valid interpretation of test results. Teachers must be responsible for the quality of the tests they develop and for selecting tests that are appropriate for the intended use. The use of high-stakes testing in progression and graduation policies is of particular concern, and guidelines are available to assist faculty members to develop fair testing policies.

The Americans with Disabilities Act of 1990 has implications for the proper assessment of students with physical and mental disabilities. This law requires educational programs to make reasonable testing accommodations for qualified individuals with learning as well as physical disabilities.

REFERENCES

American Educational Research Association, American Psychological Association, & National Council on Measurement in Education. (1999). *Standards for educational and psychological testing.* Washington, DC: American Educational Research Association.

American Nurses Association. (2010). *Nursing's social policy statement: The essence of the profession* (3rd ed.). Washington, DC: Author.

Boscher, S., & Bowles, M. (2008). The effects of linguistic modification on ESL students' comprehension of nursing course test items. *Nursing Education Perspectives, 29,* 165–172.

Boscher, S. D. (2009). Removing language as a barrier to success on multiple-choice nursing exams. In S. D. Bosher & M. D. Pharris (Eds.), *Transforming nursing education: The culturally inclusive environment* (pp. 259–284). New York, NY: Springer Publishing.

Bosek, M. S. D., & Savage, T. A. (2007). *The ethical component of nursing education.* Philadelphia, PA: Lippincott Williams & Wilkins.

Carroll, S. M. (2004). Inclusion of people with physical disabilities in nursing education. *Journal of Nursing Education, 43,* 207–212.

Giddens, J. F. (2009). Changing paradigms and challenging assumptions: Redefining quality and NCLEX-RN pass rates. *Journal of Nursing Education, 48,* 123–124.

Giddens, J. F., & Morton, N. (2010). Report card: An evaluation of a concept-based curriculum. *Nursing Education Perspectives, 31,* 372–377.

Husted, J. H., & Husted, G. L. (2007). *Ethical decision making in nursing and health care: The symphonological approach* (4th ed.). New York, NY: Springer Publishing.

Joint Committee on Testing Practices. (2004). *Code of fair testing practices in education.* Washington, DC: American Psychological Association.

Miller, M. D., Linn, R. L., & Gronlund, N. E. (2009). *Measurement and assessment in teaching* (10th ed.). Upper Saddle River, NJ: Prentice Hall.

National Council of State Boards of Nursing. (2007). *Guiding principles of nursing regulation.* Retrieved from https://www.ncsbn.org/Guiding_Principles.pdf

National Council of State Boards of Nursing. (2011). *A preferred future for prelicensure nursing program approval.* Retrieved from https://www.ncsbn.org/Report_on_Future_of_Approval.pdf

National Council of State Boards of Nursing. (2012). *2012 NCLEX® Examination candidate bulletin.* Retrieved from https://www.ncsbn.org/2012_NCLEX_Candidate_Bulletin.pdf

National Council on Measurement in Education. (1995). *Code of professional responsibilities in educational measurement.* Washington, DC: Author.

National League for Nursing. (2010). *High-stakes testing.* Retrieved from http://www.nln.org/aboutnln/reflection_dialogue/refl_dial_7.htm

National League for Nursing. (2012a). *NLN Fair testing guidelines for nursing education.* Retrieved from http://www.nln.org/facultyprograms/facultyresources/fairtestingguidelines.PDF

National League for Nursing. (2012b). *The fair testing imperative in nursing education.* Retrieved from http://www.nln.org/aboutnln/livingdocuments/pdf/nlnvision_4.pdf

Nitko, A. J., & Brookhart, S. M. (2011). *Educational assessment of students* (6th ed.). Upper Saddle River, NJ: Pearson Education.

Scanlan, J. M., & Care, W. D. (2008). Issues with grading and grade inflation in nursing education. In M. H. Oermann (Ed.), *Annual review of nursing education* (Vol. 6, pp. 173–188). New York, NY: Springer Publishing.

Spurlock, D. R. (2006). Do no harm: Progression policies and high-stakes testing in nursing education. *Journal of Nursing Education, 45,* 297–302.

U.S. Department of Education. (n.d.). *Family Educational Rights and Privacy Act (FERPA)*. Washington, DC: Family Policy Compliance Office, U.S. Department of Education. Retrieved from http://www2.ed.gov/policy/gen/guid/fpco/ferpa/index.html

Walsh, C. M., & Seldomridge, L. A. (2005). Clinical grades: Upward bound. *Journal of Nursing Education, 44*, 162–168.

SIXTEEN

Interpreting Test Scores

As a measurement tool, a test results in a score—a number. A number, however, has no intrinsic meaning and must be compared with something that has meaning to interpret its significance. For a test score to be useful for making decisions about the test, the teacher must interpret the score. Whether the interpretations are norm-referenced or criterion-referenced, a basic knowledge of statistical concepts is necessary to assess the quality of tests (whether teacher-made or published), understand standardized test scores, summarize assessment results, and explain test scores to others.

TEST SCORE DISTRIBUTIONS

Some information about how a test performed as a measurement instrument can be obtained from computer-generated test- and item-analysis reports. In addition to providing item-analysis data such as difficulty and discrimination indexes, such reports often summarize the characteristics of the score distribution. If the teacher does not have access to electronic scoring and computer software for test and item analysis, many of these analyses can be done by hand, albeit more slowly.

When a test is scored, the teacher is left with a collection of raw scores. Often these scores are recorded according to the names of the students, in alphabetical order, or by student numbers. As an example, suppose that the scores displayed in Table 16.1 resulted from the administration of a 65-point test to 16 nursing students.

Glancing at this collection of numbers, the teacher would find it difficult to answer such questions as:

1. Did a majority of students obtain high or low scores on the test?
2. Did any individuals score much higher or much lower than the majority of the students?
3. Are the scores widely scattered or grouped together?
4. What was the range of scores obtained by the majority of the students? (Nitko & Brookhart, 2011)

To make it easier to see similar characteristics of scores, the teacher should arrange them in rank order, from highest to lowest (Miller, Linn, & Gronlund, 2009), as in Table 16.2. Ordering the scores in this way makes

❑Table 16.1

LIST OF STUDENTS IN A CLASS AND THEIR RAW SCORES ON A 65-POINT TEST

STUDENT	SCORE	STUDENT	SCORE
A. Allen	53	I. Ignatius	48
B. Brown	54	J. Jimanez	55
C. Chen	52	K. Kelly	52
D. Dunlap	52	L. Lynch	42
E. Edwards	54	M. Meyer	47
F. Finley	57	N. Nardozzi	60
G. Gunther	54	O. O'Malley	55
H. Hernandez	56	P. Purdy	53

❑Table 16.2

RANK ORDER OF STUDENTS FROM TABLE 16.1 WITH RAW SCORES ORDERED FROM HIGHEST TO LOWEST

STUDENT	SCORE	STUDENT	SCORE
N. Nardozzi	60	A. Allen	53
F. Finley	57	P. Purdy	53
H. Hernandez	56	C. Chen	52
J. Jimanez	55	K. Kelly	52
O. O'Malley	55	D. Dunlap	52
B. Brown	54	I. Ignatius	48
E. Edwards	54	M. Meyer	47
G. Gunther	54	L. Lynch	42

❑Table 16.3

| FREQUENCY DISTRIBUTION OF RAW SCORES FROM TABLE 16.1 ||
RAW SCORE	FREQUENCY
61	0
60	1
59	0
58	0
57	1
56	1
55	2
54	3
53	2
52	3
51	0
50	0
49	0
48	1
47	1
46	0
45	0
44	0
43	0
42	1
41	0

it obvious that they ranged from 42 to 60, and that one student's score was much lower than those of the other students. But the teacher still cannot visualize easily how a typical student performed on the test or the general characteristics of the obtained scores. Removing student names, listing each score once, and tallying how many times each score occurs results in a frequency distribution, as in Table 16.3. By displaying scores in this way, it is easier for the teacher to identify how well the group of students performed on the exam.

The frequency distribution also can be represented graphically as a histogram. In Figure 16.1, the scores are ordered from lowest to highest along a horizontal line, left to right, and the number of asterisks above each score indicates the frequency of that score. Frequencies also can be indicated on a histogram by bars, with the height of each bar representing the frequency of the corresponding score, as in Figure 16.2.

A frequency polygon is another way to display a score distribution graphically. A dot is made above each score value to indicate the frequency with which that score occurred; if no one obtained a particular score, the dot is made on the baseline, at 0. The dots then are connected with straight

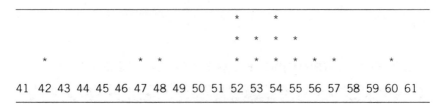

Figure 16.1   Histogram depicting frequency distribution of raw scores from Table 16.1.

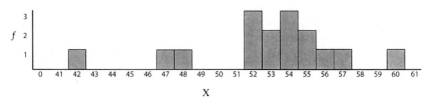

Figure 16.2   Bar graph depicting frequency distribution of raw scores from Table 16.1.
Note: X = scores; *f* = frequency.

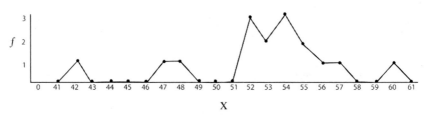

Figure 16.3   Frequency polygon depicting frequency distribution of raw scores from Table 16.1.
Note: X = scores; *f* = frequency.

lines to form a polygon or curve. Figure 16.3 shows a frequency polygon based on the histogram in Figure 16.1. Histograms and frequency polygons thus show general characteristics such as the scores that occurred most frequently, the score distribution shape, and the range of the scores.

The characteristics of a score distribution can be described on the basis of its symmetry, skewness, modality, and kurtosis. These characteristics are illustrated in Figure 16.4. A symmetric distribution or curve is one in which there are two equal halves, mirror images of each other. Nonsymmetric or asymmetric curves have a cluster of scores or a peak at one end and a tail extending toward the other end. This type of curve is said to be skewed; the direction in which the tail extends indicates whether the distribution is positively or negatively skewed. The tail of a positively skewed curve extends toward the right, in the direction of positive numbers on a

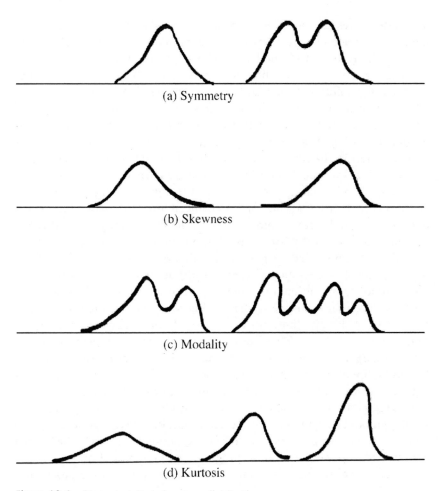

Figure 16.4   Characteristics of a score distribution.

scale, and the tail of a negatively skewed curve extends toward the left, in the direction of negative numbers. A positively skewed distribution thus has the largest cluster of scores at the low end of the distribution, which seems counterintuitive. The distribution of test scores from Table 16.1 is nonsymmetric and negatively skewed. Remember that the lowest possible score on this test was 0 and the highest possible score was 65; the scores were clustered between 43 and 60.

Frequency polygons and histograms can differ in the number of peaks they contain; this characteristic is called modality, referring to the mode or the most frequently occurring score in the distribution. If a curve has one peak, it is unimodal; if it contains two peaks, it is bimodal. A curve with many peaks is multimodal. The relative flatness or peakedness of the curve is referred to as kurtosis. Flat curves are described as platykurtic, moderate curves are said to be mesokurtic, and sharply peaked curves are referred to as leptokurtic (Waltz, Strickland, & Lenz, 2005). The histogram in Figure 16.1 is a bimodal, platykurtic distribution.

The shape of a score distribution depends on the characteristics of the test as well as the abilities of the students who were tested (Nitko & Brookhart, 2011). Some teachers make grading decisions as if all test score distributions resemble a normal curve, that is, they attempt to "curve" the grades. An understanding of the characteristics of a normal curve would dispel this notion. A normal distribution is a bell-shaped curve that is symmetric, unimodal, and mesokurtic. Figure 16.5 illustrates a normal distribution.

Many human characteristics such as intelligence, weight, and height are normally distributed; the measurement of any of these attributes in a population would result in more scores in the middle range than at either extreme. However, most score distributions obtained from teacher-made tests do not approximate a normal distribution. This is true for several reasons. The characteristics of a test greatly influence the resulting score distribution; a very difficult test tends to yield a positively skewed curve. Likewise, the abilities of the students influence the test score distribution. Regardless of the distribution of the attribute of intelligence among the human population, this characteristic is not likely to be distributed normally among a class of nursing students or a group of newly hired RNs. Because admission and hiring decisions tend to select those individuals who are most likely to succeed in the nursing program or job, a distribution of IQ scores from a class of 16 nursing students or 16 newly hired RNs would tend to be negatively skewed. Likewise, knowledge of nursing content is not likely to be normally distributed because those who have been admitted to a nursing education program or hired as staff nurses are not representative of the population in general. Therefore, grading procedures

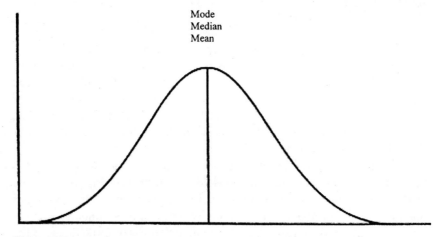

Mode
Median
Mean

Figure 16.5 The normal distribution.

that attempt to apply the characteristics of the normal curve to a test score distribution are likely to result in unwise and unfair decisions.

Measures of Central Tendency

One of the questions to be answered when interpreting test scores is, "What score is most characteristic or typical of this distribution?" A typical score is likely to be in the middle of a distribution with the other scores clustered around it; measures of central tendency provide a value around which the test scores cluster. Three measures of central tendency commonly used to interpret test scores are the mode, median, and mean.

The mode, sometimes abbreviated Mo, is the most frequently occurring score in the distribution; it must be a score actually obtained by a student. It can be identified easily from a frequency distribution or graphic display without mathematical calculation. As such, it provides a rough indication of central tendency. The mode, however, is the least stable measure of central tendency because it tends to fluctuate considerably from one sample to another drawn from the same population (Miller et al., 2009). That is, if the same 65-item test that yielded the scores in Table 16.1 were administered to a different group of 16 nursing students in the same program who had taken the same course, the mode might differ considerably. In addition, as in the distribution depicted in Figure 16.1, the mode has two or more values in some distributions, making it difficult to specify one typical score. A uniform distribution of scores has no mode; such distributions are likely to be obtained when the number of students is small, the range of scores is large, and each score is obtained by only one student.

The median (abbreviated Mdn or P_{50}) is the point that divides the distribution of scores into equal halves (Miller et al., 2009). It is a value above which fall 50% of the scores and below which fall 50% of the scores; thus it represents the 50th percentile. The median does not have to be an actual obtained score. In an even number of scores, the median is located halfway between the two middle scores; in an odd number of scores, the median is the middle score. Because the median is an index of location, it is not influenced by the value of each score in the distribution. Thus, it is usually a good indication of a typical score in a skewed distribution containing extremely high or low scores (Miller et al., 2009).

The mean often is referred to as the "average" score in a distribution, reflecting the mathematical calculation that determines this measure of central tendency. It is usually abbreviated as M or $\overline{X}$. The mean is computed by summing each individual score and dividing by the total number of scores, as in the following formula:

$$M = \frac{\Sigma X}{N} \quad \text{[Equation 16.1]}$$

where M is the mean, ΣX is the sum of the individual scores, and N is the total number of scores. Thus, the value of the mean is affected by every score in the distribution (Miller et al., 2009). This property makes it the preferred index of central tendency when a measure of the total distribution is desired. However, the mean is sensitive to the influence of extremely high or low scores in the distribution, and as such, it may not reflect the typical performance of a group of students.

There is a relationship between the shape of a score distribution and the relative locations of these measures of central tendency. In a normal distribution, the mean, median, and mode have the same value, as shown in Figure 16.5. In a positively skewed distribution, the mean will yield the highest measure of central tendency and the mode will give the lowest; in a negatively skewed distribution, the mode will be the highest value and the mean the lowest. Figure 16.6 depicts the relative positions of the three measures of central tendency in skewed distributions.

The mean of the distribution of scores from Table 16.1 is 52.75; the median is 53.5. The fact that the median is slightly higher than the mean confirms that the median is an index of location or position and is insensitive to the actual score values in the distribution. The mean, because it is affected by every score in the distribution, was influenced by the one extreme low score. Because the shape of this score distribution was negatively skewed, it is expected that the median would be higher than the mean because the mean is always pulled in the direction of the tail.

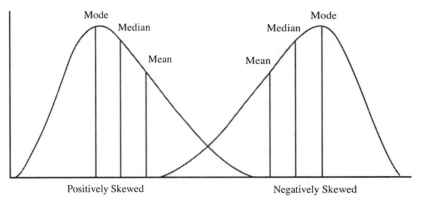

Figure 16.6 Measures of central tendency in positively and negatively skewed distributions.

Measures of Variability

It is possible for two score distributions to have similar measures of central tendency and yet be very different. The scores in one distribution may be tightly clustered around the mean, and in the other distribution, the scores may be widely dispersed over a range of values. Measures of variability are used to determine how similar or different the students are with respect to their scores on a test.

The simplest measure of variability is the range, the difference between the highest and lowest scores in the distribution. For the test score distribution in Table 16.3, the range is 18 (60 − 42 = 18). The range is sometimes expressed as the highest and lowest scores, rather than a difference score. Because the range is based on only two values, it can be highly unstable. The range also tends to increase with sample size; that is, test scores from a large group of students are likely to be scattered over a wide range because of the likelihood that an extreme score will be obtained (Miller et al., 2009).

The standard deviation (abbreviated as *SD*, *s*, or ó) is the most common and useful measure of variability. Like the mean, it takes into consideration every score in the distribution. The standard deviation is based on differences between each score and the mean. Thus, it characterizes the average amount by which the scores differ from the mean. The standard deviation is calculated in four steps:

1. Subtract the mean from each score (X − M) to compute a deviation score (*x*), which can be positive or negative.
2. Square each deviation score (x^2), which eliminates any negative values. Sum all of the squared deviation scores (Σx^2).
3. Divide this sum by the number of test scores to yield the variance.
4. Calculate the square root of the variance.

Although other formulas can be used to calculate the standard deviation, the following definitional formula represents these four steps:

$$SD = \sqrt{\frac{\Sigma x^2}{N}} \quad \text{[Equation 16.2]}$$

where *SD* is the standard deviation, Σx^2 is the sum of the squared deviation scores, and *N* is the number of scores (Miller et al., 2009).

The standard deviation of the distribution of scores from Table 16.1 is 4.1. What does this value mean? A standard deviation of 4.1 represents the average deviation of scores from the mean. On a 65-point test, 4 points is not a large average difference in scores. If the scores cluster tightly around the mean, the standard deviation will be a relatively small number; if they are widely scattered over a large range of scores, the standard deviation will be a larger number.

INTERPRETING AN INDIVIDUAL SCORE

Interpreting the Results of Teacher-Made Tests

The ability to interpret the characteristics of a distribution of scores will assist the teacher to make norm-referenced interpretations of the meaning of any individual score in that distribution. For example, how should the teacher interpret P. Purdy's score of 53 on the test whose results were summarized in Table 16.1? With a median of 53.5, a mean of 52.75, and a standard deviation of 4.1, a score of 53 is about "average." All scores between 49 and 57 fall within one standard deviation of the mean, and thus are not significantly different from one another. On the other hand, N. Nardozzi can rejoice because a score of 60 is almost two standard deviations higher than the mean; thus, this score represents achievement that is much better than that of others in the group. The teacher should probably plan to counsel L. Lynch, because a score of 42 is more than two standard deviations below the mean, much lower than others in the group.

However, most nurse educators need to make criterion-referenced interpretations of individual test scores. A student's score on the test is compared to a preset standard or criterion, and the scores of the other students are not considered. The percentage-correct score is a derived score that is often used to report the results of tests that are intended for criterion-referenced interpretation. The percentage correct is a comparison of a student's score with the maximum possible score; it is calculated by dividing the raw score by the total number of items on the test (Miller et al., 2009). Although many teachers believe that percentage-correct scores are an objective indication of how much students really know about a subject, in fact they can change significantly with the difficulty of the test items. Because percentage-correct scores are often used as a basis for assigning letter grades according to a predetermined grading system, it is important to recognize that they are determined more by test difficulty than by true quality of performance. For tests that are more difficult than they were expected to be, the teacher may want to adjust the raw scores before calculating the percentage correct on that test.

The percentage-correct score should not be confused with percentile rank, often used to report the results of standardized tests. The percentile rank describes the student's relative standing within a group and therefore is a norm-referenced interpretation. The percentile rank of a given raw score is the percentage of scores in the distribution that occur at or below that score. A percentile rank of 83, therefore, means that the student's score is equal to or higher than the scores made by 83% of the students in that group; one cannot assume, however, that the student answered 83% of the test items correctly. Because there are 99 points that divide a distribution into 100 groups of equal size, the highest percentile rank that can be obtained is the 99th. The median is at the 50th percentile. Differences between percentile ranks mean more at the highest and lowest extremes than they do near the median.

Interpreting the Results of Standardized Tests

The results of standardized tests usually are intended to be used to make norm-referenced interpretations. Before making such interpretations, the teacher should keep in mind that standardized tests are more relevant to general rather than specific instructional goals. Additionally, the results of standardized tests are more appropriate for evaluations of groups rather than individuals. Consequently, standardized test scores should not be used to determine grades for a specific course or to make a decision to hire, promote, or terminate an employee. Like most educational measures, standardized tests provide gross, not precise, data about achievement. Actual differences in performance and achievement are reflected in large score differences.

Standardized test results usually are reported in derived scores such as percentile ranks, standard scores, and norm group scores. Because all of these derived scores should be interpreted in a norm-referenced way, it is important to specify an appropriate norm group for comparison. The user's manual for any standardized test typically presents norm tables in which each raw score is matched with an equivalent derived score. Standardized test manuals may contain a number of norm tables; the norm group on which each table is based should be fully described. The teacher should take care to select the norm group that most closely matches the group whose scores will be compared to it (Miller et al., 2009). For example, when interpreting the results of standardized tests in nursing, the performance of a group of baccalaureate nursing students should be compared with a norm group of baccalaureate nursing students. Norm tables sometimes permit finer distinctions such as size of program, geographical region, and public versus private affiliation.

SUMMARY

To be meaningful and useful for decision making, test scores must be interpreted in either norm-referenced or criterion-referenced ways. Knowledge of basic statistical concepts is necessary to make valid interpretations and to explain test scores to others.

Scoring a test results in a collection of numbers known as raw scores. To make raw scores understandable, they can be arranged in frequency distributions or displayed graphically as histograms or frequency polygons. Score distribution characteristics such as symmetry, skewness, modality, and kurtosis can assist the teacher in understanding how the test performed as a measurement tool as well as to interpret any one score in the distribution.

Measures of central tendency and variability also aid in interpreting individual scores. Measures of central tendency include the mode, median, and mean; each measure has advantages and disadvantages for use. In a normal distribution, these three measures will coincide. Most score distributions from teacher-made tests do not meet the assumptions of a normal curve. The shape of the distribution can determine the most appropriate index of central tendency to use. Variability in a distribution can be described roughly as the range of scores or more precisely as the standard deviation.

Teachers can make criterion-referenced or norm-reference interpretations of individual student scores. Norm-referenced interpretations of any individual score should take into account the characteristics of the score distribution, some index of central tendency, and some index of variability. The teacher thus can use the mean and standard deviation to make judgments about how an individual student's score compares with those of others.

A percentage-correct score is calculated by dividing the raw score by the total possible score; thus it compares the student's score to a preset standard or criterion and does not take the scores of other students into consideration. A percentage-correct score is not an objective indication of how much a student really knows about a subject because it is affected by the difficulty of the test items. The percentage-correct score should not be confused with percentile rank, which describes the student's relative standing within a group and therefore is a norm-referenced interpretation. The percentile rank of a given raw score is the percentage of scores in the distribution that occurs at or below that score.

The results of standardized tests usually are reported as percentile ranks or other norm-referenced scores. Teachers should be cautious when interpreting standardized test results so that comparisons with the appropriate norm group are made. Standardized test scores should not be used to determine grades or to make personnel decisions, and results should be interpreted with the understanding that only large differences in scores indicate real differences in achievement levels.

REFERENCES

Miller, M. D., Linn, R. L., & Gronlund, N. E. (2009). *Measurement and assessment in teaching* (10th ed.). Upper Saddle River, NJ: Prentice Hall.

Nitko, A. J., & Brookhart, S. M. (2011). *Educational assessment of students* (6th ed.). Upper Saddle River, NJ: Pearson Education.

Waltz, C. F., Strickland, O. L., & Lenz, E. R. (2005). *Measurement in nursing and health research* (3rd ed.). New York, NY: Springer Publishing.

SEVENTEEN

Grading

The teacher's assessment of students provides the basis for assigning a grade for the course. The grade is a symbol reflecting the achievement of students in that course. In addition to grading the course as a whole, grades are given for individual assignments, quizzes, tests, and other learning activities completed by students throughout the course. This chapter examines the uses of grades in nursing programs, problems with grading, grading frameworks, and how to compute grades for nursing courses.

PURPOSES OF GRADES

In earlier chapters there was extensive discussion about formative and summative evaluation. Through formative evaluation the teacher provides feedback to the learner on a continuous basis. In contrast, summative evaluation is conducted periodically to indicate the student's achievement at the end of the course or at a point within the course. Summative evaluation provides the basis for arriving at grades in the course. *Grading*, or marking, is defined as the use of symbols, for instance, the letters A through F, for reporting student achievement. Grading is for summative purposes, indicating through the use of symbols how well the student performed in individual assignments, clinical practice, laboratories, and the course as a whole.

To reflect valid judgments about student achievement, grades need to be based on careful evaluation practices, reliable test results, and multiple assessment methods. No grade should be determined by one method or one assignment completed by the students; grades reflect instead a combination of various tests and other assessment methods. Along similar lines, students may complete assignments that are not included in their grade, particularly if the emphasis is on formative evaluation. Not all of the students' activities in a course, however, need to be graded. Grades serve three broad purposes: (a) instructional, (b) administrative, and (c) guidance and counseling.

Instructional Purposes

Grades for instructional purposes indicate the achievement of students in the course. They provide a measure of *what* students have learned and their competencies at the end of the course or at a certain point within it. A "pass" grade in the clinical practicum and a grade of "B" in the nursing course are examples of using grades for instructional purposes.

Administrative Purposes

The second purpose that grades serve is administrative. Grades are used for:

- admission of students to entry-level and higher degree nursing programs
- progression of students in a nursing program
- decisions about probation and whether students can continue in the program
- decisions about re-entry into a nursing program
- determining students' eligibility for graduation
- awarding scholarships and fellowships
- awarding honors and determining acceptance into honor societies such as Sigma Theta Tau International
- program evaluation studies
- reporting competency to employers

Guidance and Counseling

The third use of grades is for guidance and counseling. Grades can be used to make decisions about courses to select, including more advanced courses to take or remedial courses that might be helpful. Grades also suggest academic resources that students might benefit from such as reading, study, and test-taking workshops and support. In some situations grades assist students in making career choices, including a change in the direction of their careers.

CRITICISMS OF GRADES

Although grades serve varied purposes, there are many criticisms of them. Nitko and Brookhart (2011) identified and responded to a number of these criticisms, which are applicable to grading in nursing programs:

1. Grades are meaningless because of the diversity across nursing education programs, course faculty, clinical teachers, and preceptors.
   - Response: A consistent grading system is needed across sections of nursing courses and for grading clinical practice. It is important that full- and part-time faculty members, preceptors, and others involved in the course be oriented as to how to assess and grade each of the assignments. Clinical teachers and preceptors should discuss the clinical evaluation process and methods, how to use the clinical evaluation instrument and determine a clinical grade, and grading practices in the course.
2. A single symbol, such as an A or a pass, does not adequately represent the complex details associated with achievement in nursing courses.
   - Response: Grades are not intended to fulfill this need. They do not reflect every detail of the student's learning in a course or every accomplishment. Instead, grades are a summarization of achievements over a period of time.
3. Grades are not important.
   - Response: Although a grade is only a symbol of achievement, Nitko and Brookhart (2011) emphasized that grades are important. The many ways that grades are used to arrive at educational decisions demonstrate how important they are to students, nursing education programs, and others. In addition, grades and overall grade point average (GPA) may predict later achievement such as performance on licensure and certification examinations. Although some may argue that the most valuable outcomes of learning are intangible, grades, nevertheless, are important.
4. Self-evaluations are more important than grades.
   - Response: Developing the ability to evaluate one's own learning outcomes and competencies is essential for continued professional development. Both grades and self-evaluations are needed, not one or the other (Nitko & Brookhart, 2011).
5. Grades are unnecessary.
   - Response: In most educational settings, grades cannot be eliminated because they serve the purposes identified earlier in the chapter. A certain level of performance is essential for progression in a nursing program and for later educational decisions; grades

provide a way of determining whether students are achieving sufficiently to progress through the program.

6. Grades are ineffective motivators.
    ■ Response: For some students grades are effective motivators although for others this may not be true.
7. Low grades discourage students.
    ■ Response: Although low grades may be discouraging and stressful for students, they are essential for determining progression in a nursing program. Nursing education programs are accountable to the profession and the public for preparing graduates with knowledge and competencies for safe practice. Not all entering students have the ability to acquire this knowledge and these skills. Low grades are important for counseling students and suggesting remedial instruction; failing grades indicate that students have not met the criteria for continuing in the nursing program.
8. Grades are inflated and thus do not reflect true achievement.
    ■ Response: Both public and private colleges and universities have undergone considerable grade inflation over the last few decades, as discussed in Chapter 15. Grade inflation has become a national problem (Rojstaczer & Healy, 2012). Students are paying more for their education, and they want a reward of high grades for their "purchase." In developing a grading system, it is important for nursing faculties to be clear about the standards for each grade level in that system and to communicate these to students. Faculty also should periodically review the grades in nursing courses to assess if they are inflated, keeping in mind that nursing students are carefully selected for admission into the program and need to achieve certain grades in courses to progress. For this reason, grades in nursing courses tend to be higher than general education courses in which students are more heterogeneous.

TYPES OF GRADING SYSTEMS

There are different types of grading systems or methods of reporting grades. Most nursing education programs use a letter system for grading (A, B, C, D, E or A, B, C, D, F), which may be combined with "+" and "−". The integers 5, 4, 3, 2, and 1 (or 9 through 1) also may be used. These two systems of grading are convenient to use, yield grades that are able to be averaged within a course and across courses, and present the grade concisely.

Grades also may be indicated by percentages (100, 99, 98,...). Most programs use percentages as a basis for assigning letter grades—90 to 100%

represents an A, 80 to 89% a B, and so forth. In some nursing programs, the percentages for each letter grade are higher, for example, 92 to 100% for an A, 83 to 91% a B, 75 to 82% a C, 66 to 74% a D, and 65% and below an E or F. It is not uncommon in nursing education programs to specify that students need to achieve at least a C in each nursing course at the undergraduate level and a B or better at the graduate level. Requirements such as these are indicated in the school policies and course syllabi.

Another type of grading system is two-dimensional: pass–fail, satisfactory–unsatisfactory, or credit–no credit. For determining clinical grades, some programs add a third honors category, creating three levels: honors–pass–fail. One advantage of a two-dimensional grading system is that the grade is not calculated in the GPA. This allows students to take new courses and explore different areas of learning without concern about the grades in these courses affecting their overall GPA. This also may be viewed as a disadvantage, however, in that clinical performance in a nursing course graded on a pass–fail basis is not calculated as part of the overall course grade. A pass indicates that students met the clinical objectives or demonstrated satisfactory performance of the clinical competencies. Different systems for grading clinical practice are discussed later in the chapter.

Grade Point Average

One other dimension of a grading system involves converting the letter grade to a grade point system for calculating the grade point average or quality point average (QPA). Grades in a 4-point system are typically:

A = 4 points per credit (or unit)

B = 3 points per credit

C = 2 points per credit

D = 1 point per credit

F = 0 points per credit

If a student took two 3-credit courses and one 6-credit nursing course and received an A in one of the 3-credit courses, a C in the other, and a B in the 6-credit course, the grade point average would be:

A = 4 points/credit = 4 points × 3 credits = 12 points

C = 2 points/credit = 2 points × 3 credits = 6 points

B = 3 points/credit = 3 points × 6 credits = 18 points

$$36 \div 12 \text{ (credits)} = 3.0$$

☐Table 17.1

PLUS AND MINUS SYSTEM

LETTER GRADE	GRADE POINTS
A	4.00
A–	3.67
B+	3.33
B	3.00
B–	2.67
C+	2.33
C	2.00
C–	1.67
D+	1.33
D	1.00
D–	0.67
F	0.00

The letter system for grading also may include plus and minus grades. This is shown in Table 17.1. Although grade inflation may not decrease when plus and minus are used, these added categories allow for more differentiation for grading. The transition from whole-letter grading to adding plus and minus to grades in courses in a school of pharmacy reflected faculty members' perceptions that the plus and minus allowed for better differentiation between students' performances (Barnes & Buring, 2012).

ASSIGNING LETTER GRADES

Because most nursing education programs use the letter system for grading nursing courses, this framework will be used for discussing how to assign grades. These principles, however, are applicable to the other grading systems as well. There are two major considerations in assigning letter grades: deciding what to include in the grade and selecting a grading framework.

Deciding What to Include in the Grade

Grades in nursing courses should reflect the student's achievement and not be biased by the teacher's own values, beliefs, and attitudes. If the student did not attend class or appeared to be inattentive during lectures, this behavior should not be incorporated into the course grade unless criteria were established at the outset for class attendance and participation.

The student's grade is based on the tests and assessment methods developed for the course. Brookhart (2011) emphasized that multiple assessment methods should be used to determine the grade. The weight given to each of these in the overall grade should reflect the emphasis of the objectives and the content measured by them. Tests and other assessment methods associated with important content, for which more time was probably spent in the instruction, should receive greater weight in the course grade. For example, a midterm examination in a community health nursing course should be given more weight in the course grade than a paper that students completed about community resources for a family under their care.

How much weight should be given in the course grade to each test and other type of assessment method used in the course? The teacher begins by listing the tests, quizzes, papers, presentations, and other assessment methods in the course that should be included in the course grade. Then the teacher decides on the importance of each of these components in the overall grade for the course. Factors to consider when weighting the components of the course grade are as follows:

1. Components that assess more of the important learning outcomes and competencies should carry more weight in the course grade than those that measure only a few of the outcomes (Nitko & Brookhart, 2011).
2. Components that assess content that was emphasized in the course and for which more time was spent in the instruction should receive the most weight in the course grade (Nitko & Brookhart, 2011).
3. Components that measure the application of concepts and theories to practice and development of higher level skills should be weighted more heavily than those that focus on recall of content.
4. Components that are more difficult and time-consuming for students should receive more weight than those that are easy and require less time to complete.

Selecting a Grading Framework

To give meaning to the grades assigned, the teacher needs a grading framework or frame of reference. There are three grading frameworks used to assign meaning to grades:

1. Criterion-referenced, also referred to as grading with an absolute scale

    2. Norm-referenced or grading with a relative scale

    3. Self-referenced or grading based on the growth of the student
       (Nitko & Brookhart, 2011)

Table 17.2 illustrates these grading frameworks. Criterion- and norm-referenced evaluation methods were described in earlier chapters; these same concepts apply to grading frameworks.

CRITERION-REFERENCED GRADING

In criterion-referenced grading, grades are based on students' achievement of the outcomes of the course, the extent of content learned in the course, or how well they performed in clinical practice. Students who achieve more of the objectives, acquire more knowledge, and can perform more competencies or with greater proficiency receive higher grades. The meaning assigned to grades, then, is based on these absolute standards without regard to the achievement of other students. Using this frame of reference for grading means that it is possible for all students to achieve an A or a B in a course, if they meet the standards, or a D or F if they do not.

    This framework is appropriate for most nursing courses because they focus on outcomes and competencies to be achieved in the course. Criterion-referenced grading indicates how students are progressing toward meeting those outcomes (formative evaluation) and whether they have achieved them at the end of the course (summative evaluation). Norm-referenced grading, in contrast, is not appropriate for use in nursing courses that are based on standards or learning outcomes because it focuses on comparing students with one another, not on how they are progressing or on their achievement. For example, formative evaluation in a norm-referenced framework would indicate how each student ranks among the group rather than provide feedback on student progress in meeting the outcomes of the course and strategies for further learning.

Fixed-Percentage Method

There are several ways of assigning grades using a criterion-referenced system. One is called the fixed-percentage method. This method uses fixed ranges of percent-correct scores as the basis for assigning grades (Miller, Linn, & Gronlund, 2009). A common grading scale is 92 to 100% for an A, 83% to 91% a B, 75% to 82% a C, 66% to 74% a D, and below 65% an E or F. Each component of the course grade—written tests, quizzes, papers,

❑Table 17.2

GRADING FRAMEWORKS

GRADE	CRITERION-REFERENCED	NORM-REFERENCED	SELF-REFERENCED
A	All outcomes met Significant knowledge and cognitive skills gained Able to perform all clinical competencies at high level	Achievement/performance far exceeds average of group (e.g., other students in course, in clinical group)	Made significant progress Performed significantly better than expected
B	Met all essential outcomes and at least half of the others Important content areas learned and able to be applied to new situations Able to perform most clinical competencies at high level	Above the average of the group	Made progress and gained knowledge and skills Performed better than expected
C	All essential outcomes met; learned essential content Able to perform most clinical competencies	Average in comparison with the group	Made progress in most areas Met performance level expected by teacher
D	Only some essential outcomes met; limited understanding of content Unable to perform some essential clinical competencies	Below the average of the group	Made some gains Did not meet level of performance for which capable
F	Most outcomes not achieved; limited content learned Most clinical competencies not able to be performed	Failing achievement/performance in comparison with the group	Made no gains Performance significantly below capability

Note: Content of this table based on ideas in A. J. Nitko, & S. M. Brookhart (2011). *Educational assessment of students* (6th ed.). Upper Saddle River, NJ: Pearson Education.

case presentations, and other assignments—is given a percentage-correct score or percentage of the total points possible. For example, the student might have a score of 21 out of 25 on a quiz, or 84%. The component grades are then weighted, and the percentages are averaged to get the final grade, which is converted to a letter grade at the end of the course. With all grading systems, the students need to be informed as to how the grade will be assigned. If the fixed-percentage method is used, the students should know the scale for converting percentages to letter grades; this should be in the course syllabus with a clear explanation of how the course grade will be determined.

Computing a Composite (Single) Score for a Course

In using the fixed-percentage method, the first step, which is an important one, is to assign weights to each of the components of the grade. For example:

Paper on nursing interventions	10%
Papers critiquing issues in clinical practice	20%
Quizzes	10%
Midterm examination	20%
Portfolio	20%
Final examination	20%
	100%

In determining the composite score for the course, the student's percentage for each of the components of the grade is multiplied by the weight and summed; the sum is then divided by the sum of the weights. This procedure is shown in Table 17.3.

Generally, test scores should not be converted to grades for the purpose of later computing a final average grade. Instead, the teacher should record actual test scores and then combine them into a composite score that can be converted to a final grade.

Total-Points Method

The second method of assigning grades in a criterion-referenced system is the total-points method. In this method, each component of the grade is assigned a specific number of points, for example, a paper may be worth 100 points and midterm examination 200 points. The number of points

❏Table 17.3

FIXED-PERCENTAGE METHOD FOR GRADING NURSING COURSES

COMPONENT OF COURSE GRADE	WEIGHT
Paper on nursing interventions	10%
Papers critiquing issues in clinical practice	20%
Quizzes	10%
Midterm examination	20%
Portfolio	20%
Final examination	20%

Student	Intervention Paper (10%)	Issue Paper (20%)	Quizzes (10%)	Midterm (20%)	Portfolio (20%)	Final (20%)
Mary	85	94	98	92	94	91
Jane	76	78	63	79	70	79
Bob	82	86	89	81	80	83

Composite score for Mary:
$[10(85) + 20(94) + 10(98) + 20(92) + 20(94) + 20(91)] \div 100^* = 92.5\%$

Composite score for Jane:
$[10(76) + 20(78) + 10(63) + 20(79) + 20(70) + 20(79)] \div 100 = 75.1\%$

Composite score for Bob:
$[10(82) + 20(86) + 10(89) + 20(81) + 20(80) + 20(83)] \div 100 = 83.1\%$

*100 = sum of weights.

assigned reflects the weights given to each component within the course, that is, what each one is "worth." For example:

Paper on nursing interventions	100 points
Papers critiquing issues in clinical practice	200 points
Quizzes	100 points
Midterm examination	200 points
Portfolio	200 points
Final examination	200 points
	1,000 points

The points for each component are not converted to a letter grade; instead the grades are assigned according to the number of total points accumulated at the end of the course. At that time letter grades are assigned based on the points needed for each grade. For example:

Grade	Points
A	900–1,000
B	800–899
C	700–799
D	600–699
F	0–599

One problem with this method is that often the decision about the points to allot to each test and evaluation method in the course is made before the teacher has developed them (Nitko & Brookhart, 2011). For example, to end with 1,000 points for the course, the teacher may need 20 points for each quiz. However, in preparing one of those quizzes, the teacher finds that 10 items adequately cover the content and reflect the emphasis given to the content in the instruction. If this were known during the course planning, the teacher could assign 10 fewer points to quizzes and add another assignment worth 10 points, or could alter the points for other components of the course grade. However, when the course is already underway, changes such as these cannot be made in the grading scheme, and the teacher needs to develop a 20-point quiz even if fewer items would have adequately sampled the content. The next time the course is offered, the teacher can modify the points allotted for quizzes in the course grade.

Computing a Composite Score for a Course

In this method the composite score is the total number of points the student accumulates, and no further calculations are needed. Nitko and Brookhart (2011) cautioned teachers to be sure that the weights of the components were reflected in the points given them in the total composite. For example, if the teacher wanted the portfolio to count 20% of the course grade, and the maximum number of points for the course was 1,000, then the portfolio would be worth a maximum of 200 points (= 20% of 1,000).

NORM-REFERENCED GRADING

In a norm-referenced grading system, using relative standards, grades are assigned by comparing a student's performance with that of others in the class. Students who perform better than their peers receive higher grades

(Nitko & Brookhart, 2011). When using a norm-referenced system the teacher decides on the reference group against which to compare a student's performance. Should students be compared to others in the course? Should they be compared to students only in their section of the course? Or, to students who completed the course the prior semester or previous year? One issue with norm-referenced grading is that high performance in a particular group may not be indicative of mastery of the content or what students have learned; it reflects instead a student's standing in that group.

Grading on the Curve

Two methods of assigning grades using a norm-referenced system are (a) "grading on the curve" and (b) using standard deviations. Grading on the curve refers to the score distribution curve. In this method, students' scores are rank-ordered from highest to lowest, and grades are assigned according to the rank order. For example, the teacher may decide on the following framework for grading a test:

Top 20% of students	A
Next 20%	B
Next 40%	C
Next 15%	D
Lowest 5%	F

With this method there would always be failing grades on a test.

After the quotas are set, grades are assigned without considering actual achievement. For example, the top 20% of the students will receive an A even if their scores are close to the next group that gets a B. The students assigned lower grades may in fact have acquired sufficient knowledge in the course but unfortunately had lower scores than the other students. In these two examples, the decisions on the percentages of As, Bs, Cs, and lower grades are made arbitrarily by the teacher. The teacher determines the proportion of grades at each level; this approach is not based on a normal curve.

Another way of grading on the curve is to use the normal or bell curve for determining the percentages of each grade. The assumption of this method is that the grades of the students in the course should reflect a normal distribution. For example:

Top 10% of students	A
Next 20%	B
Next 40%	C
Next 20%	D
Lowest 10%	F

As discussed in Chapter 16, for "grading on the curve" to work correctly, student scores need to be distributed based on the normal curve. However, the abilities of nursing students tend not to be heterogeneous, especially late in the nursing education program, and therefore their scores on tests and other evaluation products are not normally distributed. They are carefully selected for admission into the program, and they need to achieve certain grades in courses and earn minimum GPAs to progress in the program. With grading on the curve, even if most students achieved high grades on a test and mastered the content, some would still be assigned lower grades.

Standard Deviation Method

The second method is based on standard deviations. With this method, the teacher determines the cut-off points for each grade. The grades are based on how far they are from the mean of raw scores for the class. To use the standard deviation method, the teacher first prepares a frequency distribution of the final scores and then calculates the mean score. With this method the teacher has a reference point (mean) and the average distance of scores from the mean (Musial, Nieminen, Thomas, & Burke, 2009, p. 318). The grade boundaries are then determined based on the standard deviation (Nitko & Brookhart, 2011). For example, the cut-off points for a "C" grade might range from one half the standard deviation below the mean to one half above the mean. To identify the "A–B" cut-off scores, the teacher adds one standard deviation to the upper cut-off number of the C range. Subtracting one standard deviation from the lower "C" cut-off provides the range for the "D–F" grades.

SELF-REFERENCED GRADING

Self-referenced grading is based on standards of growth and change in the student. With this method, grades are assigned by comparing the student's performance with the teacher's perceptions of the student's capabilities (Nitko & Brookhart, 2011). Did the student achieve at a higher level than deemed capable regardless of the knowledge and competencies acquired? Did the student improve performance throughout the course?

Table 17.2 compares self-referencing with criterion- and norm-referenced grading. One major problem with this method is the unreliability of the teacher's perceptions of student capability and growth. A second issue occurs with students who enter the course or clinical practice with a high level of achievement and proficiency in many of the clinical competencies. These students may have the least amount of growth and change but nevertheless exit the course with the highest achievement and clinical competency. Ultimately, judgments about the quality of a nursing student's performance are more important than judgments about the degree of improvement. It is difficult to make valid predictions about future performance on licensure or certification exams, or in clinical practice based on self-referenced grades. For these reasons, self-referenced grades are not widely used in nursing education programs.

GRADING CLINICAL PRACTICE

Arriving at grades for clinical practice is difficult because of the nature of clinical practice and the need for judgments about performance. Issues in evaluating clinical practice and rating performance were discussed in Chapters 13 and 14. Many teachers constantly revise their rating forms for clinical evaluation and seek new ways of grading clinical practice. Although these changes may create a fairer grading system, they will not eliminate the problems inherent in judging clinical performance.

The different types of grading systems described earlier may be used for grading clinical practice. In general these include systems using letter grades, A through F; integers, 5 through 1; and percentages. Grading systems for clinical practice also may use pass–fail, satisfactory–unsatisfactory, and met–did not meet the clinical objectives. Some programs add a third category, honors, to acknowledge performance that exceeds the level required. Pass–fail is used most frequently in nursing programs (Oermann, Yarbrough, Ard, Saewert, & Charasika, 2009). With any of the grading systems, it is not always easy to summarize the multiple types of evaluation data collected on the student's performance in a symbol representing a grade. This is true even in a pass–fail system; it may be difficult to arrive at a judgment as to pass or fail based on the evaluation data and the circumstances associated with the student's clinical, simulated, and laboratory practice.

Regardless of the grading system for clinical practice, there are two criteria to be met: (a) the evaluation methods for collecting data about student performance should reflect the outcomes and clinical competencies for which a grade will be assigned, and (b) students must understand how their clinical practice will be evaluated and graded.

Decisions about assigning letter grades for clinical practice are the same as grading any course: identifying what to include in the clinical grade and selecting a grading framework. The first consideration relates to the evaluation methods used in the course to provide data for determining the clinical grade. Some of these evaluation methods are for summative evaluation, thereby providing a source of information for inclusion in the clinical grade. Other strategies, though, are used in clinical practice for feedback only and are not incorporated into the grade.

The second consideration is the grading framework. Will achievement in clinical practice be graded from A to F? 5 to 1? Pass–fail? Or variations of these? A related question is, How will the clinical grade be included in the course grade, if at all?

Pass–Fail

Categories for grading clinical practice such as pass–fail and satisfactory–unsatisfactory have some advantages over a system with multiple levels, although there are disadvantages as well. Pass–fail places greater emphasis on giving feedback to the learner because only two categories of performance need to be determined. With a pass–fail grading system, teachers may be more inclined to provide continual feedback to learners because ultimately they do not have to differentiate performance according to four or five levels of proficiency such as with a letter system. Performance that exceeds the requirements and expectations, however, is not reflected in the grade for clinical practice unless a third category is included: honors–pass–fail.

A pass–fail system requires only two types of judgment about clinical performance. Do the evaluation data indicate that the student has met the outcomes or has demonstrated satisfactory performance of the clinical competencies to indicate a pass? Or do the data suggest that the performance of those competencies is not at a satisfactory level? Arriving at a judgment as to pass or fail is often easier for the teacher than using the same evaluation information for deciding on multiple levels of performance. A letter system for grading clinical practice, however, acknowledges the different levels of clinical proficiency students may have demonstrated in their clinical practice.

A disadvantage of pass–fail for grading clinical practice is the inability to include a clinical grade in the course grade. One strategy is to separate nursing courses into two components for grading, one for theory and another for clinical practice (designated as pass–fail), even though the course may be considered as a whole. Typically, guidelines for the course indicate that the students must pass the clinical component to pass the course. An alternative mechanism is to offer two separate courses with the clinical course graded on a pass–fail basis.

Once the grading system is determined, there are various ways of using it to arrive at the clinical grade. In one method, the grade is assigned based on the outcomes or competencies achieved by the student. To use this method, the teacher should consider designating some of the outcomes or competencies as critical for achievement. Table 17.2 provides guidelines for converting the clinical competencies into letter grades within a criterion-referenced system. For example, an A might be assigned if all of the competencies were achieved; a B might be assigned if all of the critical ones were achieved and at least half of the others were met.

For pass–fail grading, teachers can indicate that all of the outcomes or competencies must be met to pass the course, or they can designate critical behaviors required for passing the course. In both methods, the clinical evaluation methods provide the data for determining if the student's performance reflects achievement of the competencies. These evaluation methods may or may not be graded separately as part of the course grade.

Another way of arriving at the clinical grade is to base it on the evaluation methods. In this system the clinical evaluation methods become the source of data for the grade. For example:

Paper on analysis of clinical practice issue	10%
Analysis of clinical cases	5%
Conference presentation	10%
Community resource paper	10%
Portfolio	25%
Rating scale (of performance)	40%

In this illustration, the clinical grade is computed according to the evaluation methods. Observation of performance, and the rating on the clinical evaluation tool, comprise only a portion of the clinical grade. An advantage of this approach is that it incorporates into the grade the summative evaluation methods completed by the students.

If pass–fail is used for grading clinical practice, the grade might be computed as follows:

Paper on analysis of clinical practice issue	10%
Analysis of clinical cases	5%
Conference presentation	10%
Community resource paper	10%
Portfolio	25%
Clinical examination, simulations	40%
Rating scale (of performance)	Pass required

This discussion of grading clinical practice has suggested a variety of mechanisms that are appropriate. The teacher must make it clear to the students and others how the evaluation and grading will be carried out in clinical practice, through simulations, and in other settings.

Failing Clinical Practice

Teachers will be faced with determining when students have not met the outcomes of clinical practice, that is, have not demonstrated sufficient competence to pass the clinical course. There are principles that should be followed in evaluating and grading clinical practice, which are critical if a student fails a clinical course or has the potential for failing it. These principles are discussed in the text that follows.

Communicate Evaluation and Grading Methods in Writing

The evaluation methods used in a clinical course, the manner in which each will be graded if at all, and how the clinical grade will be assigned should be put in writing and communicated to the students. The practices of the teacher in evaluating and grading clinical performance must reflect this written information. In courses with preceptors, it is critical that preceptors and others involved in teaching and assessing student performance understand the outcomes of the course, the evaluation methods, how to observe and rate performance, and the preceptor's responsibilities when students are not performing adequately. Preceptors are reluctant to assign failing grades to students whose competence is questionable (Heaslip & Scammell, 2012). There is a need for faculty development especially for new and part-time teachers. As part of this development teachers should explore their own beliefs and values about grading clinical performance, the meaning of grades, and their views of "satisfactory performance" (Scanlan & Care, 2008).

Identify Effect of Failing Clinical Practicum on Course Grade

If failing clinical practice, whether in a pass–fail or a letter system, means failing the nursing course, this should be stated clearly in the course syllabus and policies. By stating it in the syllabus, which all students receive, they have it in writing before clinical learning activities begin. A sample policy statement for pass-fail clinical grading is:

> The clinical component of NUR XXX is evaluated with a Pass or Fail. A Fail in the clinical component results in failure of the course even if the theory grade is 75% or higher.

In a letter grade system, the policy should include the letter grade representing a failure in clinical practice, for example, less than a C grade. A sample policy statement for this system is:

Students must pass the clinical component of NUR XXX with the grade of "C" or higher. A grade lower than a "C" in the clinical component of the course results in failure of the course even if the theory grade is 75% or higher.

Ask Students to Sign Notes About Performance, Rating Forms, and Evaluation Summaries

Students should sign any written clinical evaluation documents—notes about the student's performance in clinical practice; rating forms (of clinical practice, clinical examinations, and performance in simulations); narrative comments about the student's performance; and summaries of conferences in which performance was discussed. Their signatures do not mean they agree with the ratings or comments, only that they have read them. Students should have an opportunity to write in their own comments. These materials are important because they document the student's performance and indicate that the teacher provided feedback and shared concerns about that performance. This is critical in situations in which students may be failing the clinical course because of performance problems.

Identify Performance Problems Early and Develop Learning Plans

Students need continuous feedback on their clinical performance. Observations made by the teacher, the preceptor, and others, as well as evaluation data from other sources should be shared with the student. They should discuss the data together. Students may have different perceptions of their performance and in some cases may provide new information that influences the teacher's judgment about clinical competencies.

When the teacher or preceptor identifies performance problems and clinical deficiencies that may affect passing the course, conferences should be held with the student to discuss these areas of concern and develop a plan for remediation. It is critical that these conferences focus on problems in performance combined with specific learning activities for addressing them. The conferences should not consist of the teacher telling the student everything that is wrong with her or his clinical performance; the student needs an opportunity to respond to the teacher's concerns and identify how to address them.

One of the goals of the conference is to develop a plan with learning activities for the student to correct deficiencies and develop competencies further. The plan should indicate that (1) completing the remedial learning activities does not guarantee that the student will pass the course, (2) one satisfactory performance of the competencies will not constitute a pass clinical grade (the improvement must be sustained), and (3) the student must demonstrate satisfactory performance of the competencies by the end of the course.

Any discussions with students at risk of failing clinical practice should focus on the student's inability to meet the clinical objectives (or outcomes) and perform the specified competencies, not on the teacher's perceptions of the student's intelligence and overall ability. In addition, opinions about the student's ability in general should not be discussed with others.

Conferences should be held in private, and a summary of the discussion should be prepared. The summary should include the date and time of the conference, who participated, areas of concern about clinical performance, and the learning plan with a timeframe for completion (Gaberson & Oermann, 2010). The summary should be signed by the teacher, the student, and any other participants. Faculty members should review related policies of the nursing education program because they might specify other requirements.

Identify Support Services

Students at risk for failing clinical practice may have other problems that are affecting their performance. Teachers should refer students to counseling and other support services and not attempt to provide these resources themselves. Attempting to counsel the student and help the student cope with other problems may bias the teacher and influence judgment of the student's clinical performance.

Document Performance

As the clinical course progresses, the teacher should give feedback to the student about performance and continue to guide learning. It is important to document the observations made, other types of evaluation data collected, and the learning activities completed by the student. The documentation should be shared routinely with students, discussions about performance should be summarized, and students should sign these summaries to confirm that they read them.

The teacher cannot observe and document the performance *only* of the student at risk for failing the course. There should be a minimum number of observations and documentation of other students in the clinical group, or the student failing the course might believe that he or she was treated differently than others in the group. One strategy is to plan an approximate number of observations of performance to be made for each student in the clinical group to avoid focusing only on the student with performance problems. However, teachers may observe students who are believed to be at risk for failure more closely, and document their observations and conferences with those students more thoroughly and frequently than is necessary for the majority of students. When observations result in feedback to students that can be used to improve performance, at-risk students usually do not object to this extra attention.

Follow Policy on Unsafe Clinical Performance

There should be a policy in the nursing program about actions to be taken if a student's work in clinical practice is unsafe. Students who are not meeting the outcomes of the course or have problems performing some of the competencies can continue in the clinical course as long as they demonstrate safe care. This is because the outcomes and clinical competencies are identified for achievement at the *end* of the course, not during it.

If the student demonstrates performance that is potentially unsafe, however, the teacher can remove the student from the clinical setting, following the policy and procedures of the nursing education program. Specific learning activities outside of the clinical setting need to be offered to help students develop the knowledge and skills they lack; simulation and practice in the skills laboratory are valuable in these situations. A learning plan should be prepared and implemented as described earlier.

Follow Policy for Failure of a Clinical Course

In all instances the teacher must follow the policies of the nursing program. If the student fails the clinical course, the student must be notified of the failure and its consequences as indicated in these policies. In some nursing education programs, students are allowed to repeat only one clinical course, and there may be other requirements to be met. If the student will be dismissed from the program because of the failure, the student must be informed of this in writing. Generally there is a specific time frame for each step in the process, which must be adhered to by the faculty, administrators, and students. It is critical that all teachers know the policies and procedures to be implemented when students have performance problems or are at-risk for failing the clinical course. These policies and procedures must be followed for all students.

GRADING SOFTWARE

A number of the procedures used to determine grades are time-consuming, particularly if the class of students is large. Although a calculator may be used, student grades can be calculated easily with a spreadsheet application such as Microsoft Excel or with an online course management system. With a spreadsheet application, teachers can enter individual scores, include the weights of each component of the grade, and compute final grades (Figure 17.1). Many statistical functions can be performed with a spreadsheet application.

Calculation Sheet

S.No	Name of Student	FORMULAS	Exam 1 (Exam) C3	Exam 2 (Exam) D3	Exam 3 (Exam) E3	Exams Total (Exam) F3=SUM(C3:E3)	Exam % G3=(F3/208)*100	Clinical Total Points (Lab) H3	Clinical % I3=(H3/906)*100	Total Points J3=(F3+H3)	Final Course % (Overall) (G3*0.6)+(I3*0.4)	Grade
1			32	32	88	152	73.08%	800	88.30%	952	79.17%	
2			27	20	90	137	65.87%	888	98.01%	1025	78.72%	
3			50	27	100	177	85.10%	900	99.34%	1077	90.79%	
4			40	38	76	154	74.04%	850	93.82%	1004	81.95%	
5			42	39	98	179	86.06%	777	85.76%	956	85.94%	
6			47	40	83	170	81.73%	890	98.23%	1060	88.33%	
7			20	40	90	150	72.12%	817	90.18%	967	79.34%	
8			48	40	87	175	84.13%	839	92.60%	1014	87.52%	
9			46	42	101	189	90.87%	856	94.48%	1045	92.31%	
10			40	43	88	171	82.21%	898	99.12%	1069	88.97%	
11			39	46	96	181	87.02%	802	88.52%	983	87.62%	
12			51	47	98	196	94.23%	852	94.04%	1048	94.15%	
13			50	48	100	198	95.19%	889	98.12%	1087	96.36%	
14			48	48	88	184	88.46%	780	86.09%	964	87.51%	
15			50	50	99	199	95.67%	807	89.07%	1006	93.03%	
16			38	50	95	183	87.98%	799	88.19%	982	88.06%	
17			43	50	99	192	92.31%	823	90.84%	1015	91.72%	
18			40	50	85	175	84.13%	856	94.48%	1031	88.27%	
19			50	47	102	199	95.67%	874	96.47%	1073	95.99%	
20			52	39	94	185	88.94%	863	95.25%	1048	91.47%	
Points Possible			52	52	104	208	100.00%	906	100.00%	1114	100.00%	
Weight			0%	0%	0%	60%	100.00%	40%	100.00%		100.00%	

Figure 17.1 Sample spreadsheet application for grading.

Online course management systems provide grade books for teachers to manage all aspects of student grades. The grades can be weighted and a final grade calculated, but usually more advanced statistical analysis cannot be done. One advantage to a course management system grade book is that students usually have online access to their own scores and grades as soon as the teacher has entered them.

There also are a number of grading software programs on the market that include a premade spreadsheet for grading purposes; these have different grading frameworks that may be used to calculate the grade and enable the teacher to carry out the tasks needed for grading. With this software the teacher can print out grading reports for the class as a whole as well as individual students. Some even calculate test statistics. Not all grading software programs are of high quality, however, and should be reviewed prior to purchase.

SUMMARY

Grading is the use of symbols, such as the letters A through F, to report student achievement. Grading is used for summative purposes, indicating how well the student met the outcomes of the course and performed in clinical practice. Grades need to be based on careful evaluation practices, valid and reliable test results, and multiple assessment methods. No grade should be determined on the basis of one method or one assignment completed by the students; grades reflect instead a combination of various tests and other assessment methods.

There are different types of grading systems or methods of reporting grades: the use of letters A–E or A–F, which may be combined with "+" and "–"; integers 5, 4, 3, 2, and 1 (or 9 through 1); percentages; and categories such as pass–fail and satisfactory–unsatisfactory. Advantages and disadvantages of pass–fail for grading clinical practice were discussed in the chapter.

Two major considerations in assigning letter grades are deciding what to include in the grade and selecting a grading framework. The weight given to each test and the evaluation method in the grade is specified by the teacher according to the emphasis of the course outcomes and the content measured by them. To give meaning to the grades assigned, the teacher needs a grading framework: criterion-referenced, also referred to as grading with absolute standards; norm-referenced, or grading with relative standards; or self-referenced, grading based on the growth of the student.

One final concept described in the chapter was grading clinical practice and guidelines for working with students who are at risk for failing a clinical course. These guidelines give direction to teachers in establishing sound grading practices and following them when working with students in clinical practice.

REFERENCES

Barnes, K. D., & Buring, S. M. (2012). The effect of various grading scales on student grade point averages. *American Journal of Pharmaceutical Education, 76*(3). Article 41. doi:10.5688/ajpe76341.

Brookhart, S. M. (2011). *Grading and learning: Practices that support student achievement.* Bloomington, IN: Solution Tree Press.

Gaberson, K. B., & Oermann, M. H. (2010). *Clinical teaching strategies in nursing* (3rd ed.). New York, NY: Springer Publishing.

Heaslip, V., & Scammell, J. M. E. (2012). Failing underperforming students: The role of grading in practice assessment. *Nurse Education in Practice, 12*, 95–100.

Miller, M. D., Linn, R. L., & Gronlund, N. E. (2009). *Measurement and assessment in teaching* (10th ed.). Upper Saddle River, NJ: Prentice Hall.

Musial, D., Nieminen, G., Thomas, J., & Burke, K. (2009). *Foundations of educational measurement.* Boston, MA: McGraw-Hill Higher Education.

Nitko, A. J., & Brookhart, S. M. (2011). *Educational assessment of students* (6th ed.). Upper Saddle River, NJ: Pearson Education.

Oermann, M. H., Yarbrough, S. S., Ard, N., Saewert, K. J., & Charasika, M. (2009). Clinical evaluation and grading practices in schools of nursing: Findings of the evaluation of learning advisory council survey. *Nursing Education Perspectives, 30*, 352–357.

Rojstaczer, S., & Healy, C. (2012). Where A is ordinary: The evolution of American college and university grading, 1940–2009. *Teachers College Record, 114*(7). Retrieved from http://www.tcrecord.org. ID Number: 16473.

Scanlan, J. M., & Care, W. D. (2008). Issues with grading and grade inflation in nursing education. In M. H. Oermann (Ed.), *Annual review of nursing education* (Vol. 6, pp. 173–188). New York, NY: Springer Publishing.

EIGHTEEN

Program Assessment

KATHLEEN B. GABERSON AND ANNA N. VIORAL

Program assessment is the process of judging the worth or value of an educational program. One purpose of program assessment is to provide data on which to base decisions about the educational program. Another purpose is to provide evidence of educational effectiveness in response to internal and external demands for accountability. With the demand for high-quality programs, development of newer models for the delivery of higher education such as Web-based instruction, and public calls for accountability, there has been a greater emphasis on systematic and ongoing program assessment. This chapter presents an overview of program assessment models and discusses assessment of selected program components, including curriculum, outcomes, and teaching.

PROGRAM ASSESSMENT MODELS

A number of models are currently used to guide program assessment activities in nursing education programs, staff education departments, and patient education programs. These models provide a framework for educators to develop an assessment plan that includes sources of data and time frames for assessment. With a planned, systematic assessment, administrators, faculty members, and others involved in the program have information for quality improvement. There are many assessment models; a few are described here.

Accreditation Models

Accreditation models such as those used by the National League for Nursing Accrediting Commission (NLNAC), Commission on Collegiate Nursing Education (CCNE), Canadian Association of Schools of Nursing for baccalaureate programs in Canada, and The Joint Commission typically use a combination of self-study and site visits to the institution by a team of peer evaluators. Program assessment based on an accreditation model is designed to assess whether the program meets external standards of quality, as evident in the accreditation criteria for each type of program.

CCNE accredits baccalaureate and master's degree nursing programs, practice-focused clinical nursing doctoral programs that award the Doctor of Nursing Practice (DNP) degree, and post-baccalaureate nurse residency programs (Commission on Collegiate Nursing Education, 2009). NLNAC accredits all levels of nursing education programs: practical; diploma; associate, baccalaureate, and master's degree; and clinical doctorate (NLNAC, 2012). Professional accreditation by organizations such as these is a voluntary, self-regulatory process that promotes self-assessment and ongoing improvement of educational programs.

Assessment of Online Programs Using an Accreditation Model

Although no specific online program accreditation standards exist, the NLNAC (2012) and the CCNE (2009) incorporate distance learning elements into their standards and criteria for quality assessment of online programs. For NLNAC accreditation, online nursing programs must demonstrate compliance with nine elements critical to effective distant education in addition to the appropriate accreditation standards for the level of program:

- Congruence with the institutional mission
- Instructional design and course delivery methods
- Competence and preparation of faculty
- Accessibility and quality of support services
- Current, relevant, and accessible learning resources
- Current, appropriate offerings relative to the delivery method
- Provision of opportunities for faculty and student interactions
- Ongoing assessment of student learning
- Processes for verifying student identity and protecting student privacy (NLNAC, 2012)

The CCNE accreditation process incorporates specific elements related to effective distance education into three of the four accreditation standards, as the following examples illustrate:

- Standard I, Program Quality, Mission and Governance: Roles of faculty members and students in program governance, including participants in distance education, are clearly defined and encourage involvement.
- Standard II, Program Quality, Institutional Commitment and Resources: Academic support services, such as library, technology, and distance education support, are adequate and support achievement of desired program outcomes.
- Standard III, Program Quality, Curriculum and Teaching–Learning Practices: Distance education teaching-learning practices and environments support individual student achievement of expected learning outcomes (CCNE, 2009).

Online nursing program assessment based on an accreditation model should therefore seek evidence that the program uses distance education effectively to facilitate achievement of program goals. Caputi (2011) suggested that program assessment should consider the extent to which the online nursing program:

- includes a definition of distance education in the program mission and governance statements;
- provides a mechanism for online students to file grievances;
- demonstrates how students contribute to the nursing program governance;
- provides time frames for adding and dropping online courses;
- notifies students of the mechanisms to report technological difficulties; and
- demonstrates how the institution offers faculty development and support related to online education, technology, and instructional design.

Decision-Oriented Models

Another type of model is decision-oriented. With these models, the goal of assessment is to provide information to decision makers for program improvement purposes. However, the existence of assessment data is no guarantee that those who are in positions to make decisions about the program will take corrective action if it is indicated (Stufflebeam & Shinkfield, 2007). Decision models focus more on using assessment as a tool to improve programs than on accountability. Decision-oriented models usually focus on internal standards of quality, value, and efficacy.

Examples of decision-oriented approaches are the Context, Input, Process, Product (CIPP) model (Stufflebeam & Shinkfield, 2007) and the Continuous Quality Improvement (CQI) model (Brown & Marshall, 2008; Deming, 1986).

The CIPP model asks: What needs to be done? (context); How should it be done? (input); Is it being done? (process); and Did it succeed? (product) (Stufflebeam & Shinkfield, 2007). *Context* assessment appraises the needs, problems, strengths, and weaknesses within a defined environment. Through *input* assessment, the system capabilities, competing strategies, work plans, and budgets of the selected approach are assessed. Input assessment ensures that the program's strategy is feasible for meeting the needs of the program and its beneficiaries. *Process* assessment focuses on providing feedback to monitor progress, identify whether the plans are being implemented as intended, and make changes as needed. *Product* assessment measures achievement of the outcomes. Product assessment is divided into (a) impact assessment (to assess if the program reached the target audience), (b) effectiveness assessment (to assess the quality and significance of the outcomes), (c) sustainability assessment (to determine the extent to which a program's contributions are continued over time), and (d) transportability assessment (to assess the extent to which a program has been or could be applied in other settings) (Stufflebeam & Shinkfield, 2007).

The CQI approach focuses on improvement of an existing process by following four phases: plan, do, study, and act (PDSA) (Deming, 1986). The CQI approach is based on the assumption that the people who are closest to the process know it best. Therefore, in education, the students, faculty, administrators, and employers of graduates should be part of the CQI effort (Brown & Marshall, 2008).

During the plan phase, CQI participants define the problems and opportunities for improvement, collect and organize data, and decide on improvement initiatives. The do phase involves identifying needed resources and implementing the planned change. During the study phase, the participants monitor the progress of the improvement initiative and observe the effects of the change. Finally, in the act phase, the improvement is modified as needed and incorporated into the program structure and policies. An important component of this phase is education of all stakeholders about the changes and then continuing to search for new opportunities for improvement. In nursing education programs, CQI is often implemented in response to the risk of failing to meet accreditation or regulatory standards. Ongoing use of this approach, however, yields valuable formative assessment data, but it requires a culture change to gain the buy-in of all participants (Brown & Marshall, 2008).

Systems-Oriented Models

Other models are systems-oriented. These examine inputs into the program such as characteristics of students, teachers, administrators, and other participants in the program, and program resources. These models also assess the operations and processes of the program as well as the context or environment within which the program is implemented. Finally, systems models examine the outcomes of the program: Are the intended outcomes being achieved? Are students, graduates, their employers, faculty, staff, and others satisfied with the program and how it is implemented? Is the program of high quality and cost effective?

Regardless of the specific model used, the process of program assessment assists various audiences or stakeholders of an educational program in judging and improving its worth or value. Audiences or stakeholders are those individuals and groups who are affected directly or indirectly by the decisions made. Key stakeholders of nursing education programs are students, faculty and staff members, partners (health care and community agencies), employers of graduates, and consumers. The purpose of the program assessment determines which audiences should be involved in generating questions or concerns to be answered or addressed. When the focus is formative, that is, to improve the program during its implementation, the primary audiences are students, teachers, and administrators. Summative assessment leads to decisions about whether a program should be continued, revised, funded, or terminated. Audiences for summative assessment include program participants, graduates, their employers, prospective students, health care and community agencies, consumers, legislative bodies, funding agencies, and others who might be affected by changes in the program.

When planning program assessment, an important decision is whether to use external or internal evaluators. External evaluators are thought to provide objectivity, but they may not know the program or its context well enough to be effective. External evaluators also add expense to the program assessment. In contrast, an internal evaluator has a better understanding of the operations and environment of the program and can provide continuous feedback to the individuals and groups responsible for the assessment. However, an internal evaluator may be biased, reducing the credibility of the assessment.

Program assessment should not be identified with any one particular approach or method. Instead, evaluators should selectively apply all useful and necessary methods to reach "defensible judgments of programs" (Stufflebeam & Shinkfield, 2007, p. 8).

When considering whether to use teacher-made or standardized assessment tools to assess program outcomes, teachers must keep in mind the qualities of effective measurement instruments, as discussed in Chapter 2. The availability of a standardized test does not ensure that teachers can make valid and reliable interpretations of the test results. Tools and other strategies for assessment should be chosen based on the outcomes to be measured.

Stufflebeam and Shinkfield (2007) cautioned against focusing entirely on assessment of outcomes because some intended outcomes may be "corrupt, dysfunctional, unimportant, [or] not oriented to the needs of the intended beneficiaries" (p. 8), and may provide feedback only at the end of a program. If the purpose of a program assessment is to contribute to program improvement, it also should examine the program goals, structure, and process as well as important "side effects" (Stufflebeam & Shinkfield, 2007, p. 8).

CURRICULUM ASSESSMENT

Curriculum assessment is not the same as program assessment. When evaluating the curriculum, the focus is on elements central to the course of studies taken by students. As such, curriculum assessment is narrower than program assessment, which includes additional elements related to institutional support for the program, administrative structure, faculty productivity, and student support services (Iwasiw, Goldenberg, & Andrusyszyn, 2009).

A number of curriculum assessment models have been used in nursing education. Over time, the focus of curriculum assessment has changed such that assessment models may be classified as first, second, third, or fourth generation, as described below:

- *First generation*: Focus on measuring to obtain student scores representing curriculum quality
- *Second generation*: Focus on describing congruence between student performance and curriculum objectives
- *Third generation*: Focus on judging the merit of performance in relation to standards
- *Fourth generation*: Focus on constructing a holistic understanding of needed improvements based on input from stakeholders (Iwasiw et al., 2009)

Curriculum elements to be assessed usually comprise:

- *Philosophical approaches*: Are they operational in teaching-learning activities and assessment approaches?

- *Curriculum outcome statements*: Do they meet professional and institutional standards? Are they appropriate to the level of the nursing education program and relevant to the healthcare context?

- *Curriculum design*: How well do the curriculum components fit together? Does the design reflect the philosophical foundation and curriculum goals? Is it congruent with the environment of the program? Are the courses logically sequenced?

- *Curriculum outcomes*: Is there evidence that students are achieving desired program outcomes (e.g., success rates on NCLEX® and certification exams)? How successful are program graduates in their positions?

- *Courses*: Are course goals congruent with curriculum goals? Are learning activities consistent with the philosophical framework and goals? Is course content current, evidence based, and logically organized?

- *Teaching-learning methods*: Are teaching strategies congruent with the philosophical framework? Do they assist students to achieve course and curriculum goals? Do they respect student diversity? How do students respond to the selected teaching methods? Are students satisfied with the quality of teaching?

- *Student achievement assessment methods*: What assessment methods are used throughout the curriculum? Are assessment approaches congruent with the philosophical framework and curriculum goals? Do they provide for demonstration of all relevant types of learning? Do they accommodate students' diverse learning styles, need for formative and summative feedback, and desire for input into the process? Do they accommodate faculty members' expertise, preferences, and academic workload?

- *Resources*: Are the human, physical, and fiscal resources sufficient to implement the curriculum? Are there sufficient numbers of appropriately credentialed faculty members to offer the curriculum as planned? Are the number of staff members and their roles and functions appropriate to support the curriculum? Are classrooms, offices, labs, and meeting rooms available? Are the rooms adequate, comfortable, and appropriately equipped? Are library holdings appropriate and sufficient? Are clinical placements available in sufficient quality and quantity?

- *Learning climate*: To what extent does the social, emotional, and intellectual atmosphere that exists within the nursing education program contribute to the quality of life of the faculty, students, and staff? To what extent are faculty members and students satisfied with their interpersonal relationships, academic freedom, and sense of community? To what extent does the learning environment promote diversity of perspective and foster responsibility and accountability?

■ *Policies*: Are academic policies appropriate, reasonable, and applied consistently? Do faculty members and students understand them? Is there a need for policies that do not yet exist? (Iwasiw et al., 2009)

As an example of a curriculum assessment approach, the faculty of one associate degree nursing program developed a conceptual model to guide its curriculum assessment and ongoing improvement. The center and focus of the model was learning, which is affected by student, faculty, resource, and curriculum factors. The development and use of this model was stimulated both by concern about curriculum outcomes, particularly NCLEX-RN® pass rates, and National League for Nursing initiatives to transform nursing education through learner-centered and concept-based curriculum approaches (Davis, 2011).

The faculty of a baccalaureate nursing program also developed a comprehensive assessment plan for its concept-based curriculum. Including both formative and summative evaluation approaches, the plan outlined a variety of data collection methods to collect evidence that desired curriculum outcomes were being met. A unique feature of this approach was the use of a small-group instructional diagnosis technique to provide midterm student input during the initial implementation of a revised or new course. If the faculty or students identified significant issues, the faculty could make necessary adjustments quickly (Giddens & Morton, 2010). In both of these examples, the faculty incorporated elements of accreditation, decision-oriented, and systems-oriented assessment models.

Although these assessment elements are important, an educational program involves more than a curriculum. The success of students in meeting the outcomes of courses and the curriculum as a whole may depend as much on the quality of the students admitted to the program or the characteristics of its faculty as it does on the sequence of courses or the instructional strategies used. Similarly, there may be abundant evidence that graduates meet the goals of the curriculum, but those graduates may not be satisfied with the program or may be unable to pass licensure or certification examinations.

Assessment of Online Courses

One element of curriculum assessment focuses on the courses that are offered within the curriculum. Online course assessment involves many of the same criteria used to assess courses offered in traditional classrooms, but additional elements specific to the online environment must also be evaluated, such as technology, accessibility, instructional design, content, and interactive activities (O'Neil, Fisher, & Newbold, 2009). These elements of course evaluation are included in the International Association for K-12 Online Learning (iNACOL) guidelines and recommendations for evaluating online courses (Pape, Wicks, & the iNACOL Quality Standards for Online Programs Committee, 2011). Although developed for elementary and secondary education programs, many, if not all, of the standards also apply to online courses in higher education. Table 18.1 provides a summary of the iNACOL standards. Potential methods for collecting this information

◻Table 18.1

iNACOL NATIONAL STANDARDS FOR QUALITY ONLINE COURSES

STANDARD	PERFORMANCE CRITERIA
Content	Course goals or objectives clearly state in measurable terms what the participants will know or be able to do at the end of the course
	Course components (objectives or goals, assessments, instructional methods, content, assignments, and technology) are appropriately rigorous
	Information literacy skills are integrated into the course
	A variety of learning resources and materials are available to students before the course begins (e.g., textbooks, browsers, software, tutorials, orientation)
	Information is provided to students about how to communicate with the online instructor
	A code of conduct, including netiquette standards, and expectations for academic integrity are posted
Instructional design	Course offers a variety of instructional methods
	Course is organized into units or lessons
	An overview for each unit or lesson describes objectives, activities, assignments, assessments, and resources
	Course activities engage students in active learning (e.g., collaborative learning groups, student-led review sessions, games, concept mapping, case study analysis)
	A variety of supplemental resources is clearly identified in the course materials
Student assessment	Methods for assessing student performance or achievement align with course goals or objectives
	The course provides frequent or ongoing formative assessments of student learning
	Feedback tools are built into the course to allow students to view their progress
	Assessment materials provide flexibility to assess students in variety of ways
	Assessment rubrics are provided for each graded assignment

(continued)

Table 18.1 *(continued)*

STANDARD	PERFORMANCE CRITERIA
Technology	The course uses consistent navigation methods requiring minimal training
	Students can use icons, graphics, and text to move logically through the course
	Media are available in multiple formats for ease of access and use to meet diverse student needs (e.g., video, podcast)
	All technology requirements (hardware, software, browser, etc.) and prerequisite technology skills are specified in the course descriptions before the course begins
	The course syllabus clearly states the copyright or licensing status including permission to share when applicable
	Course materials and activities are designed to facilitate access by all students
	Student information is protected as required by the Family Educational Rights and Privacy Act
Course evaluation and support	A combination of students, instructors, content experts, instructional designers, and outside reviewers review the course for effectiveness using multiple data collection methods (e.g., course evaluations, surveys, peer review)
	The course is updated annually with the date posted on the course management system and all course documents
	The course provider offers technical support and course management assistance to the students and course instructor 24 hours a day, 7 days a week

Adapted from International Association for K-12 Online Learning. (2011). *National Standards for Quality Online Courses (Version 2)*. Retrieved from http://www.inacol.org/research/nationalstandards/iNACOL_CourseStandards_2011.pdf

include student and teacher end-of-course evaluations, interviews or focus groups with students and teachers (electronically if necessary), and peer evaluation of online courses by other faculty members.

In some ways online courses are isolated and hidden from the view of faculty members and administrators who are not directly involved in teaching them, limiting the role that these colleagues can play in course evaluation. Unlike courses that are taught in traditional classrooms, faculty peers and administrators cannot walk by an open classroom door for a quick informal observation of activities, easily obtain and review hard copies of student assignments and instructor feedback to the students, or critique a printed copy of a course examination and the test and item analysis that pertains to it. Because course activities may take place within a course management system that controls access to course documents and features such as a discussion board, assignment drop box, and grade book, faculty peer reviewers and administrators must make arrangements to enter the course site to assess elements such as the course design and components, congruence of learning activities with intended course outcomes, availability of learning resources and materials, and ways in which student performance is assessed. Also, if course learning activities are conducted asynchronously, such as posting comments to a discussion board, it is difficult for an outside reviewer to assess such elements as the pace of the learning activities and the timing of instructor feedback to students.

TEACHING

Another area of assessment involves appraising the effectiveness of the teacher. This assessment addresses the quality of teaching in the classroom and clinical setting and other dimensions of the teacher's role, depending on the goals and mission of the nursing education program. These other roles may include scholarship and research; service to the nursing program, college or university, community, and nursing profession; and clinical practice. It is beyond the scope of this book to examine the multiple dimensions of faculty member evaluation in nursing; however, a brief discussion is provided about assessing the quality of teaching in the classroom and the clinical setting.

The National League for Nursing's "Core Competencies of Nurse Educators with Task Statements" (2005) describe the knowledge, skills, and attitudes required for effectiveness in the role of nurse educator as identified in research-based literature. Each competency statement is followed by a description of tasks that exemplify it. Three of the core competencies focus on effective performance in the role of teacher; these are listed below with several examples of their associated task statements:

Competency 1—Facilitate learning: Implements a variety of teaching strategies, communicates effectively, shows enthusiasm for teaching and nursing, demonstrates interest in learners, demonstrates personal attributes that facilitate learning, maintains a professional practice knowledge base

Competency 2—Facilitate learner development and socialization: Identifies individual learning needs and styles, provides appropriate learning resources, creates learning environments that promote socialization to the role of nurse

Competency 3—Use assessment and evaluation strategies: Uses a variety of methods to assess and evaluate learning, gives timely and constructive feedback to learners, demonstrates skill in design and use of assessment tools (NLN, 2005)

The research in nursing education suggests five qualities of effective teaching in nursing: (a) knowledge of the subject matter, (b) clinical competence, (c) teaching skill, (d) interpersonal relationships with students, and (e) personal characteristics. These findings are consistent with studies about teacher effectiveness in other fields (Gaberson & Oermann, 2010).

Knowledge of Subject Matter

An effective teacher is an expert in the content area, has an understanding of theories and concepts relevant to nursing practice, and assists students in applying these to patient care (Gaberson & Oermann, 2010). Teachers need to keep current with nursing and other interventions, new developments in their areas of expertise, and research. In their analysis of student evaluations of faculty performance, Wolf, Bender, Beitz, Wieland, and Vito (2004) found that being knowledgeable and scholarly were identified as strengths of good teachers. However, knowledge of the subject matter is not sufficient; the teacher must be able to communicate that knowledge to students.

Competence in Clinical Practice

If teaching in the clinical setting, the teacher has to be competent in clinical practice (Gaberson & Oermann, 2010). Tang, Chou, and Chiang (2005) concluded that the clinical competence of the teacher was one of the most important characteristics of effective clinical teaching in nursing. The best teachers are expert practitioners who know how to care for patients, can make sound clinical judgments, have expert clinical skills, and can guide students in developing those skills.

An interesting finding of a comparative study of teaching quality among tenured and sessional (e.g., employed on a time-limited contract) nursing faculty members was the higher ratings of sessional teachers by first- and second-year students as compared to ratings by third-year students (Salamonson, Halcomb, Andrew, Peters, & Jackson, 2010). One explanation of this finding was that sessional faculty members were more likely than tenured faculty members to be concurrently employed in nursing and therefore to maintain clinical currency, an importance characteristic of effective teaching (Andrew, Halcomb, Jackson, Peters, & Salamonson, 2010).

Skills in Teaching

The teacher also needs to know how to teach. Berg and Lindseth (2004) found in their study of 171 baccalaureate nursing students that teaching methods, presentation of course materials, and personality were the three main characteristics of an effective teacher, according to the students. Competencies in teaching involve the ability to:

- identify students' learning needs,
- plan instruction,
- present material (or "content") effectively,
- explain concepts and ideas clearly,
- demonstrate procedures effectively, and
- use sound assessment practices.

The research suggests that the teacher's skills in clinical evaluation are particularly important to teaching effectiveness. Evaluating learners fairly, having clear expectations and communicating those to students, correcting mistakes without embarrassing students, and giving immediate feedback are important teacher behaviors (Gaberson & Oermann, 2010).

Positive Relationships With Learners

Another important characteristic is the ability of the teacher to establish positive relationships with students as a group in the classroom, online environment, and clinical setting, and with students on an individual basis. Effective teaching qualities in this area include showing respect for and confidence in students, being honest and direct, supporting students, and being approachable (Gaberson & Oermann, 2010). Effective teachers treat students fairly and create an environment of mutual respect between educator and student.

In their study of teaching quality among sessional and tenured teachers, Salamonson et al. (2010) proposed that one explanation for the higher ratings of sessional faculty members by first- and second-year students might be that sessional teachers may identify more strongly with students and this close identification with students may help them learn more in their classes (Andrew et al., 2010).

Personal Characteristics of Teacher

Effective teaching also depends on the personal characteristics of the teacher. Characteristics in this area include enthusiasm, patience, having a sense of humor, friendliness, integrity, perseverance, courage, and willingness to admit mistakes (Gaberson & Oermann, 2010; Tang et al., 2005). In the study by Berg and Lindseth (2004), in which teaching methods, presentation of course materials, and personality were the three primary characteristics of effective teaching, personality was found to be the most important one.

In Salamonson et al.'s (2010) comparison of student-rated teaching quality among sessional and tenured teachers, one explanation proposed for the higher ratings of sessional faculty members by first- and second-year students was that sessional teachers "are more enthusiastic and vibrant than their tenured colleagues" (p. 428) and that students learned more as a result. However, the relative importance of personal characteristics appeared to shift to a greater appreciation for a broad professional nursing knowledge base, a strength of tenured teachers, among third-year students.

Personal characteristics that convey caring about students also support caring as a core value in nursing. In one study, online baccalaureate nursing students from five universities identified 12 behavioral attributes of online nurse educators that support student perceptions of caring (Sitzman, 2010). The investigator synthesized these 12 attributes into 5 categories: clarity and expertise, timeliness, empathic presence, full engagement, and accessibility. Most students preferred instructors who could manage the online process and content so that students understood what they needed for successful learning (Sitzman, 2010).

HOW TO EVALUATE TEACHING EFFECTIVENESS

Teaching effectiveness data are available from a variety of sources. These include: students, peers, administrators, and others involved in the educational experience such as preceptors.

Student Ratings

Student evaluations are a necessary but insufficient source of information. Because students are the only participants other than the teacher who are consistently present during the teaching–learning process, they have a unique perspective of the teacher's behavior over time. Students can make valid and reliable interpretations about the teacher's use of teaching methods, fairness, interest in students, and enthusiasm for the subject. Student ratings of overall teaching effectiveness are moderately correlated with independent measures of student learning and achievement (Davis, 2007).

There are limitations, though, to the use of student ratings. These ratings can be affected by class size, with smaller classes tending to rate teacher effectiveness higher than larger classes. Student ratings can also be influenced by the type of course format; for example, discussion courses tend to receive higher ratings than do lecture courses (Davis, 2007). Students have a tendency to rate required and elective courses in their own field of study higher than courses they are required to take outside their majors. Lastly, it is questionable whether students can evaluate the accuracy, depth, and scope of the teacher's knowledge because they do not have expertise in the content to make this judgment. Characteristics such as these are best evaluated by peers from one's own nursing education program or other institutions because those individuals have expertise in the content area.

Many colleges and universities have a standard form for student evaluation of teaching that is used in all courses across the institution. These forms generally ask students to rate the teacher's performance in areas of: (a) presentation and teaching skills, (b) interactions with students as a group and individually, (c) breadth of coverage of content, and (d) assessment and grading practices. Students also may be asked to provide a rating of the overall quality of the faculty member's teaching in the course, the extent of their own learning in the course, and the workload and difficulty of the course. Table 18.2 lists typical areas that are assessed by students on these forms.

Table 18.2

TYPICAL AREAS ASSESSED ON STUDENT EVALUATION OF TEACHING FORMS

Presentation or Teaching Skills
Organized course well
Gave clear explanations
Used examples, illustrations, and other methods to promote understanding of content
Was well prepared for class
Was enthusiastic about content and teaching
Stimulated students' interest in subject
Motivated students to do best work
Used learning activities, readings, and assignments that facilitated understanding of course content
Had realistic appreciation of time and effort for students to complete assignments and course work

Interactions With Students Individually and in Groups
Encouraged student participation and discussion
Showed respect for students' views and opinions
Was readily available to students (e.g., questions after class, by e-mail, by appointment)

Breadth of Coverage of Subject Matter
Demonstrated knowledge of course content
Presented different views and perspectives as appropriate

Assessment and Grading Practices
Communicated student responsibilities clearly
Explained course assignments, assessment methods, and grading procedures
Was fair in assessment and grading
Provided prompt and valuable feedback

(continued)

Table 18.2 (continued)

Overall Course Evaluation

Course difficulty (e.g., rated on scale of *too difficult* to *too elementary*)
Workload in course (e.g., rated on scale of *too heavy* to *too light*)
Course pace (e.g., rated on scale of *too fast* to *too slow*)
Extent of learning in course (e.g., rated on scale of *a great deal* to *nothing new*)
Overall course rating (e.g., rated on scale of *excellent* to *poor*)

Overall Teacher Evaluation

Overall quality of faculty member's teaching (e.g., rated on scale of *excellent* to *poor*)

These general forms, however, do not assess teacher behaviors important in the clinical setting. Faculty members can add questions on clinical teaching effectiveness to these general forms or can develop a separate tool for students to use in assessing teacher performance in clinical courses. Sample questions for evaluating the effectiveness of the clinical teacher are found in Table 18.3.

Students may complete teacher evaluations in class, administered by someone other than the teacher and without the teacher present in the

☐Table 18.3

SAMPLE QUESTIONS FOR EVALUATING EFFECTIVENESS OF CLINICAL TEACHERS

Clinical Teacher Evaluation

Purpose: These questions are intended for use in evaluating teacher effectiveness in courses with a clinical component. The questions are to be used in conjunction with the college or university student evaluation of teaching form.

Clinical Teaching Items

Did the teacher:

1. Encourage students to ask questions and express diverse views in the clinical setting?
2. Encourage application of theoretical knowledge to clinical practice?
3. Provide feedback on student strengths and weaknesses related to clinical performance?
4. Develop positive relationships with students in the clinical setting?
5. Inform students of their professional responsibilities?
6. Facilitate student collaboration with members of health care teams?
7. Facilitate learning in the clinical setting?
8. Strive to be available in the clinical setting to assist students?

Was the instructor:

9. An effective clinical teacher?

room, or they can be placed online. With an online course evaluation system, it is critical that students' anonymity and confidentiality be protected and that students have the computer capabilities to access the system. In many institutions, student services can be accessed online, and student evaluation of teaching forms can be made available at those sites. At Oregon State University, for example, students log on, navigate to the Student Online Services page, choose Student Records, and then select Online Course Evaluation (Oregon State University, 2012).

Assessment of teaching in online courses: Many colleges and universities use the same instruments for student evaluation of teaching both in traditional courses and online courses. However, because of the unique features of online courses, including reliance on technology for course delivery, the asynchronous nature of some or all learning activities, and physical separation of teacher and students, additional elements may be added to the student evaluation of teaching to reflect these differences or an entirely different instrument may be used. For example, students in online courses may assess the instructor's skill in using the course management system and other technology, facilitating online discussions and other interactions among students, and responding to student questions and comments within a reasonable period of time.

As with online course assessment, iNACOL standards and guidelines developed for assessing the quality of online teaching in K-12 education (Pape et al., 2011) may be adapted for use in higher education settings, including nursing education programs. Table 18.4 presents iNACOL standards and criteria that may be used to develop instruments for student assessment of online teaching.

A common challenge to administering online surveys for student assessment of teaching, however, is a response rate lower than that usually achieved when surveys are distributed to students in traditional courses during a regular class period by someone other than the teacher and without the teacher present. As previously discussed, the low response rate may be attributed to student concern about whether their responses will be anonymous or whether the teacher will be able to identify the source of specific ratings and comments, especially if surveys are administered within the online course site. One potential solution is to make electronic student assessment of teaching available from college or university websites that are separate from course management systems and specific course sites, as discussed above.

Peer Review

Another source of data for evaluating teacher effectiveness comes from peers. Peer review is a form of assessment in which instructors give

☐Table 18.4

iNACOL NATIONAL STANDARDS FOR QUALITY ONLINE TEACHING

STANDARD	PERFORMANCE CRITERIA
The online instructor:	The online instructor provides a learning environment that enables students to meet identified learning outcomes by:
Creates learning activities to enable student success	Using an array of online tools for communication, productivity, collaboration, assessment, presentation, and content delivery
	Incorporating multimedia and visual resources into online modules
Uses a range of technologies to support student learning	Performing basic troubleshooting skills and addressing basic technical issues of online students
Designs strategies to encourage active learning, interaction, participation, and collaboration in the online environment	Using online instructional strategies based on current research and practice (e.g., discussion, student-directed learning, collaborative learning, lecture, project-based learning, discussion forum, group work)
	Promoting student success through clear expectations, prompt responses, and regular feedback
Guides legal, ethical, and safe behavior related to technology use	Providing "netiquette" guidelines in the syllabus
	Establishing criteria for appropriate online behavior for both teacher and students
Demonstrates competence in creating and implementing assessments in online learning environments	Updating knowledge and skills of evolving technology that support online students' learning styles
	Addressing the diversity of student academic needs Recognizing and addressing the inappropriate use of electronically accessed data or information

Adapted from International Association for K-12 Online Learning. (2011). *National Standards for Quality Online Courses (Version 2)*. Retrieved from http://www.inacol.org/research/national-standards/iNACOL_CourseStandards_2011.pdf

feedback about teaching and learning to one another. Combined with other sources of information such as student learning outcomes, teacher self-assessment, and student feedback, peer review of teaching can be an important component of assessment of teaching. Peer review offers a perspective of another instructor who knows the course content and who has experience working with students at that level of the educational program (Center for Instructional Development and Research, n.d.). One form of peer evaluation is observing the teacher in the classroom, clinical setting, or laboratory. Observations of teaching performance are best used for formative evaluation because there are too many variables that can influence the reliability of these observations. The faculty member making the observation may not be an expert in that content or clinical practice area and may have limited understanding of how that particular class or practice experience fits into the overall course. Observations can be influenced too easily by personal feelings, positive or negative, about the colleague.

Peer evaluation of teaching can be conducted for online courses as well as in more traditional settings. By reviewing course materials and visiting course Web sites as guest users, peer evaluators of teaching in online courses can look for evidence that teachers demonstrate application of the following principles of effective instruction, such as:

- How quickly and thoroughly does the teacher respond to student questions?
- Does the teacher use group assignments, discussion boards, or peer critique of assignments to promote interaction and collaboration among students?
- Does the teacher use assignments that require the active involvement of students in their own learning?
- Does the teacher provide prompt, meaningful feedback on assignments posted to a course website or submitted via e-mail?
- Is there evidence that students are actively engaged and spend an appropriate amount of time on course tasks?
- Does the teacher have realistically high standards for achievement of course objectives and communicate them to students?
- Does the teacher accommodate a variety of learning modes, views, abilities, and preferences?
- Is the online course well organized, with easy-to-locate course material and clear directions?
- Is the Web design for the course inviting, are graphics used appropriately, and is color used in an appealing way?

Peers can review course syllabi, instructional materials, teaching strategies, learning activities, discussion board questions, tests, and other documents developed for courses; materials developed for clinical teaching and clinical learning activities; grants, publications, and similar materials documenting the teacher's scholarship; the teaching portfolio (see below); and other materials. This review can be used for formative purposes, to give suggestions for further development, or for summative purposes, to make decisions about contract renewal, tenure, promotion, and merit pay increases (personnel decisions).

To be most effective, peer review of teaching should take place within a context of continuous improvement of the teaching–learning process. It must be supported by adequate resources for faculty development, mentoring, and modeling of effective teaching by master teachers (Center for Instructional Evaluation and Research, n.d.).

Teaching Portfolio

Another approach to documenting teaching effectiveness is the use of a teaching portfolio or dossier. More than just a curriculum vitae, the portfolio is a collection of teacher-selected materials or artifacts that describe the faculty member's teaching activities in the classroom, the online environment, clinical practice, the simulation center, and other settings where the instruction took place. The materials included in the portfolio should be highly selective and organized to create a cohesive professional narrative.

Teaching portfolios may serve a specific purpose, such as for teaching improvement (formative assessment) or promotion or tenure review (summative assessment). A career portfolio might be assembled and used to seek a faculty position. While some portfolios are assembled from printed materials, an electronic format is becoming widely used (University of Michigan School of Nursing, 2012).

A teaching portfolio should contain materials that illustrate the faculty member's teaching effectiveness, such as syllabi, teaching strategies, sample tests, student assignments, and online materials, to name a few. The portfolio also includes the faculty member's philosophy of teaching, which should be reflected in the documents in the portfolio. Table 18.5 lists materials typically included in a portfolio for personnel decisions, such as contract renewal, tenure, promotion, and merit pay increases.

⬜Table 18.5

SUGGESTED CONTENT OF A TEACHING PORTFOLIO

Material From the Faculty Member

Personal philosophy of teaching

Statement about teaching goals

Description of teaching responsibilities (e.g., classroom instruction, online teaching, clinical instruction)

List of courses taught with dates

Course syllabus, sample teaching strategies, materials, assignments, online activities and discussion board questions, tests, instructional media, and other documents from one or more courses (documents should reflect the types of courses taught, e.g., classroom, online, clinical, laboratory, seminar)

An edited 5-minute videotape of a class or a segment from an online course

Teaching awards and recognition of teaching effectiveness (by alumni, clinical agency personnel, others)

Table 18.5 *(continued)*

Material From Students

Samples of student papers, good and poor, with teacher's written comments; other products of student learning

Unsolicited letters from students, alumni, and clinical agency staff who work with students addressing the faculty member's teaching effectiveness (a few that are carefully selected)

Material From Colleagues and Administrators

Peer evaluation of teaching materials

Other Documents

Self-appraisal and teaching goals (short and long term)

Appendices

Portfolios for instructional improvement include these same materials, but also identify areas of teaching that need improvement and efforts to further develop teaching skills such as workshops attended. In this type of teaching portfolio, peer and administrator evaluations of teaching, a self-evaluation of strengths and weaknesses, and other documents that demonstrate areas for improvement and steps taken can be included. However, these are not appropriate for a teaching portfolio that will be used for personnel decisions.

SUMMARY

Program assessment is the process of judging the worth or value of an educational program for the purposes of making decisions about the program or to provide evidence of its effectiveness in response to demands for accountability. A number of models can be used for program assessment, including accreditation, decision-oriented, and systems-oriented approaches. Accreditation models are designed to determine whether a program meets external standards of quality and typically use a combination of self-study and site visits to the institution by an assessment team. Current accreditation criteria reflect the importance of evaluating program outcomes in an effort to ensure quality and increase accountability. Decision-oriented models usually focus on internal standards of quality, value, and efficacy to provide information for making decisions about the program. Systems-oriented approaches consider the inputs, processes or operations, and outputs or outcomes of an educational program.

The process of program assessment assists various audiences or stakeholders of an educational program in judging its worth. Audiences or stakeholders are individuals and groups who are affected directly or indirectly by the decisions made, such as students, teachers, employers, clinical agencies, and the public. An important decision when planning a program assessment is whether to use external or internal evaluators or both.

One area of program assessment involves determining the quality of teaching in the classroom and clinical setting and other dimensions of the teacher's role, depending on the goals and mission of the nursing program. The literature suggests five characteristics and qualities of effective teaching in nursing: (a) knowledge of the subject matter, (b) clinical competence, (c) teaching skill, (d) interpersonal relationships with students, and (e) personal characteristics. Teaching effectiveness data are available from a variety of sources, including students, faculty peers, and administrators. The use of a teaching portfolio as a way to document teaching effectiveness is another approach that allows the teacher to select and comment on items that reflect implementation of a personal philosophy of teaching.

The chapter also discussed modifications of program assessment approaches for online nursing education programs or courses. Standards for assessing online courses and online teaching were described.

REFERENCES

Andrew, S., Halcomb, E. J., Jackson, D., Peters, K., & Salamonson, Y. (2010). Sessional teachers in a BN program: Bridging the divide or widening the gap? *Nurse Education Today, 30*, 453–457.

Berg, C. L., & Lindseth, G. (2004). Students' perspectives of effective and ineffective nursing instructors. *Journal of Nursing Education, 43*, 565–568.

Brown, J. F., & Marshall, B. L. (2008). Continuous quality improvement: An effective strategy for improvement of program outcomes in a higher education setting. *Nursing Education Perspectives, 4*, 205–211.

Caputi, L. (2011). Program approval and accreditation. In T. J. Bristol & J. Zerwekh (Eds.), *Essentials of e-learning for nurse educators* (pp. 295–307). Philadelphia, PA: F. A. Davis.

Center for Instructional Development and Research. (n. d.). *Consultation: Peer review of teaching.* University of Washington, Seattle, WA. Retrieved from http://depts.washington.edu/cidrweb/consulting/peer-review.html

Commission on Collegiate Nursing Education. (2009). *Standards for accreditation of baccalaureate and graduate degree nursing programs.* Retrieved from http://www.aacn.nche.edu/Accreditation/pdf/standards09.pdf

Davis, B. G. (2007). *Tools for teaching. Student rating forms.* University of California Berkeley. Retrieved October 31, 2008, from http://teaching.berkeley.edu/bgd/ratingforms.html

Davis, B. W. (2011). A conceptual model to support curriculum review, revision, and design in an associate degree nursing program. *Nursing Education Perspectives, 32*, 389–394.

Deming, W. E. (1986). *Out of the crisis.* Cambridge, MA: Massachusetts Institute of Technology, Center for Advanced Engineering Study.

Gaberson, K. B., & Oermann, M. H. (2010). *Clinical teaching strategies in nursing* (3rd ed.). New York, NY: Springer Publishing.

Giddens, J. F., & Morton, N. (2010). Report card: An evaluation of a concept-based curriculum. *Nursing Education Perspectives, 31*, 371–377.

Iwasiw, C., Goldenberg, D., & Andrusyszyn, M.-A. (2009). *Curriculum development in nursing education* (2nd ed.). Boston, MA: Jones & Bartlett.

National League for Nursing. (2005). *Core competencies of nurse educators with task statements*. Retrieved from http://www.nln.org/facultyprograms/pdf/corecompetencies.pdf

National League for Nursing Accreditation Commission. (2012). *NLNAC accreditation manual*. Retrieved from http://www.nlnac.org/manuals/NLNACManual2008.pdf

O'Neil, C. A., Fisher, C. A., & Newbold, S. K. (2009). *Developing an online course: Best practices for nurse educators* (2nd ed.). New York, NY: Springer Publishing.

Oregon State University. (2012). *Online course evaluations: Student evaluation of teaching*. Retrieved from http://ecampus.oregonstate.edu/soc/start/onlinecourse-evaluation.htm

Pape, L., Wicks, M., & the iNACOL Quality Standards for Online Programs Committee. (2011). *National standards for quality online programs*. Vienna, VA: International Association for K-12 Online Learning. Retrieved from http://www.eric.ed.gov/PDFS/ED509638.pdf

Salamonson, Y., Halcomb, E. J., Andrew, S., Peters, K., & Jackson, D. (2010). A comparative study of assessment grading and nursing students' perceptions of quality in sessional and tenured teachers. *Journal of Nursing Scholarship, 42*, 423–429.

Sitzman, K. (2010). Student-preferred caring behaviors for online nursing education. *Nursing Education Perspectives, 31*, 171–178.

Stufflebeam, D. L., & Shinkfield, A. J. (2007). *Evaluation theory, models, and applications*. San Francisco, CA: Jossey-Bass.

Tang, F., Chou, S., & Chiang, H. (2005). Students' perceptions of effective and ineffective clinical instructors. *Journal of Nursing Education, 44*, 187–192.

University of Michigan School of Nursing. (2012). *Faculty portfolios*. Retrieved from http://www.nursing.umich.edu/about-our-school/computing-technology/electronic-portfolios/faculty-portfolios

Wolf, Z. R., Bender, P. J., Beitz, J. M., Wieland, D. M., & Vito, K. O. (2004). Strengths and weaknesses of faculty teaching performance reported by undergraduate and graduate nursing students: A descriptive study. *Journal of Professional Nursing, 20*, 118–128.

APPENDICES ❑

A □

Code of Fair Testing

Practices in Education

PREPARED BY THE JOINT COMMITTEE ON TESTING PRACTICES

The Code of Fair Testing Practices in Education (*Code*) is a guide for professionals in fulfilling their obligation to provide and use tests that are fair to all test takers regardless of age, gender, disability, race, ethnicity, national origin, religion, sexual orientation, linguistic background, or other personal characteristics. Fairness is a primary consideration in all aspects of testing. Careful standardization of tests and administration conditions helps to ensure that all test takers are given a comparable opportunity to demonstrate what they know and how they can perform in the area being tested. Fairness implies that every test-taker has the opportunity to prepare for the test and is informed about the general nature and content of the test, as appropriate to the purpose of the test. Fairness also extends to the accurate reporting of individual and group test results. Fairness is not an isolated concept, but must be considered in all aspects of the testing process.

The *Code* applies broadly to testing in education (admissions, educational assessment, educational diagnosis, and student placement) regardless of the mode of presentation, so it is relevant to conventional paper-and-pencil tests, computer-based tests, and performance tests. It is not designed to cover employment testing, licensure or certification testing, or other types of testing outside the field of education. The *Code* is directed primarily at professionally developed tests used in formally administered testing programs. Although the *Code* is not intended to cover tests made by teachers for use in their own classrooms, teachers are encouraged to use the guidelines to help improve their testing practices.

The *Code* addresses the roles of test developers and test users separately. Test developers are people and organizations that construct tests, as well as those who set policies for testing programs. Test users are people and agencies that select tests, administer tests, commission test development services, or make decisions on the basis of test scores. Test-developer and test-user roles may overlap, for example, when a state or local education agency commissions test development services, sets policies that control the test development process, and makes decisions on the basis of the test scores.

Many of the statements in the *Code* refer to the selection and use of existing tests. When a new test is developed, when an existing test is modified, or when the administration of a test is modified, the *Code* is intended to provide guidance for this process.

The *Code* is not intended to be mandatory, exhaustive, or definitive, and may not be applicable to every situation. Instead, the *Code* is intended to be aspirational and is not intended to take precedence over the judgment of those who have competence in the subjects addressed.

The *Code* provides guidance separately for test developers and test users in four critical areas:

A. Developing and Selecting Appropriate Tests
B. Administering and Scoring Tests
C. Reporting and Interpreting Test Results
D. Informing Test Takers

A. DEVELOPING AND SELECTING APPROPRIATE TESTS

Test Developers	Test Users
Test developers should provide the information and supporting evidence that test users need to select appropriate tests.	Test users should select tests that meet the intended purpose and that are appropriate for the intended test takers.
A-1. Provide evidence of what the test measures, the recommended uses, the intended test takers, and the strengths and limitations of the test, including the level of precision of the test scores.	A-1. Define the purpose for testing, the content and skills to be tested, and the intended test takers. Select and use the most appropriate test based on a thorough review of available information.
A-2. Describe how the content and skills to be tested were selected and how the tests were developed.	A-2. Review and select tests based on the appropriateness of test content, skills tested, and content coverage for the intended purpose of testing.
A-3. Communicate information about a test's characteristics at a level of detail appropriate to the intended test users.	A-3. Review materials provided by test developers and select tests for which clear, accurate, and complete information is provided.
A-4. Provide guidance on the levels of skills, knowledge, and training necessary for appropriate review, selection, and administration of tests.	A-4. Select tests through a process that includes persons with appropriate knowledge, skills, and training.

Test Developers	Test Users
A-5. Provide evidence that the technical quality, including reliability and validity, of the test meets its intended purposes.	A-5. Evaluate evidence of the technical quality of the test provided by the test developer and any independent reviewers.
A-6. Provide to qualified test users representative samples of test questions or practice tests, directions, answer sheets, manuals, and score reports.	A-6. Evaluate representative samples of test questions or practice tests, directions, answer sheets, manuals, and score reports before selecting a test.
A-7. Avoid potentially offensive content or language when developing test questions and related materials.	A-7. Evaluate procedures and materials used by test developers, as well as the resulting test, to ensure that potentially offensive content or language is avoided.
A-8. Make appropriately modified forms of tests or administration procedures available for test takers with disabilities who need special accommodations.	A-8. Select tests with appropriately modified forms or administration procedures for test takers with disabilities who need special accommodations.
A-9. Obtain and provide evidence on the performance of test takers of diverse subgroups, making significant efforts to obtain sample sizes that are adequate for subgroup analyses. Evaluate the evidence to ensure that differences in performance are related to the skills being assessed.	A-9. Evaluate the available evidence on the performance of test takers of diverse subgroups. Determine to the extent feasible which performance differences may have been caused by factors unrelated to the skills being assessed.

B. ADMINISTERING AND SCORING TESTS

Test Developers	Test Users
Test developers should explain how to administer and score tests correctly and fairly.	Test users should administer and score tests correctly and fairly.
B-1. Provide clear descriptions of detailed procedures for administering tests in a standardized manner.	B-1. Follow established procedures for administering tests in a standardized manner.
B-2. Provide guidelines on reasonable procedures for assessing persons with disabilities who need special accommodations or those with diverse linguistic backgrounds.	B-2. Provide and document appropriate procedures for test takers with disabilities who need special accommodations or those with diverse linguistic backgrounds. Some accommodations may be required by law or regulation.
B-3. Provide information to test takers or test users on test question formats and procedures for answering test questions, including information on the use of any needed materials and equipment.	B-3. Provide test takers with an opportunity to become familiar with test question formats and any materials or equipment that may be used during testing.

Test Developers	Test Users
B-4. Establish and implement procedures to ensure the security of testing materials during all phases of test development, administration, scoring, and reporting.	B-4. Protect the security of test materials, including respecting copyrights and eliminating opportunities for test takers to obtain scores by fraudulent means.
B-5. Provide procedures, materials, and guidelines for scoring the tests, and for monitoring the accuracy of the scoring process. If scoring the test is the responsibility of the test developer, provide adequate training for scorers.	B-5. If test scoring is the responsibility of the test user, provide adequate training to scorers and ensure and monitor the accuracy of the scoring process.
B-6. Correct errors that affect the interpretation of the scores and communicate the corrected results promptly.	B-6. Correct errors that affect the interpretation of the scores and communicate the corrected results promptly.
B-7. Develop and implement procedures for ensuring the confidentiality of scores.	B-7. Develop and implement procedures for ensuring the confidentiality of scores.

C. REPORTING AND INTERPRETING TEST RESULTS

Test Developers	Test Users
Test developers should report test results accurately and provide information to help test users interpret test results correctly.	Test users should report and interpret test results accurately and clearly.
C-1. Provide information to support recommended interpretations of the results, including the nature of the content, norms or comparison groups, and other technical evidence. Advise test users of the benefits and limitations of test results and their interpretation. Warn against assigning greater precision than is warranted.	C-1. Interpret the meaning of the test results, taking into account the nature of the content, norms or comparison groups, other technical evidence, and benefits and limitations of test results.
C-2. Provide guidance regarding the interpretations of results for tests administered with modifications. Inform test users of potential problems in interpreting test results when tests or test administration procedures are modified.	C-2. Interpret test results from modified test or test administration procedures in view of the impact those modifications may have had on test results.
C-3. Specify appropriate uses of test results and warn test users of potential misuses.	C-3. Avoid using tests for purposes other than those recommended by the test developer unless there is evidence to support the intended use or interpretation.
C-4. When test developers set standards, provide the rationale, procedures, and evidence for setting performance standards or passing scores. Avoid using stigmatizing labels.	C-4. Review the procedures for setting performance standards or passing scores. Avoid using stigmatizing labels.

Test Developers	Test Users
C-5. Encourage test users to base decisions about test takers on multiple sources of appropriate information, not on a single test score.	C-5. Avoid using a single test score as the sole determinant of decisions about test takers. Interpret test scores in conjunction with other information about individuals.
C-6. Provide information to enable test users to accurately interpret and report test results for groups of test takers, including information about who were and who were not included in the different groups being compared, and information about factors that might influence the interpretation of results.	C-6. State the intended interpretation and use of test results for groups of test takers. Avoid grouping test results for purposes not specifically recommended by the test developer unless evidence is obtained to support the intended use. Report procedures that were followed in determining who were and who were not included in the groups being compared and describe factors that might influence the interpretation of results.
C-7. Provide test results in a timely fashion and in a manner that is understood by the test taker.	C-7. Communicate test results in a timely fashion and in a manner that is understood by the test taker.
C-8. Provide guidance to test users about how to monitor the extent to which the test is fulfilling its intended purposes.	C-8. Develop and implement procedures for monitoring test use, including consistency with the intended purposes of the test.

D. INFORMING TEST TAKERS

Test developers or test users should inform test takers about the nature of the test, test taker rights and responsibilities, the appropriate use of scores, and procedures for resolving challenges to scores.

D-1. Inform test takers in advance of the test administration about the coverage of the test, the types of question formats, the directions, and appropriate test-taking strategies. Make such information available to all test takers.

D-2. When a test is optional, provide test takers or their parents/guardians with information to help them judge whether a test should be taken—including indications of any consequences that may result from not taking the test (e.g., not being eligible to compete for a particular scholarship)—and whether there is an available alternative to the test.

D-3. Provide test takers or their parents/guardians with information about rights test takers may have to obtain copies of tests and completed answer sheets, to retake tests, to have tests rescored, or to have scores declared invalid.

D-4. Provide test takers or their parents/guardians with information about responsibilities test takers have, such as being aware of the intended purpose and uses of the test, performing at capacity, following directions, and not disclosing test items or interfering with other test takers.

D-5. Inform test takers or their parents/guardians how long scores will be kept on file and indicate to whom, under what circumstances, and in what manner test scores and related information will or will not be released. Protect test scores from unauthorized release and access.

D-6. Describe procedures for investigating and resolving circumstances that might result in canceling or withholding scores, such as failure to adhere to specified testing procedures.

D-7. Describe procedures that test takers, parents/guardians, and other interested parties may use to obtain more information about the test, register complaints, and have problems resolved.

Under some circumstances, test developers have direct communication with the test-takers and/or control of the tests, testing process, and test results. In other circumstances the test users have these responsibilities.

The *Code* is intended to be consistent with the relevant parts of the Standards for Educational and Psychological Testing (American Educational Research Association [AERA], American Psychological Association [APA], and National Council on Measurement in Education [NCME], 1999). The *Code* is not meant to add new principles over and above those in the Standards or to change their meaning. Rather, the *Code* is intended to represent the spirit of selected portions of the Standards in a way that is relevant and meaningful to developers and users of tests, as well as to test takers and/or their parents or guardians. States, districts, schools, organizations, and individual professionals are encouraged to commit themselves to fairness in testing and safeguarding the rights of test takers. The *Code* is intended to assist in carrying out such commitments.

The *Code* has been prepared by the Joint Committee on Testing Practices, a cooperative effort among several professional organizations. The aim of the Joint Committee is to act, in the public interest, to advance the quality of testing practices. Members of the Joint Committee include the American Counseling Association (ACA), the AERA, the APA, the American Speech-Language-Hearing Association (ASHA), the National Association of School Psychologists (NASP), the National Association of Test Directors (NATD), and the NCME.

Note: The membership of the Working Group that developed the *Code of Fair Testing Practices in Education* and of the Joint Committee on Testing Practices that guided the Working Group is as follows:

Peter Behuniak, PhD

Lloyd Bond, PhD

Gwyneth M. Boodoo, PhD

Wayne Camara, PhD

Ray Fenton, PhD

John J. Fremer, PhD (Co-Chair)

Sharon M. Goldsmith, PhD

Bert F. Green, PhD

William G. Harris, PhD

Janet E. Helms, PhD

Stephanie H. McConaughy, PhD

Julie P. Noble, PhD

Wayne M. Patience, PhD

Carole L. Perlman, PhD

Douglas K. Smith, PhD
(deceased)

Janet E. Wall, EdD (Co-Chair)

Pat Nellor Wickwire, PhD

Mary Yakimowski, PhD

Lara Frumkin, PhD, of the APA
served as staff liaison.

National League for Nursing
Fair Testing Guidelines for
Nursing Education

Developed by the National League for Nursing (NLN) Presidential Task Force on High-Stakes Testing, the Fair Testing Guidelines for Nursing Education are based on the League's core values of caring, integrity, diversity, and excellence, and on widely accepted testing principles. Fair, in this context, means that all test-takers are given comparable opportunities to demonstrate what they know and are able to do in the learning area being tested (Code of Fair Testing Practices in Education, 2004).

These guidelines have been formulated within the context of an overall need for testing. We acknowledge that faculty are fully committed to assessing students' abilities and to assuring that they are competent to practice nursing. Faculty are also cognizant that current approaches to learning assessment are limited and imperfect.

The NLN supports the belief that tests and evaluative measures are used not only to evaluate student achievement but, as importantly, to support student learning, and evaluate and improve teaching and program effectiveness. Within this framework, the standards for testing in high stakes situations are consistent with general practices for ethical and fair testing practices.

The NLN Fair Testing Guidelines for Nursing Education value students' perspectives and backgrounds and acknowledge the role of faculty in their implementation.

    I. General Guidelines
        A. Faculty have an ethical obligation to ensure that both tests and the decisions based on tests are valid, supported by solid evidence, consistent across their programs, and fair to all test takers

regardless of age, gender, disability, race, ethnicity, national origin, religion, sexual orientation, linguistic background, testing style and ability, or other personal characteristics.

B. Faculty have the responsibility to assess students' abilities and assure that they are competent to practice nursing, while recognizing that current approaches to learning assessment are limited and imperfect.

C. Multiple sources of evidence are required to evaluate basic nursing competence. Multiple approaches for assessment of knowledge and clinical abilities are particularly critical when high-stakes decisions (such as progression or graduation) are based on the assessment.

D. Tests and other evaluative measures are used not only to evaluate students' achievements, but, as importantly, to support student learning, improve teaching and guide program improvements.

E. Standardized tests must have comprehensive testing, administration, and evaluation information readily available to faculty before they administer, grade, distribute results, or write related policies for test results. Faculty have the responsibility to review and incorporate these materials in communications to students about standardized testing and its consequences.

F. Faculty and schools of nursing have an ethical obligation to protect every student's right to privacy by maintaining appropriate confidentiality related to the testing process and to test results.

II. Test Development and Implementation

    A. Selecting Appropriate Tests

        1. Standardized tests must show evidence of reliability, content and predictive validity, and evidence of fairness and equity as shown by test performance across test-taking subgroups based on culture, race, or gender.

        2. Tests should be appropriate to their purpose and have good technical quality.

        3. Tests should be screened for offensive content or scenarios.

        4. Tests should be reviewed regularly for content accuracy and relevance to practice.

        5. Test vendors should provide technical manuals that provide information on the test's blueprint, test development procedures, psychometric testing, and norms.

    B. Informing Test Takers

        1. Students should be notified as early as possible about the nature and content of the test and any consequences of taking the test (i.e., how test scores will be used).

        2. Students should be informed about the test's different modalities (print, web, verbal) and available accommodations.

3. A process should be implemented to document that students have read, understood, and accepted the guidelines.

C. Administering and Scoring Tests

1. Detailed test administration procedures should be clearly outlined ahead of time and adhered to (time frame, use of books/notes).
2. Scoring procedures for evaluative measures (clinical performance, simulation, case analysis, etc.) should be delineated.
3. Interrater reliability should be regularly assessed.
4. Psychometric analysis should be used when possible to assure that the test is valid and internally consistent.
5. Methods of protecting the integrity of test items for standardized tests or other forms of testing, in which the items will be used in more than one context, should be clearly defined.

D. Reporting/Interpreting Test Results

1. Detailed norming information on standardized tests should be provided.
2. On tests used for predictive purposes, periodic evaluation of predictive validity should be included.
3. More than one mode of learning assessment should be used to make high stakes decisions.

III. Recommendations to Achieve a Fair Testing Environment

A. Convene a culturally and demographically representative group of faculty, students, and administrators to review your program's current high stakes testing plans and policies.

Through the input of a diverse group of people affected by testing policies, new understanding about high stakes tests and their consequences can be mutually discovered. All members of your review group should feel free to share their knowledge about the tests, their perceptions of how tests are used and their intended purposes, and the consequences of any change to testing policy.

B. As a faculty, undertake a thoughtful and comprehensive review of the factors leading to the development and implementation of high stakes testing in your program.

Program quality encompasses more than what is measured by licensure exam pass rates. The nursing education literature and stories from students and faculty alike reveal that high stakes tests are often quickly implemented in response to both internal and external pressures. The feeling of *having done something* can unintentionally divert faculty attention from other systems-related issues that bear on NCLEX-RN® pass rates and other measures of program quality. Factors such as admissions policies, instructional effectiveness, remediation and study requirements, and course-level assessments are all valid aspects of the educational process for review and improvement.

C. Invite faculty or other experts with experience using high stakes tests to provide feedback on how high stakes tests are best used within the context of national guidelines, ethical considerations, and regulatory requirements.

Faculty members from other disciplines such as psychology, educational assessment, and psychometrics may have a longer history of using high stakes tests in their educational practice. This could also be an opportunity to seek legal review of testing policies. This step is often overlooked during policy development but is increasingly important as schools seek to avoid costly and time consuming legal battles, and the negative publicity that ensues.

D. Until more formal studies are done, seek out and learn the practices of schools that have not needed to implement high-stakes testing, or that use tests in non-high stakes ways, but still achieve excellent NCLEX-RN pass rates.

Across the nation—likely in every state—there are nursing education programs that maintain high NCLEX-RN pass rates. These programs admit very diverse students from a range of educational backgrounds, provide outstanding educational experiences, and have high retention rates. Students graduate from these programs, successfully pass the licensing exam, and enter the nursing workforce well prepared. Much could be learned about the effective practices and characteristics of these schools; their strengths are worthy of study and possible replication.

E. Develop a communications plan for students and faculty that conveys essential information about your testing policy and practices.

Reassure students and faculty that local testing policies are aligned with NLN Fair Testing Guidelines, that there is strong psychometric support for using tests in fair and effective ways, and that testing policy, like other components of the overall assessment plan, considers the input of a variety of constituents, including students, faculty, and program leaders.

Code of Fair Testing Practices in Education. (2004). Washington, DC: Joint Committee on Testing Practices. http://www.apa.org/science/programs/testing/fair-code.aspx. Reprinted by permission of the National League for Nursing, New York, NY, 2012. Copyright, National League for Nursing, 2012.

Code of Professional Responsibilities

in Educational Measurement

Prepared by the
NCME Ad Hoc Committee on the Development of a Code of Ethics:
Cynthia B. Schmeiser, ACT—Chair
Kurt F. Geisinger, State University of New York
Sharon Johnson-Lewis, Detroit Public Schools
Edward D. Roeber, Council of Chief State School Officers
William D. Schafer, University of Maryland

PREAMBLE AND GENERAL RESPONSIBILITIES

As an organization dedicated to the improvement of measurement and evaluation practice in education, the National Council on Measurement in Education (NCME) has adopted this Code to promote professionally responsible practice in educational measurement. Professionally responsible practice is conduct that arises from either the professional standards of the field, general ethical principles, or both.

The purpose of the Code of Professional Responsibilities in Educational Measurement, hereinafter referred to as the Code, is to guide the conduct of NCME members who are involved in any type of assessment activity in education. NCME is also providing this Code as a public service for all individuals who are engaged in educational assessment activities in the hope that these activities will be conducted in a professionally responsible manner. Persons who engage in these activities include local educators such as classroom teachers, principals, and superintendents; professionals such as school psychologists and counselors; state and national technical, legislative, and policy staff in education; staff of research, evaluation, and testing organizations; providers of test preparation services; college and university faculty and administrators; and professionals in business and industry who design and implement educational and training programs.

This Code applies to any type of assessment that occurs as part of the educational process, including formal and informal, traditional and alternative techniques for gathering information used in making educational decisions at all levels. These techniques include, but are not limited to, large-scale assessments at the school, district, state, national, and international levels; standardized tests; observational measures; teacher-conducted assessments; assessment support materials; and other achievement, aptitude, interest, and personality measures used in and for education.

Although NCME is promulgating this Code for its members, it strongly encourages other organizations and individuals who engage in educational assessment activities to endorse and abide by the responsibilities relevant to their professions. Because the Code pertains only to uses of assessment in education, it is recognized that uses of assessments outside of educational contexts, such as for employment, certification, or licensure, may involve additional professional responsibilities beyond those detailed in this Code.

The Code is intended to serve an educational function: to inform and remind those involved in educational assessment of their obligations to uphold the integrity of the manner in which assessments are developed, used, evaluated, and marketed. Moreover, it is expected that the Code will stimulate thoughtful discussion of what constitutes professionally responsible assessment practice at all levels in education.

SECTION 1: RESPONSIBILITIES OF THOSE WHO DEVELOP ASSESSMENT PRODUCTS AND SERVICES

Those who develop assessment products and services, such as classroom teachers and other assessment specialists, have a professional responsibility to strive to produce assessments that are of the highest quality. Persons who develop assessments have a professional responsibility to:

1.1 ensure that assessment products and services are developed to meet applicable professional, technical, and legal standards
1.2 develop assessment products and services that are as free as possible from bias due to characteristics irrelevant to the construct

being measured, such as gender, ethnicity, race, socioeconomic status, disability, religion, age, or national origin

1.3 plan accommodations for groups of test takers with disabilities and other special needs when developing assessments

1.4 disclose to appropriate parties any actual or potential conflicts of interest that might influence the developers' judgment or performance

1.5 use copyrighted materials in assessment products and services in accordance with state and federal law

1.6 make information available to appropriate persons about the steps taken to develop and score the assessment, including up-to-date information used to support the reliability, validity, scoring and reporting processes, and other relevant characteristics of the assessment

1.7 protect the rights of privacy of those who are assessed as part of the assessment development process

1.8 caution users, in clear and prominent language, against the most likely misinterpretations and misuses of data that arise out of the assessment development process

1.9 avoid false or unsubstantiated claims in test preparation and program support materials and services about an assessment or its use and interpretation

1.10 correct any substantive inaccuracies in assessments or their support materials as soon as feasible

1.11 develop score reports and support materials that promote the understanding of assessment results

SECTION 2: RESPONSIBILITIES OF THOSE WHO MARKET AND SELL ASSESSMENT PRODUCTS AND SERVICES

The marketing of assessment products and services, such as tests and other instruments, scoring services, test preparation services, consulting, and test interpretive services, should be based on information that is accurate, complete, and relevant to those considering their use. Persons who market and sell assessment products and services have a professional responsibility to:

2.1 provide accurate information to potential purchasers about assessment products and services and their recommended uses and limitations

2.2 not knowingly withhold relevant information about assessment products and services that might affect an appropriate selection decision

2.3 base all claims about assessment products and services on valid interpretations of publicly available information

2.4 allow qualified users equal opportunity to purchase assessment products and services

2.5 establish reasonable fees for assessment products and services

2.6 communicate to potential users, in advance of any purchase or use, all applicable fees associated with assessment products and services

2.7 strive to ensure that no individuals are denied access to opportunities because of their inability to pay the fees for assessment products and services

2.8 establish criteria for the sale of assessment products and services, such as limiting the sale of assessment products and services to those individuals who are qualified for recommended uses and from whom proper uses and interpretations are anticipated

2.9 inform potential users of known inappropriate uses of assessment products and services and provide recommendations about how to avoid such misuses

2.10 maintain a current understanding about assessment products and services and their appropriate uses in education

2.11 release information implying endorsement by users of assessment products and services only with the users' permission

2.12 avoid making claims that assessment products and services have been endorsed by another organization unless an official endorsement has been obtained

2.13 avoid marketing test preparation products and services that may cause individuals to receive scores that misrepresent their actual levels of attainment

SECTION 3: RESPONSIBILITIES OF THOSE WHO SELECT ASSESSMENT PRODUCTS AND SERVICES

Those who select assessment products and services for use in educational settings, or help others do so, have important professional responsibilities to make sure that the assessments are appropriate for their intended use. Persons who select assessment products and services have a professional responsibility to:

3.1 conduct a thorough review and evaluation of available assessment strategies and instruments that might be valid for the intended uses

3.2 recommend and/or select assessments based on publicly available documented evidence of their technical quality and utility rather than on insubstantial claims or statements

3.3 disclose any associations or affiliations that they have with the authors, test publishers, or others involved with the assessments under consideration for purchase and refrain from participation if such associations might affect the objectivity of the selection process

3.4 inform decision makers and prospective users of the appropriateness of the assessment for the intended uses, likely consequences of use, protection of examinee rights, relative costs, materials and services needed to conduct or use the assessment, and known limitations of the assessment, including potential misuses and misinterpretations of assessment information

3.5 recommend against the use of any prospective assessment that is likely to be administered, scored, and used in an invalid manner for members of various groups in our society for reasons of race, ethnicity, gender, age, disability, language background, socioeconomic status, religion, or national origin

3.6 comply with all security precautions that may accompany assessments being reviewed

3.7 immediately disclose any attempts by others to exert undue influence on the assessment selection process

3.8 avoid recommending, purchasing, or using test preparation products and services that may cause individuals to receive scores that misrepresent their actual levels of attainment

SECTION 4: RESPONSIBILITIES
OF THOSE WHO ADMINISTER ASSESSMENTS

Those who prepare individuals to take assessments and those who are directly or indirectly involved in the administration of assessments as part of the educational process, including teachers, administrators, and assessment personnel, have an important role in making sure that the assessments are administered in a fair and accurate manner. Persons who prepare others for, and those who administer, assessments have a professional responsibility to:

4.1 inform the examinees about the assessment prior to its administration, including its purposes, uses, and consequences; how the assessment information will be judged or scored; how the results will be distributed; and examinees' rights before, during, and after the assessment

4.2 administer only those assessments for which they are qualified by education, training, licensure, or certification

4.3 take appropriate security precautions before, during and after the administration of the assessment

4.4 understand the procedures needed to administer the assessment prior to administration

4.5 administer standardized assessments according to prescribed procedures and conditions and notify appropriate persons if any nonstandard or delimiting conditions occur

4.6 not exclude any eligible student from the assessment

4.7 avoid any conditions in the conduct of the assessment that might invalidate the results

4.8 provide for and document all reasonable and allowable accommodations for the administration of the assessment to persons with disabilities or special needs

4.9 provide reasonable opportunities for individuals to ask questions about the assessment procedures or directions prior to and at prescribed times during the administration of the assessment

4.10 protect the rights to privacy and due process of those who are assessed

4.11 avoid actions or conditions that would permit or encourage individuals or groups to receive scores that misrepresent their actual levels of attainment

SECTION 5: RESPONSIBILITIES OF THOSE WHO SCORE ASSESSMENTS

The scoring of educational assessments should be conducted properly and efficiently so that the results are reported accurately and in a timely manner. Persons who score and prepare reports of assessments have a professional responsibility to:

5.1 provide complete and accurate information to users about how the assessment is scored, such as the reporting schedule, scoring process to be used, rationale for the scoring approach, technical characteristics, quality control procedures, reporting formats, and the fees, if any, for these services

5.2 ensure the accuracy of the assessment results by conducting reasonable quality control procedures before, during, and after scoring

5.3 minimize the effect on scoring of factors irrelevant to the purposes of the assessment

5.4 inform users promptly of any deviation in the planned scoring and reporting service or schedule and negotiate a solution with users

5.5 provide corrected score results to the examinee or the client as quickly as practicable should errors be found that may affect the inferences made on the basis of the scores

5.6 protect the confidentiality of information that identifies individuals as prescribed by state and federal law

5.7 release summary results of the assessment only to those persons entitled to such information by state or federal law or those who are designated by the party contracting for the scoring services

5.8 establish, where feasible, a fair and reasonable process for appeal and rescoring the assessment

SECTION 6: RESPONSIBILITIES OF THOSE WHO INTERPRET, USE, AND COMMUNICATE ASSESSMENT RESULTS

The interpretation, use, and communication of assessment results should promote valid inferences and minimize invalid ones. Persons who interpret, use, and communicate assessment results have a professional responsibility to:

6.1 conduct these activities in an informed, objective, and fair manner within the context of the assessment's limitations and with an understanding of the potential consequences of use

6.2 provide to those who receive assessment results information about the assessment, its purposes, its limitations, and its uses necessary for the proper interpretation of the results

6.3 provide to those who receive score reports an understandable written description of all reported scores, including proper interpretations and likely misinterpretations

6.4 communicate to appropriate audiences the results of the assessment in an understandable and timely manner, including proper interpretations and likely misinterpretations

6.5 evaluate and communicate the adequacy and appropriateness of any norms or standards used in the interpretation of assessment results

6.6 inform parties involved in the assessment process how assessment results may affect them

6.7 use multiple sources and types of relevant information about persons or programs whenever possible in making educational decisions

6.8 avoid making, and actively discourage others from making, inaccurate reports, unsubstantiated claims, inappropriate interpretations, or otherwise false and misleading statements about assessment results

6.9 disclose to examinees and others whether and how long the results of the assessment will be kept on file, procedures for appeal and rescoring, rights examinees and others have to the assessment information, and how those rights may be exercised

6.10 report any apparent misuses of assessment information to those responsible for the assessment process

6.11 protect the rights to privacy of individuals and institutions involved in the assessment process

SECTION 7: RESPONSIBILITIES OF THOSE WHO EDUCATE OTHERS ABOUT ASSESSMENT

The process of educating others about educational assessment, whether as part of higher education, professional development, public policy discussions, or job training, should prepare individuals to understand and engage in sound measurement practice and to become discerning users of tests and test results. Persons who educate or inform others about assessment have a professional responsibility to:

7.1 remain competent and current in the areas in which they teach and reflect that in their instruction

7.2 provide fair and balanced perspectives when teaching about assessment

7.3 differentiate clearly between expressions of opinion and substantiated knowledge when educating others about any specific assessment method, product, or service

7.4 disclose any financial interests that might be perceived to influence the evaluation of a particular assessment product or service that is the subject of instruction

7.5 avoid administering any assessment that is not part of the evaluation of student performance in a course if the administration of that assessment is likely to harm any student

7.6 avoid using or reporting the results of any assessment that is not part of the evaluation of student performance in a course if the use or reporting of results is likely to harm any student

7.7 protect all secure assessments and materials used in the instructional process

7.8 model responsible assessment practice and help those receiving instruction to learn about their professional responsibilities in educational measurement

7.9 provide fair and balanced perspectives on assessment issues being discussed by policymakers, parents, and other citizens

SECTION 8: RESPONSIBILITIES OF THOSE WHO EVALUATE EDUCATIONAL PROGRAMS AND CONDUCT RESEARCH ON ASSESSMENTS

Conducting research on or about assessments or educational programs is a key activity in helping to improve the understanding and use of assessments and educational programs. Persons who engage in the evaluation of educational programs or conduct research on assessments have a professional responsibility to:

8.1 conduct evaluation and research activities in an informed, objective, and fair manner

8.2 disclose any associations that they have with authors, test publishers, or others involved with the assessment and refrain from participation if such associations might affect the objectivity of the research or evaluation

8.3 preserve the security of all assessments throughout the research process as appropriate

8.4 take appropriate steps to minimize potential sources of invalidity in the research and disclose known factors that may bias the results of the study

8.5 present the results of research, both intended and unintended, in a fair, complete, and objective manner

8.6 attribute completely and appropriately the work and ideas of others

8.7 qualify the conclusions of the research within the limitations of the study

8.8 use multiple sources of relevant information in conducting evaluation and research activities whenever possible

8.9 comply with applicable standards for protecting the rights of participants in an evaluation or research study, including the rights to privacy and informed consent

Standards for Teacher Competence in

Educational Assessment of Students

Developed by the American Federation of Teachers
National Council on Measurement in Education
National Education Association

1. Teachers should be skilled in choosing assessment methods appropriate for instructional decisions.
2. Teachers should be skilled in developing assessment methods appropriate for instructional decisions.
3. Teachers should be skilled in administering, scoring, and interpreting the results of both externally produced and teacher produced assessment methods.
4. Teachers should be skilled in using assessment results when making decisions about individual students, planning teaching, developing curriculum, and school improvement.
5. Teachers should be skilled in developing valid student grading procedures that use student assessments.
6. Teachers should be skilled in communicating assessment results to students, parents, other lay audiences, and other educators.
7. Teachers should be skilled in recognizing unethical, illegal, and otherwise inappropriate assessment methods and uses of assessment information.

From: Standards for Teacher Competence in Educational Assessment of Students. Developed by American Federation of Teachers, National Council on Measurement in Education, and National Education Association, 1990. This is not copyrighted material. Reproduction and dissemination are encouraged. Retrieved July 30, 2012, from http://buros.org/standards-teacher-competence-educational-assessment-students.

Educational Assessment Knowledge

and Skills for Teachers

I. Teachers should understand learning in the content area they teach.

II. Teachers should be able to articulate clear learning intentions that are congruent with both the content and depth of thinking implied by standards and curriculum goals, in such a way that they are attainable and assessable.

III. Teachers should have a repertoire of strategies for communicating to students what achievement of a learning intention looks like.

IV. Teachers should understand the purposes and uses of the range of available assessment options and be skilled in using them.

V. Teachers should have the skills to analyze classroom questions, test items, and performance assessment tasks to ascertain the specific knowledge and thinking skills required for students to do them.

VI. Teachers should have the skills to provide effective, useful feedback on student work.

VII. Teachers should be able to construct scoring schemes that quantify student performance on classroom assessments into useful information for decisions about students, classrooms, schools, and districts. These decisions should lead to improved student learning, growth, or development.

VIII. Teachers should be able to administer external assessments and interpret their results for decisions about students, classrooms, schools, and districts.

IX. Teachers should be able to articulate their interpretations of assessment results and their reasoning about the educational decisions based on assessment results to the educational populations they serve (student and his/her family, class, school, community).

X. Teachers should be able to help students use assessment information to make sound educational decisions.

XI. Teachers should understand and carry out their legal and ethical responsibilities in assessment as they conduct their work.

From: Brookhart, S. M. (2011). Educational assessment knowledge and skills for teachers. *Educational Measurement: Issues and Practice, 30*, 3–12. Reprinted by permission, John Wiley and Sons, 2012.

Index